热敏灸学

陈日新 谢丁一 著

人民卫生出版社
·北京·

图书在版编目（CIP）数据

热敏灸学 / 陈日新，谢丁一著. —北京：人民卫生出版社，2023.9

ISBN 978-7-117-35235-2

Ⅰ.①热… Ⅱ.①陈… ②谢… Ⅲ.①艾灸 Ⅳ.①R245.81

中国国家版本馆 CIP 数据核字（2023）第 172822 号

人卫智网	www.ipmph.com	医学教育、学术、考试、健康，购书智慧智能综合服务平台
人卫官网	www.pmph.com	人卫官方资讯发布平台

热敏灸学
Reminjiuxue

著　　者：陈日新　谢丁一
出版发行：人民卫生出版社（中继线 010-59780011）
地　　址：北京市朝阳区潘家园南里 19 号
邮　　编：100021
E - mail：pmph @ pmph.com
购书热线：010-59787592　010-59787584　010-65264830
印　　刷：北京顶佳世纪印刷有限公司
经　　销：新华书店
开　　本：710×1000　1/16　印张：27
字　　数：442 千字
版　　次：2023 年 9 月第 1 版
印　　次：2023 年 11 月第 1 次印刷
标准书号：ISBN 978-7-117-35235-2
定　　价：169.00 元

打击盗版举报电话：**010-59787491**　E-mail：WQ @ pmph.com
质量问题联系电话：**010-59787234**　E-mail：zhiliang @ pmph.com
数字融合服务电话：**4001118166**　E-mail：zengzhi @ pmph.com

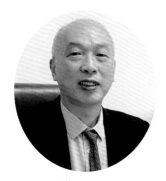

陈日新

　　江西中医药大学首席教授、主任中医师、博士研究生导师，全国名中医，全国老中医药专家学术经验继承工作指导老师，全国中医药高等学校教学名师，全国优秀教师，全国卫生系统先进工作者，全国优秀科技工作者，全国创新争先奖状获得者，江西省有突出贡献人才。国家中医药管理局热敏灸重点研究室主任，中国针灸学会副会长，中国针灸学会灸养专业委员会主任委员，世界中医药学会联合会热敏灸专业委员会会长，江西省针灸学会会长，江西省热敏灸学会理事长，享受国务院政府特殊津贴。热敏灸技术发明人，热敏灸小镇创始人，热敏灸机器人首创者，获国家科学技术进步奖二等奖 1 项、江西省科学技术进步奖一等奖 2 项及二等奖 2 项、教育部科学技术进步奖二等奖 1 项、世界中医药学会联合会中医药国际贡献奖二等奖 1 项（均为第一完成人）。

　　长期从事腧穴敏化与灸疗规律的研究，近年来发表论文 200 余篇，其中 SCI 论文 31 篇。出版热敏灸专著 11 部，其中英文版 2 部、日文版 3 部。主持承担了国家重点基础研究发展计划（973 计划）、国家自然科学基金、江西省重大创新项目等科研课题 20 余项，发现了灸疗过程中的灸疗热敏现象及其规律，突破了长期以来对腧穴的传统认识，揭示了腧穴敏化态新内涵，创立了热敏灸新技术，大幅度提高了灸疗临床疗效，已在国内外广泛推广应用。

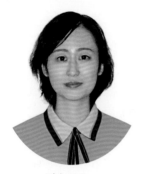

谢丁一

　　医学博士、副教授，中国针灸学会灸养专业委员会副主任委员兼秘书长，世界中医药学会联合会热敏灸专业委员会副会长兼秘书长，江西省热敏灸学会副理事长兼秘书长。主编论著 3 部，发表学术论文 38 篇，其中 SCI 6 篇。参与制定、主持发布了世界中联国际组织标准《热敏灸技术操作规范》。获得国家科学技术进步奖二等奖 1 项、江西省科学技术进步奖一等奖 1 项及二等奖 2 项、教育部科学技术进步奖二等奖 1 项、世界中医药学会联合会中医药国际贡献奖二等奖 1 项、江西省高等学校科技成果奖一等奖 1 项。

前　言

　　热敏灸的研究源于临床灸疗热敏现象的发现。在 20 世纪 80 年代，当时全国针灸临床灸法萎缩，"但见针刺病，不闻艾绒香"。江西中医药大学灸疗科研团队在临床艾灸过程中陆续发现了一组神奇的灸感现象：局部不（微）热远部热、表面不（微）热深部热、非热感觉等。当这些现象发生时，灸疗疗效似乎明显提高，然而现代医学不能解释这些现象，这就引起了团队的极大兴趣与重视。于是陈日新教授带领研究团队普查了神经系统、运动系统、消化系统、呼吸系统、生殖系统等近 20 种病症后发现，这些患者在艾灸时都能不同程度地产生上述特殊灸感现象，尤其以寒证、湿证、瘀证、虚证患者居多，急性病和慢性病均可出现，出现率高达 70% 以上，当疾病好转或痊愈后，这种灸感现象消失，而健康人出现率仅为 10%。当艾灸出现这些特殊灸感现象后，气至病所率明显提高，表明上述特殊灸感现象的出现具有普遍性、与疾病状态的高度相关性及气至病所率的高效性。至此，团队认识了热敏现象出现的基本规律，大家非常振奋，似乎看到了振兴灸法、提高疗效的一道曙光。

　　然而产生上述特殊灸感的"位点"与教科书中经穴、奇穴、阿是穴的位置并不重合，并且呈现位置"动态"性、"旁开"的特征。产生特殊灸感的位点是穴位吗？如果是穴位，它不在已知穴位位置上；如果不是穴位，疗效却比已知穴位好。这时现有的穴位理论与临床实践发生了矛盾，引发了陈日新团队的困惑与深深思考，意识到这很可能是建立新的灸学理论与提高灸疗疗效的突破口。带着"穴位是什么"的困惑，团队直溯《黄帝内经》求解。穴位是什么？《灵枢·九针十二原》云："所言节者，神气之所游行出入也，非皮肉筋骨也。"这就是说，腧穴不是指一般的皮肉筋骨等有其特定的形态结构及固定不变的位置，而是神气游行出入的动态的功能变化部位。动态的功能态穴位如何精准定位？《灵枢·背腧》论述："欲得而验之，按其处，应在中而痛解，乃其俞也。"说明腧穴具有"按其处而应（腧穴特殊反应）"的敏感特征及"欲得而验之"的动态特征。《灵枢·五邪》列举临床病例论述腧穴的上述特征："咳动肩背，取之膺中外腧，背三节之傍，以手疾按之，快然乃刺之。"再次说明穴位具有状态之别，而不仅仅是部位之别。更令陈日新团队惊讶的是：《黄帝内经》对穴位的论述竟然与在临床灸疗实践中的观察完全一致！我们深感到，中医经典对现代临床的重要指导作用。可以得出结论，艾灸过程中产生特殊灸感的位点不但是穴位，而且是符合《黄帝内经》中穴位原始定义的正宗穴位，是提高灸疗疗效的特异性穴位。正因如此，我们仿佛感觉到灸疗研究插上了一双腾飞的翅膀，经典支持，临床疗效支撑！

团队抓住"灸位"与"灸量"两个关键技术环节，创立了热敏灸技术：探感定位，辨敏施灸，量因人异，敏消量足。这是一项全新的灸法技术，穴位已不是一个固化的坐标位点，而是一个动态的功能位点；灸时也不是千人一律的 10~15 分钟，而是个体化与标准化结合的灸时标准；灸疗适应证也不是用寒热虚实来判断，而是以机体是否开启热敏穴位为判断指征；灸感也不是皮肤温热而无灼痛，而是局部不（微）热远部热，表面不（微）热深部热，非热感觉等；辨证施灸已不能满足临床需求了，而是需要辨敏施灸；灸效也不是与热灸强度、热灸时间有关，而是与热敏灸强度、热敏灸时间有关。一句话，热敏灸从理论到技术，再到疗效都完全不一样了。2006 年 10 月 28 日，热敏灸技术通过江西省科学技术厅组织的成果鉴定，中国工程院院士石学敏教授任主任委员，评价意见为：热敏灸属原始创新，达到国际领先水平。中国著名针灸学家魏稼教授评价："新灸法无论理论、技术和疗效都是针灸发展史上的里程碑，将改写中国针灸学篇章。"时任卫生部副部长兼国家中医药管理局局长的佘靖对"腧穴热敏化艾灸新疗法"给予了充分肯定，并批示"希望认真抓落实，形成'北看天津针，南看江西灸'的格局"。2010 年热敏灸受邀参展上海世界博览会，联合国国际信息发展组织罗马总干事丹尼尔·巴瑞奥在热敏灸启航仪式上郑重宣布，将热敏灸列为重点推广的国际合作项目。

临床实践是检验中医理论的唯一标准。为了检验热敏灸的疗效，我们采用大样本、多中心、中央随机对照临床试验方法，分别以腰椎间盘突出症（急性期）、膝关节骨性关节炎（肿胀型）、支气管哮喘（慢性持续期）患者为研究对象，围绕选取热敏穴位施灸是否优于辨证选穴，以及根据施灸过程中穴位消敏程度确定每穴的个体化施灸时间是否优于常规固定施灸时间这两个关键问题，对比其疗效差异。结果表明，辨敏施灸疗效明显优于辨证施灸，以消敏时间为度的个体化与标准化结合的施灸时间标准也明显优于常规固定施灸时间标准。热敏灸技术的创立开启了一条源于经典、基于临床、继承创新、提高疗效的灸疗发展新路。

基础研究是科技发展的重要基石。团队建立了行业内协同创新、跨学科协同创新与国际协同创新平台，进行了热敏灸生物学基础的系列研究。应用红外热断层成像技术及温度觉定量测定技术，证实了热敏穴位局部能量代谢明显增强；应用高密度脑电、功能性磁共振与神经计算技术，证实了热敏穴位的客观性、效应特异性，揭示了相关脑区功能连接度与穴位热敏化发生密切相关；首次建立了灸疗热敏动物模型，采用分子生物学技术，提示了热敏现象的产生与大脑神经网络可塑性变化有关。

理论对实践具有积极和深远的指导作用。在基于临床实践发现穴位热敏现象和经典理论依据支撑的基础上，2006 年我们出版了《腧穴热敏化艾灸新疗法》专著，首次提出了腧穴敏化论新观点。2011 年，根据新的研究进展，在《中国针灸》发表论文《岐伯归来——论"腧穴敏化状态说"》，再次阐述腧穴敏化新观点。2016 年，根据新的研究成果，又发表了《再论"腧穴敏化状态说"》论文，从循证评价、基础研究与理论构建三方面论述腧穴敏化状态说。2015 年腧穴敏化论引起科技部重视，首次设立腧穴敏化研究为国家自然科学基金中医重大项目研究。基于艾灸热敏化腧穴能高效激发经气的系列研究结果，2008 年在《中国针灸》发表论文提出了"灸之要，气至而有效"新理念，阐述了艾灸也能激发针刺类得气，艾灸必须激发得气才能提高灸疗疗效及艾灸如何激发得气等新观点，完善了"刺之要，气至而有效"的针灸理论。该篇论文获得 2012 年度"中国百篇最具影响国内学术论文"的殊荣，影响深远。作者根据临床上腧穴敏化状态不仅可以帮助选穴定位，还能帮助施灸定量及判断艾灸适应证的规律，2013 年再次出版热敏灸专著，总结并提出了"辨敏施灸"新概念，形成了一个新的贯穿施灸全过程的诊疗模式，发展了传统"辨证施灸"的理论。这些灸疗新概念已经写入"十二五"规划教材《实验针灸学》，对提高灸疗疗效具有重大的指导意义。2018 年在《中国针灸》发表论文《热敏灸得气灸感量表的研制与初步评价》，进一步量化了得气的评估。2019 年在《中国针灸》发表论文《试论艾灸得气》，提出了艾灸得气新概念，即艾灸得气是指一组与疗效相关的、舒适的透热、扩热、传热、深部热、远部热等感受，而不是局部的、表面的热感，填补了艾灸得气理论的空白。至此，热敏灸形成了一个完整的灸疗新体系，丰富了传承数千年的灸疗理论内涵，促进了灸疗学术发展的新跨越、技术水平的大提升。2016 年世界中医药学会联合会热敏灸专业委员会发布了热敏灸技术标准，2018 年提升为世界中医药学会联合会国际组织标准，2019 年由中医古籍出版社正式出版发行，引领着灸疗学的新发展。

人才培养是热敏灸学科持续发展的重要保证。2011 年江西中医学院成立了全国首个灸学院，专门培养本科生及硕士、博士研究生灸学人才，以满足热敏灸高级人才的社会需求。2015 年与葡萄牙传统医学院合作，创办了热敏灸系，专门培养葡萄牙语国家热敏灸技术人才，同时为国外 20 多个国家与地区培养了大量热敏灸技术人才。

理论的突破，技术的创新，带来了灸疗疗效的大幅度提高。热敏灸在治疗过敏性病症、脊柱关节痛症、功能性胃肠病症、妇科病症、男性前列腺病症及强身健体保健等方面有独特优势。2011 年 9 月，在江西南昌开办了全球首家热敏灸医院，2012 年 12 月开办了江西热敏灸医院高安分院，2014 年组建江西省中医康复（热敏灸）联盟，目前省内已有 55 家联盟分院；在省外建立了 10 家分院，在山东博兴建立了热敏灸肿瘤康复基地；在国外开办了葡萄牙分院、瑞典分院、瑞士分院，标志着热敏灸成果的临床规模转化。目前全国已有 27 个省、市、自治区的 500 余家医院广泛应用热敏灸技术。美国、日本、德国、新西兰、澳大利亚、瑞典、瑞士、葡萄牙等 20 多个国家的针灸师来我院学习热敏灸技术，国际辐射效应进一步发挥。

热敏灸技术不仅有很好的医疗作用，而且在国民强身健体、促进慢病康复、居家养老等方面的优势也日益凸显。2017 年 12 月在山东省潍坊市峡山区太保庄建设了全球首家热敏灸小镇，2018 年建设了江西高阜热敏灸小镇，标志着热敏灸走进千家万户，向探索有中国特色、中医特色国民健康新模式迈出新的一步，为热敏灸助力精准扶贫、健康中国提供了可行性、可复制性、刚需性、精准性、高效性的样板。2020 年出版了《热敏常灸出奇效：慢病康复新选择》艾灸新法专著，介绍了短程热敏灸未曾开发的新天地，开创了一条有中国特色、中医特色的慢病康复、强身健体新途径。

2020 年初，热敏灸积极参与抗击新冠疫情的战斗，在全国率先进入隔离病房，取得显著疗效，并支援湖北省蕲春县人民医院实现清零目标。该临床成果在《中国针灸》杂志网络首发，临床团队出版了专著《热敏灸防治疫病理论与实践：应对新冠肺炎方案》，阐明了热敏灸得气是治疗新型冠状病毒感染取得显著疗效的关键技术。

本书是全新的灸法理论与临床专著，具有以下特点：①介绍了基于临床、源于经典、继承创新、提高疗效的热敏灸研究思路与历程；②展示了基于腧穴敏化与艾灸得气新理论建立的辨敏施灸诊疗新体系；③示范了中医临床研究的一般规律，即发现现象、肯定现象、总结规律、验证疗效、升华理论、回归临床。本书分为五章内容。第一章是理论篇，介绍了不同于常规艾灸的四个新概念，构建了热敏灸理论新体系，是作者长期临床实践的总结与升华。第二章是技术篇，详细阐述了热敏灸操作方法、作用与特点、适应病症、注意事项及常用穴位热敏灸感，这些均是提高灸疗疗效的关键。第三章是治疗篇，重点介绍了作者有临床体会的 30 个疾病，既包括常见病，也有疑难病症，病名基本上采用现代医学名称，每种病症分临床表现、灸法治则、治疗方案、验案举例。第四章是保健篇，重点介绍了确有效果的 15 个保健项目，每个项目从保健对象、自我判断、热敏探查、施灸手法、建议灸量、灸后防护、验案举例 7 个方面进行介绍。第五章是抗疫篇，简要介绍了热敏灸参与抗击新冠疫情的概况，阐述了热敏灸治疗新冠肺炎临床思路、热敏灸防治新冠肺炎临床方案、热敏灸治疗新冠肺炎临床疗效以及病案举例。

32 年的研究，仅仅发现穴位秘密的冰山一角，即穴位热敏化，灸疗疗效已明显提高。我们深信热敏灸蕴藏着人类调动本能、治疗疾病的秘密，将继续发现、开发并应用这些秘密，为人类的健康造福！

多年来，热敏灸研究得到了国家重点基础研究发展计划（973 计划）、国家自然科学基金、国家中医药管理局研究课题、江西省科技厅重大专项的支持，在此致以最诚挚的感谢。同时也向长期以来付出辛勤劳动的许多同事及在本书文字处理与绘图中给予帮助的李海燕同志，表示深深的谢意。

著者

2020 年 8 月

目 录

第一章
理论篇 ——————————————————————

第二章
技术篇 ————————————

第三章
治疗篇 ————————————————————

第四章
保健篇 ————————————————

第五章
抗疫篇 ——————————————————

第一章

理论篇

　　热敏灸是采用点燃的艾材产生的艾热悬灸热敏穴位，激发透热、传热、扩热、非热觉、喜热、身烘热、面红（或额汗出）、肢端热、胃肠蠕动反应、皮肤扩散性潮红等艾灸得气活动，并施以个体化的饱和消敏灸量，从而提高艾灸疗效的一项新灸法。陈日新团队基于临床、源于经典、继承创新，历经32年的系统研究，建立了全新的灸疗理论体系、技术体系、临床操作规范，大幅度提高了灸疗疗效，继承和发展了传统灸疗学，显著提升了中国灸学的社会服务能力。本篇介绍热敏灸理论的"腧穴敏化""艾灸得气""消敏灸量"及"辨敏施灸"四个重要新概念，它是热敏灸技术体系与临床操作规范的指导。

第一节　"腧穴敏化"新概念

一、腧穴敏化的含义

长期以来，人们认为腧穴是脏腑经络之气输注于体表的特殊部位，它既是疾病的反映点，又是针灸的施术部位[1]。江西中医药大学陈日新团队基于 18 年的临床研究成果，于 2006 年出版《腧穴热敏化艾灸新疗法》专著[2]，首次正式提出"腧穴敏化"新概念，认为：人体腧穴存在敏化态和静息态两种功能态，当人体处于疾病状态时，体表腧穴发生敏化，敏化的类型多种多样，而腧穴热敏化是腧穴敏化的一种新类型，处在热敏态的腧穴对外界相关刺激呈现"小刺激大反应"。2011 年又撰文在《中国针灸》明确提出并全面论述腧穴敏化的学术观点：腧穴的本质属性具有功能状态之别，而不仅仅是固定部位之别[3]。2016 年依据新的研究成果，从循证评价、基础研究与理论构建 3 个方面再次论述"腧穴敏化"新概念[4]，强调以腧穴敏化为腧穴研究的切入点与突破口，对我们重新认识腧穴，进一步夯实针灸学理论基石，提高针灸疗效、催发临床新的生命力及可能发现新的体表 – 内脏生命调控规律具有十分重要的意义。

二、腧穴敏化的古代文献依据

"腧穴敏化"概念的提出并非只是依据现代临床的发现，早在《黄帝内经》中就有腧穴敏化现象的相关记载。《灵枢·九针十二原》述："所言节者，神气之所游行出入也，非皮肉筋骨也。"这就是说，腧穴不是指一般的皮肉筋骨等有其特定的形态结构及固定不变的位置，而是神气游行出入的、动态的、功能变化的部位。《灵枢·背腧》论述："胸中大俞在杼骨之端，肺俞在三椎之傍，心俞在五椎之傍，膈俞在七椎之傍，肝俞在九椎之傍，脾俞在十一椎之傍，肾俞在十四椎之傍，皆挟脊相去三寸所。则欲得而验之，按其处，应在中而痛解，乃其俞也。"这段经文表明：腧穴具有"通过按压等方法会产生特殊感应"的敏感特征。《灵枢·五邪》再次列举临床病例论述腧穴的敏感特征："咳动肩背，取之膺中外腧，背三节之傍，以手疾按之，快然乃刺之。"这段经文再次告诉我们：腧穴具有"按之快然"的敏化特征。唐代孙思邈《备急千金要方·针灸上·灸例》记载："有阿是之法，言人有病痛，即令捏其上，若里当其处，不问孔穴，即得便快成（或）痛处，即云阿是。灸刺皆验，故曰阿是穴也。"这就是大家熟知的"阿是"现象，即一种以压力刺激诱发的腧穴力敏现象。由此可见，《黄帝内经》等古代文献对腧穴的论述与临床实践中的发现完全一致，腧穴不仅仅有部位之别，而且具有"敏化"与"静息"两种功能状态之别。

三、腧穴热敏现象与临床规律

腧穴敏化的类型多种多样，除了上述唐代孙思邈《备急千金要方》描述的"阿是"力敏现象，陈日新团队系统研究了腧穴热敏现象。腧穴热敏现象是指当手持艾条悬灸患者某个腧穴时，患者会产生一些深部热、远部热等特殊感觉，而艾灸患者这个腧穴的邻近部位或另外某个体表部位时，患者没有这种特殊感觉产生，仅仅有局部与表面的热感。这些特殊感觉，又称热敏灸感，产生热敏灸感的腧穴称为热敏态腧穴（简称热敏腧穴）[5]。热敏腧穴对艾热刺激产生"小刺激大反应"，是灸疗的特异性穴位。热敏灸感包括以下 10 类：透热、扩热、传热、非热觉、皮肤扩散性潮红、面红（或额汗出）、胃肠蠕动、肢端热、身烘热、喜热。

透热：灸热从施灸部位皮肤表面直接向深部组织穿透，甚至直达胸、腹腔，或施灸部位的皮肤不（或微）热，而皮肤下深部组织甚至胸腹腔脏器感觉甚热，这种现象又称表面不（微）热深部热；

扩热：灸热以施灸部位为中心向周围扩散；

传热：灸热从施灸部位开始沿某一路线向远部传导，甚至到达疾病部位，或施灸部位不（或微）热，而远离施灸的部位感觉甚热，这种现象又称局部不（微）热远部热；

非热觉：施灸部位或远离施灸部位产生酸、胀、压、重、痛、麻、冷等非热感觉；

皮肤扩散性潮红：施灸部位的皮肤呈现均匀的向四周扩散性的潮红；

面红（或额汗出）：施灸躯干四肢部位的穴位，面部皮肤潮红或额部、颈项部微汗出；

胃肠蠕动：施灸中自觉胃部紧缩感或腹中肠鸣；

肢端热：施灸中自觉四肢末端或掌心、足心逐渐温热；

身烘热：施灸中自觉全身或上半身由里而表的阵阵温热、欲汗出或微汗出；

喜热：施灸中自觉舒适感、舒畅感，甚至身体轻松感。

以上 10 类热敏灸感或单独出现或多种同时出现，因病位、病性、病情、施灸穴位的不同，热敏灸感的类型也不同。对神经系统、运动系统、消化系统、呼吸系统、生殖系统等 20 种疾病患者进行艾灸腧穴观察，上述 10 类热敏灸感均能出现。寒证、湿证、瘀证、虚证者居多，急性病和慢性病均可出现。团队深入研究发现腧穴发生热敏化有以下临床规律[5]。

（一）腧穴热敏现象具有普遍性

通过对颈椎病、腰椎间盘突出症、膝关节骨性关节炎、肌筋膜疼痛综合征、支气管哮喘、慢性支气管炎、非溃疡性消化不良、功能性便秘、肠易激综合征、排卵障碍性不孕、慢性盆腔炎、痛经、周围性面瘫等 20 种疾病及健康人对照的穴位热敏普查的研究，结果表明，在疾病状态下，腧穴热敏现象的出现率为 70%，明显高于健康人的 10%。寒证、湿证、瘀证、虚证中居多，急性病和慢性病均可出现。疾病痊愈后腧穴热敏出现率降为 15% 左右。表明人体在疾病状态下，体表腧穴发生热敏具有普遍性，与疾病高度相关。

（二）腧穴热敏部位具有动态性

以周围性面瘫、腰椎间盘突出症、膝关节骨性关节炎、肌筋膜疼痛综合征、支气管哮喘、痛经、排卵障碍性不孕等 7 种疾病患者为研究对象，将 469 个热敏穴位与经穴作对比研究，结果表明，腧穴热敏部位随病情变化而变化。动态的热敏腧穴与部位固定的经穴重合率仅为 48.76%，与压痛点的重合率为 34.75%，表明热敏腧穴的出现部位仅可以经穴或压痛点为参照坐标系来粗定位，而准确定位必须以热敏灸感为标准。

（三）腧穴热敏的分布与病症具有相关性

腧穴发生热敏有一定的分布规律，如腹泻型肠易激综合征患者热敏腧穴在天枢、命门穴区出现率最高，其次为大肠俞、足三里、关元穴区；慢性前列腺炎患者热敏腧穴在中极、命门、关元、阴陵泉、三阴交等穴区出现率最高；慢性盆腔炎患者热敏腧穴在腰阳关、关元、子宫、次髎、三阴交、阴陵泉等穴区出现率最高；原发性痛经患者热敏腧穴在关元、子宫、次髎、三阴交等穴区出现率最高；原发性三叉神经痛患者热敏腧穴在下关、四白、夹承浆、风池、鱼腰等穴区出现率最高。

（四）艾灸热敏腧穴产生经气传导具有高效性

热敏腧穴在艾热刺激下，呈现对艾热刺激的高敏性，表现为透热、扩热、传热、非热觉、皮肤扩散性潮红、面红（或额汗出）、胃肠蠕动、肢端热、身烘热、喜热等10种热敏现象。通过对周围性面瘫、三叉神经痛、颈椎病、腰椎间盘突出症、膝关节骨性关节炎、肌筋膜疼痛综合征、慢性支气管炎、支气管哮喘、非溃疡性消化不良、功能性便秘、肠易激综合征、排卵障碍性不孕、原发性痛经和勃起功能障碍共14种病症、540例患者的临床检测，艾灸热敏腧穴激发经气传导的出现率达94.0%，而艾灸非热敏腧穴的经气传导出现率仅约23.5%，二者有非常显著的统计学差异。以上腧穴发生热敏的数据表明，热敏腧穴对艾热刺激产生"小刺激，大反应"，极易激发经气感传，气至病所，具有提高灸疗疗效的巨大潜力。

四、腧穴热敏的客观特征

腧穴热敏的判断多根据患者的主观描述，但是通过红外热成像、温度觉定量测定等现代科学技术手段可以在一定程度上反映腧穴热敏的现象与特征。

（一）腧穴热敏现象的体表红外辐射特征

人体是一个天然的生物发热体，由于解剖结构、组织代谢、血液循环及神经功能状态不同，机体各部位温度不同，形成不同的热像图。医用红外热像仪其实质是一种全身温度分布扫描仪，通过扫描接收人体内的能量分布、强度、形态、走势，全面真实地反映人体的健康状态。正常的机体功能状态有正常的热像图，异常的机体功能状态有异常的热像图，比较两者异同，结合临床就可以帮助辅助诊断病情。

应用红外热成像技术研究发现：支气管哮喘（慢性持续期）患者[6-8]，其热敏腧穴具有高红外辐射强度特点，并形成以热敏腧穴为中心的一定范围高红外辐射强度区域，如肺俞穴区发生热敏时，红外热成像呈高温态；红外法与灸感法比较，其敏感性为69%、特异性为64%、准确率为66.7%。腰椎间盘突出症患者[9-10]热敏腧穴的红外辐射强度以高温区为主，且艾灸热敏腧穴的传热长径显著高于非热敏腧穴；艾灸热敏态命门穴区后，产生明显的沿腰部正中纵向扩散（督脉）或横向扩散的红外辐射增强区域，与灸感法比较，其敏感性为88.1%，特异性为80.0%，准确性为85.5%。对原发性痛经患者[11]关元穴位进行敏化后，红外辐射的温度降低。与艾灸相比，其敏感性率为76.6%，发散率为70.1%，准确率为74.6%。在对关元穴区进行艾灸后，红外辐射区域在纵向和横向上都显著扩展。与灸感法相比，其敏感性为78.7%，特异性为83.3%，准确性为80.3%。艾灸心气虚患者的内关穴区红外辐射强度多数显示高温特征，艾灸内关穴后发现热敏化的内关穴区产生明显的沿前臂内侧纵向扩散的红外辐射增强区[12]。

以上研究结果表明热敏腧穴产生的扩热、传热等热敏现象在一定程度上可被红外热成像客观显示，受试者的主观感觉与红外热成像明显相关，从而可应用红外热成像技术探索不同病症热敏腧穴的分布规律，指导热敏灸临床治疗。采用红外热断层成像技术已经探明了腰椎间盘突出症、痛经、支气管哮喘等21种病症热敏腧穴高发区（图1-1-1），在高发区内进行细定位，极大缩减了热敏灸探感定位时间，提高了探查效率。

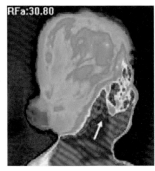 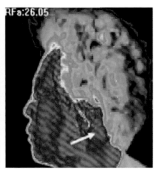 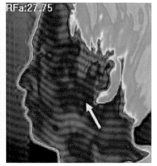

偏头痛患者风池穴　　　　面瘫患者翳风穴　　　　面肌痉挛患者下关穴

图1-1-1　21种病症的穴位热敏高发区分布典型图例

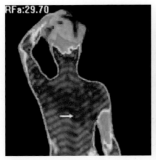

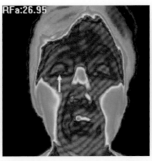

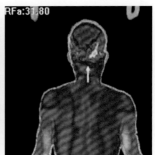

失眠患者心俞穴 三叉神经痛患者四白穴 脑梗死患者风府穴

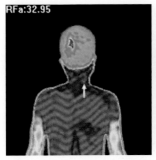

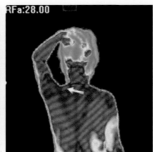

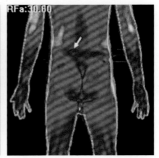

颈椎病患者颈夹脊穴 肩周炎患者肩井穴 腰肌劳损患者大肠俞穴

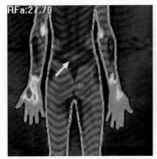

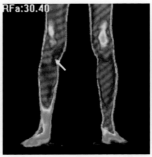

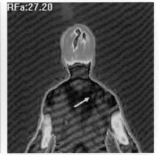

腰椎间盘突出症患者 膝关节炎患者阴陵泉穴 背肌筋膜炎患者膏肓穴
腰阳关穴

图 1-1-1 21 种病症的穴位热敏高发区分布典型图例（续）

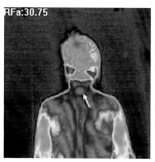

哮喘患者大椎穴

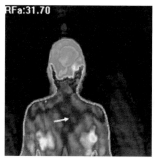

慢性支气管炎患者肺俞穴

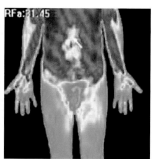

胃溃疡患者水分穴

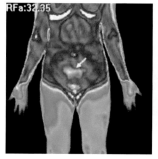

非溃疡性消化不良患者
关元穴

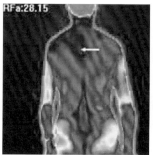

冠心病患者心俞穴

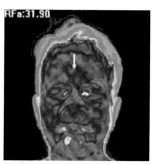

过敏性鼻炎患者印堂穴

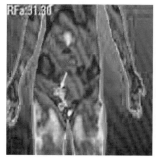

盆腔炎症患者子宫穴

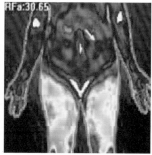

肠易激综合征患者天枢穴

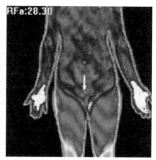

痛经患者中极穴

图 1-1-1 21 种病症的穴位热敏高发区分布典型图例（续）

（二）腧穴热敏的温度觉阈值特征

感觉定量检测是一种测定特定感觉的技术，可用于定量测定振动觉、温度觉（冷和暖）和痛觉（冷痛觉及热痛觉）等的阈值。温度感觉阈值可以反映被测皮肤部位对温度感知的敏感性。采用温度觉定量测定技术，以腰椎间盘突出症、神经根型颈椎病、膝关节骨性关节炎等患者为研究对象[13-15]，发现腰椎间盘突出症患者腰阳关穴、腰俞穴、关元俞穴热敏组热觉阈值、热痛阈值和热耐痛阈值分别显著高于同一穴位非热敏组（$P<0.01$）。在此基础上，对热敏态关元俞穴给予40℃、42℃温控激发，结果显示，与热敏态关元俞穴激发温度为40℃时比较，42℃时灸感强度更强，效应期时间更长，潜伏期时间更短（$P<0.01$，$P<0.05$）。神经根型颈椎病患者大椎穴、肩井穴、肩髃穴热敏组热觉阈值、热痛阈值和热耐痛阈值分别明显高于同一穴位非热敏组，差异均具有统计学意义（$P<0.05$）。与热敏态肩井穴激发温度为40℃时比较，42℃时灸感强度更强，潜伏期时间更短，效应期时间更长，差异均具有统计学意义（$P<0.05$）。膝关节骨性关节炎患者热敏组三个穴位（血海、内膝眼和阴陵泉）的热觉阈值、热痛阈值和热耐痛阈值均高于非热敏组同名穴位的相应测量值，差异均具有统计学意义（$P<0.01$）。结果表明：热敏态腧穴与非热敏态腧穴具有不同温度觉特征，热敏态腧穴的热觉阈、热痛阈、热耐痛阈值均高于非热敏态腧穴，这与临床上热敏态腧穴具有喜热的特征是一致的。并且不同的激发温度，热敏灸感出现的灸感强度、潜伏期、效应期时间不同，42℃为临床较佳激发温度。（见表1-1-1～表1-1-11）

表 1-1-1　腰阳关穴两组温度觉阈值的比较（$\bar{x} \pm s$）

组别	例数	热觉阈值 /℃	热痛阈值 /℃	热耐痛阈值 /℃
热敏组	26	37.61 ± 0.65 •	44.46 ± 1.67 •	48.31 ± 0.62 •
非热敏组	14	36.12 ± 0.78	42.79 ± 1.84	46.67 ± 0.84

注：•表示与非热敏组比较，$P<0.01$。

表 1-1-2 　腰俞穴两组温度觉阈值的比较（$\bar{x} \pm s$）

组别	例数	热觉阈值 /℃	热痛阈值 /℃	热耐痛阈值 /℃
热敏组	23	37.44 ± 0.67●	44.86 ± 1.24●	48.92 ± 0.74●
非热敏组	17	36.05 ± 0.74	43.13 ± 1.84	46.91 ± 0.82

注：●表示与非热敏组比较，$P < 0.01$。

表 1-1-3 　关元俞穴两组温度觉阈值的比较（$\bar{x} \pm s$）

组别	例数	热觉阈值 /℃	热痛阈值 /℃	热耐痛阈值 /℃
热敏组	24	36.71 ± 0.94●	44.71 ± 1.48●	48.43 ± 0.62●
非热敏组	16	35.64 ± 1.04	43.08 ± 1.52	46.67 ± 0.81

注：●表示与非热敏组比较，$P < 0.01$。

表 1-1-4 　热敏态关元俞穴不同温度激发情况比较（$\bar{x} \pm s$）

激发温度	例数	灸感强度	潜伏期时间 /min	效应期时间 /min
42℃	24	4.32 ± 2.21●	10.56 ± 2.86★	11.72 ± 2.93●
40℃	24	2.81 ± 1.44	41.55 ± 18.37	5.15 ± 3.07

注：●表示两组比较，$P < 0.01$；★表示两组比较，$P < 0.05$。

表 1-1-5 　大椎穴两组温度觉阈值的比较（$\bar{x} \pm s$）

组别	例数	热觉阈值 /℃	热痛阈值 /℃	热耐痛阈值 /℃
热敏组	24	37.66 ± 1.14*	44.45 ± 1.87*	47.73 ± 0.63*
非热敏组	16	36.11 ± 1.13	42.93 ± 1.23	46.23 ± 1.17

注：与非热敏组比较，*$P < 0.05$。

表 1-1-6 　肩井穴两组温度觉阈值的比较（$\bar{x} \pm s$）

组别	例数	热觉阈值 /℃	热痛阈值 /℃	热耐痛阈值 /℃
热敏组	22	37.56 ± 1.35*	44.96 ± 1.59*	48.16 ± 0.53*
非热敏组	18	36.32 ± 1.41	42.85 ± 1.75	46.33 ± 0.52

注：与非热敏组比较，*$P < 0.05$。

表 1-1-7　肩髃穴两组温度觉阈值的比较（$\bar{x} \pm s$）

组别	例数	热觉阈值 /℃	热痛阈值 /℃	热耐痛阈值 /℃
热敏组	25	38.96 ± 1.66[*]	44.49 ± 1.59[*]	48.54 ± 0.57[*]
非热敏组	15	37.31 ± 2.01	42.78 ± 1.92	46.75 ± 0.63

注：与非热敏组比较，[*]$P < 0.05$。

表 1-1-8　热敏态肩井穴不同温度激发情况比较（$\bar{x} \pm s$）

激发温度	例数	灸感强度	潜伏期时间 /min	效应期时间 /min
42℃	22	5.21 ± 2.50[*]	12.15 ± 3.22[*]	14.22 ± 3.83[*]
40℃	22	3.55 ± 1.26	36.31 ± 12.74	10.28 ± 3.53

注：与激发温度40℃组比较，[*]$P < 0.05$。

表 1-1-9　血海穴两组温度觉阈值的比较（$\bar{x} \pm s$）

组别	例数	热觉阈值 /℃	热痛阈值 /℃	热耐痛阈值 /℃
热敏组	25	38.21 ± 2.03[★]	44.47 ± 1.86[★]	48.59 ± 0.74[★]
非热敏组	21	36.76 ± 1.93	42.91 ± 2.05	46.95 ± 1.14

注：[★]表示与非热敏组比较，$P < 0.01$。

表 1-1-10　内膝眼穴两组温度觉阈值的比较（$\bar{x} \pm s$）

组别	例数	热觉阈值 /℃	热痛阈值 /℃	热耐痛阈值 /℃
热敏组	26	37.47 ± 1.77[★]	44.55 ± 1.63[★]	47.48 ± 0.47[★]
非热敏组	20	35.92 ± 1.69	42.72 ± 1.94	45.53 ± 0.41

注：[★]表示与非热敏组比较，$P < 0.01$。

表 1-1-11　阴陵泉穴两组温度觉阈值的比较（$\bar{x} \pm s$）

组别	例数	热觉阈值 /℃	热痛阈值 /℃	热耐痛阈值 /℃
热敏组	27	37.30 ± 2.23[★]	44.39 ± 1.92[★]	47.76 ± 0.58[★]
非热敏组	19	36.06 ± 1.86	42.63 ± 1.88	45.91 ± 0.72

注：[★]表示与非热敏组比较，$P < 0.01$。

五、热敏腧穴提高疗效的临床证据

腧穴热敏规律的研究结果表明，腧穴存在状态之别，即静息态与敏化态，敏化态穴位对外界艾热刺激呈现"小刺激大反应"，由此我们认为，腧穴状态不同，效应必然不同，热敏腧穴的灸效优于非热敏（静息态）腧穴。有学者分别观察了采用热敏腧穴与非热敏腧穴治疗过敏性鼻炎、原发性痛经、慢性腰肌劳损、慢性前列腺炎、膝关节骨性关节炎、腰椎间盘突出症、神经根型颈椎病、肌筋膜疼痛综合征、枕神经痛、跟痛症 10 种病症的显效率，结果显示，热敏腧穴组的显效率平均提高了 38.2%，选取热敏腧穴治疗可以显著提高临床疗效[16]。

（一）艾灸不同功能态腧穴治疗腰椎间盘突出症（急性期）的临床疗效研究 [17-20]

由江西中医药大学附属医院牵头，组织 4 家医院采用大样本、多中心、中央随机对照试验方法联合开展了艾灸不同功能态腧穴治疗腰椎间盘突出症（急性期）的临床疗效研究。各分中心受试对象的随机分配采用中心随机化方法，由中国中医科学院中医临床基础医学研究所统一控制，随机分为试验组（热敏腧穴悬灸治疗组）、对照 A 组（非热敏腧穴悬灸对照组）、对照 B 组（西药加针刺对照组），分组结果采用"药物临床试验中央随机分配交互式语音操作系统 V1.00（中央随机分配系统）"通过语音电话、网络进行发布。

1. 治疗方案

（1）试验组

1）热敏腧穴的探查：①环境：检测室保持安静，室内温度保持在 24 ~ 30℃；②体位：选择舒适、充分暴露病位的体位；③探查工具：江西省中医院生产，规格：直径 22mm×长度 160mm 特制精艾绒艾条；④探查方法：选择俯卧或侧卧体位，充分暴露腰部，用点燃的艾条在患者双侧大肠俞与腰俞构成的三角区域（大肠俞–腰俞–对侧大肠俞区域内），距离皮肤 3cm 左右施行温和灸，当患者感受到艾热发生透热（艾热从施灸部位皮肤表面直接向深部组织穿透）、扩热（以施灸点为中心向周围扩散）、传热（灸热从施灸点开始循某一方向传导）和非热觉中的一种或一种以上感觉时，即为发生腧穴热敏现象，该探查穴点为热敏腧穴。重复上述步骤,直至所有的热敏腧穴被探查出。

2)热敏腧穴的悬灸方法:在上述热敏化强度最强的穴位实施艾条温和悬灸,每天2次,每次艾灸时间以热敏灸感消失为度(上限60min,下限30min),共治疗4天;第5天开始每天1次,连续治疗10次;共治疗18次(共14天)。前7天为1个疗程,后7天为1个疗程,第1个疗程结束后如痊愈可不进入第2个疗程。

(2)**对照A组**:在大肠俞、阿是穴、委中(均为患侧)实施温和悬灸,每次每穴15min,3穴共45min,每天2次,共治疗4天;第5天开始每天1次,连续治疗10次;共治疗18次(共14天)。前7天为1个疗程,后7天为1个疗程,第1个疗程结束后如痊愈可不进入第2个疗程。

(3)**对照B组**:①西药:患者入院后第1天即开始使用20%甘露醇250ml,静脉滴注,每天1次;同时口服双氯芬酸钠肠溶片75mg,每天2次,饭后服用;3天后停用甘露醇,仅口服双氯芬酸钠肠溶片。②针刺:患者入院后第1天开始配合针刺治疗,以足太阳、足少阳经穴为主。取穴:大肠俞、腰夹脊、环跳、委中、阳陵泉、悬钟、丘墟,平补平泻法(腰部取双侧同名穴,下肢取患侧穴位),每次留针30min,每天1次。

西药加针刺共治疗14天,患者住院期间严格卧硬板床休息。前7天为1个疗程,后7天为1个疗程,第1个疗程结束后如痊愈可不进入第2个疗程。

2.**观察指标、观察周期与时点** 采用改良日本骨科协会腰痛评分表(M-JOA)。评分表总分为30分,病情程度分级:轻度者总分≤10分,10分<中度者总分≤20分,20分<重度者总分≤30分。改善率=[(治疗前分值−治疗后分值)/治疗前分值]×100%。所选病例均满足治疗前临床症状评分积分值>10。

观察周期为14天,随访观察6个月。观察时点分别为治疗前、治疗1个疗程后、治疗结束后即刻及治疗结束后6个月。

3.**研究结果** 共纳入合格受试者456例。其中试验组、对照A组、对照B组分别完成152例。试验完成后失访脱落共26例,占5.70%。患者的性别、年龄、体重等人口学特征具有可比性($P>0.05$)。腰椎间盘突出症患者中,M-JOA评分量表总分、各项因子以及病情严重程度等基线资料均具有可比性($P>0.05$)。

(1)**M-JOA评分量表总分**:如表1-1-12所示,治疗7天,即1个疗程时，3组比较有非常显著性差异（$P<0.01$）；治疗14天，即结束后，3组比较有非常显著性差异（$P<0.01$）。随访6个月后，3组比较有非常显著性差异（$P<0.01$）。试验结果表明，选取热敏态腧穴施灸治疗腰椎间盘突出症（急性期）对M-JOA评分的改善优于传统选穴施灸。

表 1-1-12　M-JOA 评分量表总分比较（$\bar{x} \pm s$）

观测时点	组别		
	试验组	对照 A 组	对照 B 组
治疗前	18.6 ± 3.8	17.5 ± 3.3	17.2 ± 4.4
治疗 7 天	9.8 ± 4.1 ★◆	12.6 ± 3.8 ★	13.2 ± 5.5 ★
治疗 14 天	3.8 ± 2.6 ★●	7.9 ± 3.0 ★	8.5 ± 2.9 ★
随访 6 个月	3.7 ± 2.2 ★●	8.9 ± 3.1 ★	10.1 ± 2.9 ★

注：★表示与治疗前比较 $P<0.01$，◆表示与对照组比较 $P<0.05$，●表示与对照组比较 $P<0.01$。

（2）治疗结束后 3 组间临床整体疗效比较： 如表 1-1-13 所示，治疗结束后，3 组愈显率比较具有非常显著性差异（$P<0.01$）。结果表明，选取热敏腧穴施灸治疗腰椎间盘突出症（急性期）的临床整体疗效优于传统选穴施灸。

表 1-1-13　3 组间临床整体疗效比较

组别	例数	治愈（治愈率 /%）	显效（显效率 /%）	有效（有效率 /%）	无效（无效率 /%）	愈显数（愈显率 /%）
试验组	152	46（30.26）	80（52.63）	20（13.16）	6（3.95）	126（82.89）
对照 A 组	152	20（13.16）	56（36.84）	67（44.07）	9（5.93）	76（50.00）
对照 B 组	152	26（17.10）	58（38.16）	57（37.50）	11（7.24）	84（55.26）

4. 研究结论　试验组的 M-JOA 评分、临床整体疗效均明显优于对照组，选取热敏腧穴治疗腰椎间盘突出症（急性期）的疗效明显优于传统选穴施灸。

（二）艾灸不同功能态腧穴治疗膝关节骨性关节炎（肿胀型）的临床疗效研究[21-23]

由江西中医药大学附属医院牵头，组织 4 家医院同样采用大样本、多中心、中央随机对照试验方法联合开展了艾灸不同功能态腧穴治疗膝关节骨性关节炎（肿胀型）的临床疗效研究。

1. 治疗方案

（1）**热敏腧穴悬灸治疗组**

1）热敏腧穴的探查：①环境：检测室保持安静，室内温度保持在 24 ~ 30℃；②体位：选择舒适、充分暴露病位的体位；③探查工具：江西省中医院生产，规格：直径 22mm × 长度 160mm 特制精艾绒艾条；④探查方法：选择仰卧体位，充分暴露膝关节，用点燃的艾条在患者膝关节周围（阴陵泉 – 阳陵泉 – 梁丘 – 血海穴组成的区域内），距离皮肤 3cm 左右施行温和灸，当患者感受到艾热发生透热（艾热从施灸部位皮肤表面直接向深部组织穿透）、扩热（以施灸点为中心向周围扩散）、传热（灸热从施灸点开始循某一方向传导）和非热觉中的一种或一种以上感觉时，即为发生腧穴热敏现象，该探查穴点为热敏腧穴。重复上述步骤，直至所有的热敏穴位被探查出。

2）热敏腧穴的悬灸方法：首先在上述热敏化强度最强的穴位实施艾条温和悬灸，每天 2 次，每次施灸时间以上述热敏化高发区内所有热敏穴热敏灸感消失为度（上限 60min，下限 30min），共治疗 5 天，第 6 天开始每天 1 次，连续治疗 25 次，共治疗 35 次（共 30 天），治疗前、治疗结束后及 6 个月后进行疗效评价。

（2）**非热敏腧穴悬灸对照组（对照 A 组）**：在内、外膝眼，鹤顶实施温和悬灸，每天 2 次，每次每穴 15min，3 穴共 45min，共治疗 5 天，第 6 天开始每天 1 次，连续治疗 25 次，共治疗 35 次（共 30 天），治疗前、治疗结束后及 6 个月后进行疗效评价。

（3）**西药对照组（对照 B 组）**：每 6 天给患侧膝关节腔内注射玻璃酸钠 2ml，共注射 5 次，治疗前、治疗结束后及 6 个月后进行疗效评价。

2. 观察指标、观察周期与时点　参照《中药新药临床研究指导原则》（2002 年版），按疼痛、活动与疼痛的关系、功能障碍相关的特殊检查分项就其程度进行评分。按下列标准评估膝关节骨性关节炎的轻重程度：轻度＜5分；中度5～9分；重度＞9分。本课题所选病例均满足治疗前临床症状评分积分值≥5。

临床控制：症状消失，功能活动正常，临床症状评分减少≥95%；

显效：症状基本消失，关节功能基本正常，能参加正常活动和工作，临床症状评分减少≥70%、＜95%；

有效：疼痛基本消失，关节屈伸活动基本正常，参加活动或工作能力有改善，临床症状评分减少≥30%、＜70%；

无效：未达到有效标准，临床症状评分减少不足30%。

观察周期为30天，随访观察6个月。观察时点分别为治疗前、治疗结束后即刻、治疗结束后6个月。

3. 研究结果

（1）**膝关节GPCRND-KOA评分量表总分**：如表1-1-14所示，治疗结束后，3组比较有显著性差异（$P<0.05$）。随访6个月后，3组比较有非常显著性差异（$P<0.01$）。结果表明，选取热敏腧穴施灸治疗膝关节骨性关节炎（肿胀型）优于传统选穴施灸。

表1-1-14 GPCRND-KOA评分量表总分比较（$\bar{x} \pm s$）

观测时点	组别		
	试验组	对照A组	对照B组
治疗前	11.2 ± 3.3	11.3 ± 3.2	12.1 ± 2.9
治疗30天	2.8 ± 1.8 ★◆	4.9 ± 2.8 ★	5.6 ± 2.1 ★
随访6个月	3.6 ± 1.6 ★●	6.4 ± 1.5 ★	7.0 ± 1.9 ★

注：★表示与治疗前比较$P<0.01$，◆表示与对照组比较$P<0.05$，●表示与对照组比较$P<0.01$。

（2）**膝关节周径比较**：如表1-1-15所示，治疗结束后，3组比较有显著性差异（$P<0.05$）。随访6个月后，3组比较有显著性差异（$P<0.05$）。结果表明，选取热敏腧穴施灸对膝关节骨性关节炎肿胀的改善作用优于传统选穴施灸。

表 1-1-15　3 组间膝关节周径比较（$\bar{x} \pm s$）　　　单位: cm

观测时点	组别		
	试验组	对照 A 组	对照 B 组
治疗前	41.2 ± 3.2	42.2 ± 3.2	41.3 ± 2.7
治疗 30 天	36.8 ± 2.7○◆	38.3 ± 2.6	38.6 ± 2.2
随访 6 个月	35.7 ± 1.8○◆	37.4 ± 1.6○	37.2 ± 1.4○

注：○表示与治疗前比较 $P < 0.05$，◆表示与对照组比较 $P < 0.05$。

（3）**治疗结束后 3 组间临床整体疗效比较**：如表 1-1-16 所示，治疗结束后，3 组愈显率比较具有显著性差异（$P < 0.05$）。结果表明，选取热敏腧穴施灸治疗膝关节骨性关节炎（肿胀期）的临床整体疗效优于传统选穴施灸。

表 1-1-16　3 组间临床整体疗效比较

组别	例数	治愈（治愈率 /%）	显效（显效率 /%）	有效（有效率 /%）	无效（无效率 /%）	愈显数（愈显率 /%）
试验组	144	31（21.52）	69（47.92）	40（27.78）	4（2.78）	100（69.44）
对照 A 组	144	16（11.11）	50（34.72）	62（43.05）	16（11.12）	66（45.83）
对照 B 组	144	14（9.72）	63（43.75）	52（36.11）	15（10.42）	77（53.47）

　　4. 研究结论　试验组的 GPCRND-KOA 评分、关节周径、临床整体疗效明显优于对照组，选取热敏腧穴治疗膝关节骨性关节炎（肿胀期）的疗效明显优于传统选穴施灸。

　　（三）艾灸热敏腧穴治疗支气管哮喘（慢性持续期）的临床疗效研究 [24-25]

　　由江西中医药大学附属医院牵头，组织 12 家医院采用大样本、多中心、中央随机对照试验方法联合开展了艾灸热敏腧穴治疗支气管哮喘（慢性持续期）的临床疗效研究。各分中心受试对象的随机分配采用中心随机化方法，由中国中医科学院中医临床基础医学研究所统一控制，随机分为试验组（热敏腧穴悬灸治疗组）、对照组（西药对照组），分组结果采用

"药物临床试验中央随机分配交互式语音操作系统 V1.00（中央随机分配系统）"通过语音电话、网络进行发布。

1. 治疗方案

（1）试验组

1）热敏腧穴的探查：①环境：检测室保持安静，室内温度保持在24~30℃；②体位：选择舒适、充分暴露病位的体位；③探查工具：江西省中医院生产，规格：直径22mm×长度160mm特制精艾绒艾条；④探查方法：选择俯卧或侧卧体位，充分暴露胸背部，用点燃的艾条在患者双侧肺俞、膈俞，距离皮肤3cm左右施行温和灸，当患者感受到艾热发生透热（艾热从施灸部位皮肤表面直接向深部组织穿透）、扩热（以施灸点为中心向周围扩散）、传热（灸热从施灸点开始循某一方向传导）和非热觉中的一种或一种以上感觉时，即为发生腧穴热敏现象，该探查穴点为热敏腧穴。重复上述步骤，直至所有的热敏腧穴被探查出。

2）热敏腧穴的悬灸方法：在上述热敏化强度最强的穴位实施艾条温和悬灸，每次艾灸时间以热敏灸感消失为度（上限60min，下限30min），在第1个月的前8天，每天1次，剩余的22天共治疗12次。第2、3个月，每个月治疗15次。

（2）对照组：患者入院后第1天即开始使用沙美特罗替卡松粉吸入剂（沙美特罗50μg/氟替卡松250μg），每次1吸，每天2次，持续90天。

2. 观察指标、观察周期与时点　主要观察指标为治疗前，治疗后15天、30天、60天和90天的哮喘控制测试（asthma control test，ACT）问卷。ACT评分包括5个问题：活动受限，呼吸困难，夜间症状，药物使用情况和过去4个星期的发作频率。计分从1（最差）至5（最佳），最高得分为25分。次要观察指标是第1秒用力呼气容积（forced expiratory volume in one second，FEV_1），最大呼气流量（maximal expiratory flow，MEF），发作频率和不良反应。

3. 研究结果　本临床研究共纳入合格受试者288例。其中试验组、对照组分别完成144例。试验完成后失访、脱落共11例，占3.82%。患者的年龄、性别、哮喘持续时间和ACT评分具有可比性（$P>0.05$）。

（1）ACT评分比较：如表1-1-17所示，治疗3个月后得分（$P=0.0002$）和在6个月的随访期间得分（$P=0.00003$），有显著性差异。图1-1-2显示两组的平均ACT分数在治疗半个月至随访6个月期间持续增加。在对照组中，ACT 评分在 3 个月和 6 个月的随访期间保持稳定，并且患者在随访期间继续逐渐减少服用药物的剂量。

表 1-1-17　两组不同时间点 ACT 评分比较（$\bar{x} \pm s$）

观察时点	组别		t 值	P 值
	试验组	对照组		
治疗前	15.10 ± 4.05	15.70 ± 3.78	1.30	0.19
治疗半个月	17.86 ± 3.69	18.54 ± 4.13	−1.18	0.14
治疗 1 个月	19.54 ± 3.68	19.81 ± 3.99	−0.31	0.56
治疗 2 个月	20.65 ± 3.22	20.98 ± 3.27	−0.52	0.39
治疗 3 个月	21.60 ± 2.77	21.20 ± 3.61	3.15	0.000 2
随访 3 个月	21.35 ± 2.75	20.47 ± 3.58	2.68	0.000 9
随访 6 个月	21.29 ± 2.88	20.35 ± 3.72	4.42	0.000 03

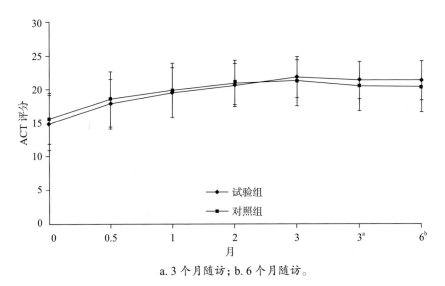

a. 3 个月随访；b. 6 个月随访。

图 1-1-2　两组不同时间点 ACT 评分比较

（2）**发作频率比较**：如表 1-1-18 所示，热敏灸组治疗 3 个月后哮喘发作的频率大大低于对照组（$P = 0.000\ 17$），在 6 个月的随访期间，两组之间仍存在明显差异（$P = 0.047$）。

表 1-1-18　两组不同时间点发作频率比较（$\bar{x} \pm s$）

观察时点	组别		t 值	P 值
	试验组	对照组		
治疗前	4.53 ± 1.02	4.36 ± 1.13	0.21	0.18
治疗 3 个月	0.81 ± 0.29	1.28 ± 0.25	3.56	0.000 17
随访 6 个月	0.59 ± 0.25	1.12 ± 0.33	1.74	0.047

（3）中医症状比较：采用 ITT 分析，比较两组中医症状，分别在治疗 1 个月时、3 个月治疗结束时以及治疗结束 6 个月后有统计学意义。为了便于进一步分析，将其中中医症状各项因子在治疗前积分值为 2 分的例数抽提出来，对其在 3 个月治疗结束时积分值提高了 2 分的记为"显效"，比治疗前提高 1 分的记为"有效"，积分前后无变化的记为"无效"。结果显示，两组中医症状显效率比较均有统计学意义（见表 1-1-19 ~ 表 1-1-23）。数据分析提示：热敏灸在改善患者中医症状方面，如寐差、易于感冒、倦怠无力、畏寒、胸闷等，有一定疗效优势。

表 1-1-19　3 个月治疗结束时两组寐差显效率比较

组别	例数	显效	显效率	两组比较 P 值
试验组	33	18	54.5%	<0.01
对照组	35	16	45.7%	

表 1-1-20　3 个月治疗结束时两组易于感冒显效率比较

组别	例数	显效	显效率	两组比较 P 值
试验组	42	18	42.9%	<0.01
对照组	48	10	20.8%	

表 1-1-21　3 个月治疗结束时两组倦怠无力显效率比较

组别	例数	显效	显效率	两组比较 P 值
试验组	27	14	51.9%	<0.01
对照组	32	6	18.8%	

表 1-1-22　**3 个月治疗结束时两组畏寒显效率比较**

组别	例数	显效	显效率	两组比较 P 值
试验组	48	24	50.0%	<0.01
对照组	43	17	39.5%	

表 1-1-23　**3 个月治疗结束时两组胸闷显效率比较**

组别	例数	显效	显效率	两组比较 P 值
试验组	42	17	40.5%	<0.01
对照组	40	9	22.5%	

4. 研究结论　治疗 3 个月后和随访期间，试验组与对照组的 ACT 评分和肺功能在治疗前后存在显著差异，表明具有等效性。热敏灸在减少发作频率、改善患者中医症状方面，如寐差、倦怠无力、畏寒、胸闷、易于感冒等有明显疗效优势。

（四）艾灸不同功能态腧穴治疗神经根型颈椎病的临床疗效研究

临床上温和灸治疗神经根型颈椎病时选择热敏腧穴优于非热敏腧穴。例如：唐福宇等[26]将神经根型颈椎病患者分为热敏灸组与传统艾灸组（各 60 例），热敏灸组在百会、颈夹脊、大椎、至阳、手三里、阳陵泉等穴位附近或皮下有硬结、条索状物等反应物部位探查热敏腧穴进行热敏灸，传统艾灸组在以上部位辨证选取两个腧穴进行温和灸，每天治疗 1 次，7 天为 1 疗程。结果显示，热敏灸组有效率为 86.70%，传统艾灸组有效率为 63.30%；3 个月随访，热敏组有效率为 82.70%，传统艾灸组有效率为 63.3%。李冠豪等[27]在颈背部及上肢区域寻找热敏穴施热敏灸与在夹脊穴、风池、肩外俞等穴位温和灸治疗作对比，二者愈显率分别为 63.30%、40.00%，差异有统计学意义（$P<0.05$）。谢炎烽等[28]在颈夹脊、百会、大椎、至阳、手三里等穴区探查热敏穴施热敏灸治疗，相同穴区辨证取穴采用温和灸治疗进行疗效对比，结果显示，选择热敏腧穴施灸疗效更好。

第二节　"艾灸得气"新概念

一、艾灸得气的含义

得气是针刺学中的一个重要概念，《灵枢·九针十二原》曰"刺之要，气至而有效"，可见得气与否与疗效密切相关。得气，近又称"针感"，是指当针刺入腧穴后，通过施用捻转、提插等手法，使针刺部位产生特殊的感觉和反应。这种经气感应产生时，患者会在针下出现相应的酸、麻、胀、重等感觉，并可沿着一定的部位、向一定方向扩散传导，同时，医生会感到针下有徐和或沉紧的感觉[1]。然而，得气概念在灸疗学中，几乎是一个空白。陈日新执着研究艾灸 18 年，发现与系统研究了腧穴热敏现象，分析了灸疗过程中热敏现象与针刺得气现象的临床类同性，在《中国针灸》提出了"灸之要，气至而有效"新概念[29]，指出艾灸能够产生针刺类得气，也必须产生得气才能提高疗效。艾灸得气的表现是：透热、扩热、传热、局部不（微）热远部热、表面不（微）热深部热、非热觉，而不仅仅是施灸局部热、表面热。在此基础上，通过对《黄帝内经》得气原始定义的溯源，结合现代临床研究，2019 年陈日新在《中国针灸》正式提出了"艾灸得气"新概念[30]，即艾灸得气是指一组与疗效密切相关的、舒适的透热、扩热、传热等感应。艾灸得气新概念的提出不仅指导临床提高了灸疗疗效，而且丰富发展了灸疗学理论。

二、得气的古代文献依据

对得气概念的正确认识，应该溯源其原始定义。"得气"一词，首见于《素问·离合真邪论》，"吸则内针，无令气忤。静以久留，无令邪布。吸则转针，以得气为故。"这段论述提出了"得气"的概念，示范了针刺"得气"的操作手法，指出了施展针刺手法的目的是"以得气为故"。得气，在《黄帝内经》中又称"气至"，《灵枢·九针十二原》进一步论述了"得气"的内涵、表现与特征："刺之要，气至而有效。效之信，若风之吹云，明乎若见苍天。"这段经文首先指出了"得气"是一个与疗效有关的概念，即"气至而有效"；接着用了一个天气变化的例子论述了"得气"的表现与特征，即"效之信，若风之吹云，明乎若见苍天"。试想从天空乌云密布，马上就要下大雨，到一阵风吹过，突然云开日见，一片蔚蓝天空出现在眼前，心神是何等的豁然开朗、愉悦舒适。《黄帝内经》中这个举例不仅说明了针刺得气之后的速效、特效，而且描述了得气时舒适愉悦的心身感受。因此，笔者认为：《内经》"得气"概念的原始定义与内涵是指针刺产生的一种与疗效有关的，愉悦与舒适的心身感应与体验，而不仅仅是指针刺产生的躯体感应。可见，《内经》中原始定义的"得气"概念内涵包括三个要素：一是针刺激发的躯体感应，二是伴发的舒适的心神感受，三是以前二者为基础的疗效反应。在这里，笔者将这三个要素称为《内经》"得气"概念三特征，即：舒适的躯体与心神感应及病痛缓解的疗效反应。然而，艾灸得气在《黄帝内经》中几乎是空白，直到清·吴谦《医宗金鉴·刺灸心法要诀》论述"凡灸诸病，必火足气到，始能求愈"，说明灸法和针刺一样需要得气，"气到"才能取得更好疗效。那么"气到"的表现是什么？历代医家也有一些观察，如《黄帝明堂灸经》说："灸穴不中，即火气不能远达，而病未能愈矣。"《备急灸法·骑竹马灸法》云"觉火气游走，周遍一身，蒸蒸而热"，"其艾火即随流注先至尾闾，其热如蒸，又透两外肾，俱觉蒸热，移时复流足涌泉穴，自下而上，渐渐周遍一身，奇功异效盖原于此也"。《针灸大成·取灸痔漏法》云："痔疾未深，止灸长强甚效……觉一团火气通入肠至胸，乃效。"《医学入门·炼脐法》中指出："艾火灸之，无时损易，壮其热气，或自上而下，自下而上，一身热透。患人必倦沉如醉，灸至五六十壮，遍身大汗，上至泥丸宫，下至涌泉穴。如此，则骨髓风寒暑湿，五劳七伤尽皆拔除。苟不汗则病未愈，再于三五日后又灸，灸至汗出为度。"由此可见，《黄帝内经》等古代文献对艾灸得气现象已有零星描述，但缺乏系统论述。

三、艾灸得气的临床特征

《针灸学》教科书在论述悬灸操作时有这样一段话：使患者局部有温热感而无灼痛为宜，至皮肤出现红晕为度[1]。这显然与《内经》中原始定义的"得气"内涵三要素不同。陈日新团队基于长期的灸疗实践，发现人体在疾病状态下，相关腧穴会发生热敏化，热敏腧穴对艾热刺激产生"小刺激、大反应"，如透热、扩热、传热、局部不（微）热远部热、表面不（微）热深部热、非热觉等热敏灸感[2,5,31]，而非热敏腧穴对艾热仅产生局部和表面的热感。进一步的研究表明，热敏灸感的出现伴随着舒适情感的产生，并且显著提高疗效[29,32]。可见，艾灸热敏腧穴能够激发《内经》原始定义的"得气"，表现为透热、扩热、传热等躯体感应，舒适、愉悦、喜热的心神感受及显著提高灸疗疗效三个方面，符合《内经》"得气"概念三特征。

由于艾灸得气对艾灸疗效的重要性，艾灸得气条目的系统筛查与量化就显得尤为重要。艾灸得气的量化评估必须以得气条目为基础，而得气条目的基础是灸感条目，因此首先对灸感条目进行科学、系统的筛查，这是对艾灸得气条目系统筛查、量化及艾灸得气量表研制的前提。陈日新团队从古籍、文献和医患访谈中对灸感条目进行了系统筛查研究，编制了热敏灸感条目专家问卷调查表，并运用国际常用的德尔菲法对热敏灸感条目进行科学、系统的筛查研究。结果表明，通过文献分析与访谈，所得灸感初始条目为40条，再通过两轮德尔菲法问卷调查分析与专家积极程度、意见的集中程度、协调程度、权威程度等指标的评估，最终筛查出热敏灸感条目25条。在此基础上，笔者团队为了进一步筛查与量化艾灸得气条目，通过专家问卷、患者问卷以及核心小组专家讨论，采用主观评价法对热敏灸感条目进行筛选并量化，对灸感条目25条层层筛选后剩余得气条目10条，建立了艾灸得气条目的量表初稿[33-34]。这10条的得气量表条目分别是：透热、扩热、传热、非热觉、皮肤扩散性潮红、面红（或额汗出）、胃肠蠕动、肢端热、身烘热、喜热（舒适感）。通过探索性因子分析（主要成分）检测量表的结构效度及使用克朗巴赫系数评估量表的内部一致性，对上述条目进行了初步评价。共纳入患者121例，其中回收有效量表110份，共计110例，超过条目数的5倍，符合样本要求。计算KMO值 = 0.679，Bartlett球形度检验值为229.478，自由度为36，$P = 0.00$，说明适合进行因子分析。采用探索性因子分析（主要成分）检测量表的结构效度，经最大变异法转轴后，提取4个公因子，其累积方差贡献率为73.924%，陡坡图也显示提取4个公因子可以采纳，条目的因子负荷量大于0.4被认为具有这一因子的特征（见表1-2-1）。肢端热、身烘热、喜热为因子1，为涉及全身舒适情感体验；皮肤扩散性潮红、面红（或额汗出）、胃肠蠕动反应为因子2，为自主神经反应；透热、扩热、传热为因子 3，为灸感的热觉感传；非热觉不归类为前三者任何一因子，而单独为因子 4，是除热觉外的其他感觉。前 3 个维度的内在一致性系数均大于 0.6，分别为：全身舒适情感体验 0.773，自主神经反应 0.665，热觉感传 0.677。这说明各因子内部一致性较好，信度可以接受，条目可靠。令作者惊讶的是：上述经临床采集与数学计算后得到的三个因子恰与《内经》"得气"概念的三特征殊途同归，一一对应：一是热觉感传对应躯体感应，二是全身舒适情感体验对应舒适心神感应，三是自主神经反应对应疗效反应。

表 1-2-1　热敏灸得气灸感条目因子分析 – 因子负荷矩阵

条目	因子 1 全身舒适情感体验	因子 2 自主神经反应	因子 3 热感传	因子 4 非热觉
肢端热	**0.822**	0.133	—	−0.157
身烘热	**0.807**	0.204	—	0.247
舒适感	**0.791**	—	0.323	0.103
皮肤扩散性潮红	0.163	**0.827**	—	—
面红（或额汗出）	0.229	**0.736**	—	−0.367
胃肠蠕动反应	—	**0.719**	—	0.308
透热	—	—	**0.870**	—
扩传热	0.190	—	**0.845**	—
非热觉	0.106	—	—	**0.917**

注：SPSS 软件设置中因子负荷小于 0.1 则不显示，用"—"表示。

在上述研究的基础上，对上述艾灸得气条目进行量化，构建了艾灸得气量表，分为 A、B、C 3 个部分计分[3]。

A 部分包括透热、传热、非热觉 3 项，每项计分均由灸感出现的空间位置与灸感强度的乘积所得。灸感出现的空间位置分为 4 个等级，即：无（0）；指向病所但未超过一半（1）；指向病所超过一半，但未到达病所（2）；到达病所（3）。灸感强度也分为 4 个等级，即：无（0）；轻度（1）；

中度（2）；明显（3）。

B 部分为扩热，计分同样是由灸感出现的空间位置与灸感强度的乘积所得。灸感出现的空间位置分 4 个等级：灸感长径＜2.5 倍艾条直径（0）；灸感长径≥2.5 倍且＜5 倍艾条直径（1）；灸感长径≥5 倍且＜10 倍艾条直径（2）；灸感长径≥10 倍艾条直径（3）。灸感强度分级与 A 部分相同。

C 部分包括喜热、身烘热、面红（或额汗出）、肢端热、胃肠蠕动反应、皮肤扩散性潮红 6 项，由于这 6 项无空间位置的变化，故只计算灸感强度，分 4 个等级，即：无（0）；轻度（1）；中度（2）；明显（3）。

量表按照 A、B、C 的顺序计分，若 A 中传热项为 0，可进入 B 计分，若 A 中传热项不为 0，则直接跳至 C 计分。A、B、C 得分之和即为量表总分（见表 1-2-2）。

表 1-2-2　**热敏灸得气灸感量表** V1.0

热敏灸得气灸感量表 V1.0							
A 表							
A 表项	灸感出现的空间位置（X）				灸感强度（Y）		
	无（0）	指向病所，但未超过一半（1）	指向病所，超过一半，但未到达病所（2）	到达病所（3）	无（0）	轻度（1）	中度（2）	明显（3）
透热 T = X × Y								
传热 C = X × Y								
非热觉 F = X × Y								
A 总分 = T + C + F								

续表

B 表								
B 表项	灸感出现的空间位置（X）				灸感强度（Y）			
	灸感长径 < 2.5 倍 艾条直径 （0）	灸感长径 ≥2.5 倍 且＜5 倍 艾条直径 （1）	灸感长径 ≥5 倍且 ＜10 倍 艾条直径 （2）	灸感长径 ≥10 倍 艾条直径 （3）	无 （0）	轻度 （1）	中度 （2）	明显 （3）
扩热 $K = X \times Y$								
B 总分 = K								

C 表				
C 表项	计分等级			
	无（0）	轻度（1）	中度（2）	明显（3）
舒适感 S1				
身烘热 S2				
面红（额汗出）M				
肢端热 Z				
胃肠蠕动反应 W				
皮肤扩散性潮红 P				
C 总分 = S1 + S2 + M + Z + W + P				
量表总分 W = A + B + C				

使用说明：

1.本表按照 A、B、C 表的顺序计分，若 A 表中传热项为 0，可进入 B 项计分，若 A 表中传热项不为 0，则直接跳至 C 表计分。

2.本表仅适用于热敏穴位。

四、艾灸得气的客观显示

（一）艾灸得气现象高密度脑电的客观显示

人类感觉是外界刺激投射到大脑意识领域而产生的。大脑神经细胞的基本活动是电活动。廖斐斐等[35-37]通过 EGI 128 导高密度脑电系统记录慢性腰背痛患者静息态、艾灸中及艾灸后脑电信号，结果显示：腧穴热敏现象伴随显著头皮脑电活动改变，主要体现在出现热敏现象时的 theta，alpha 和 beta 频段功率频谱密度增高。脑电地形图提示 theta 和 beta 频段功率频谱密度（power spectral density，PSD）变化以额顶区为主，而 alpha 频段则为广泛性变化。此外，热敏现象伴随 theta 和 beta 频段相位同步化也显著增强，而未出现热敏现象的患者以上变化均不明显。结果表明，在热敏位点艾灸过程中，大脑神经网络中确有明显不同的电活动产生，并且这种电活动有明显的调节紊乱功能的作用。

黄仙保等[38]观察了艾灸膝关节骨性关节炎患者外膝眼穴得气时脑电功率频谱密度特征变化。结果提示，艾灸热敏外膝眼穴过程中与灸后、灸前比较，平均功率频谱密度明显增加区域集中在双侧额区、顶区、枕区。并且在整个脑电能量中 alpha、beta 频段所占比重较大，而非得气状态下脑电信号变化较少，这有可能成为艾灸得气现象的客观判断指标之一。

（二）艾灸得气现象动物模型的客观显示

艾灸得气通常是施灸时患者的自我感觉，也可通过高密度脑电等技术客观反映。艾灸得气现象能否在动物上客观重现，对于其发生机制的生物学基础研究具有重要意义[39-41]。

1. **大脑中动脉线栓法建立大鼠缺血再灌注模型（MCAO/R）**　将浓度 3% 的戊巴比妥钠以 30mg/kg 剂量腹腔注射使大鼠麻醉。使用直肠探头监测中心体温，用加热灯和加热垫将温度保持在（37±0.5）℃。使用腔内线栓法实现大脑中动脉闭塞。简单地说就是从颈部正中切开，分离颈总动脉、颈内动脉和颈外动脉。用 4-0 号丝线结扎颈外动脉远端，再用 4-0 号丝线结扎颈总动脉近端。另一根丝线松散地扎在颈总动脉分叉处。用一根头部圆润，直径 0.205mm、长 5cm 的鱼线由颈总动脉插入，轻轻向前推进至大脑中动脉起始部（距离颈总动脉分叉处 18mm）。缠绕在颈总动脉上的丝线扎紧以阻止血流。经过 2 小时栓塞后，鱼线从大脑中动脉的起始部抽出，使脑部血液再灌注。

2. **脑缺血再灌注大鼠悬灸治疗**　实验过程中，将大鼠放置于一个特制的笼中，使大鼠保持一种舒适的体位，使其情绪稳定。用艾条（专门用于动物实验，长 12cm、直径 0.6cm，由江西省中医院生产）放置在离去毛皮肤的大椎穴约 3cm 高度处进行悬灸。悬灸于再灌注 6 小时后进行。共治疗 7 天，每天悬灸 1 次。根据悬灸时间分为 15 分钟和 40 分钟两组。

3. **大鼠尾温的测量**　在每次悬灸之前和之后应用热断层扫描成像（TTM）仪器分别探测大鼠背部纵轴的红外线温热信息。小于 0.05℃的温度变化均用 TTM 机记录下来。因应用 TTM 机探测的尾部温度为相对值，在 40 分钟治疗过程中，用电子数字温度计，每 2 分钟精确测量大鼠尾部中点的温度。测量环境保持安静，室温维持在（25±2）℃。实验开始之前需先将大鼠放置于笼中 30 分钟。

4. **大鼠神经学评估**　实验成员以外的测试者应用改良神经系统严重程度量表，分别在缺血再灌注后 0 小时、1 天、3 天和 7 天后进行神经学评估。简单地讲，这一量表的评分主要是通过评估动物的轻偏瘫实验（包括抓住大鼠尾巴将其提起或将大鼠放置于平板上），感觉缺失实验（定位，本体感觉），平衡木实验（包括将大鼠放置于窄的平衡横木上时大鼠对位置和姿势的反应以及掉落时间），反射缺失实验（包括听力反射、角膜反射和惊恐反射）和异常活动（包括抽搐、肌阵挛、肌张力障碍）等获得的神经功能缺损评分。该评分等级为 18 分制（正常为 0 分；最大功能缺损为 18 分），无法完成任务或反射缺失则加 1 分。

5. **热敏灸动物模型的建立**

（1）**悬灸 40 分钟能使部分脑缺血再灌注模型大鼠尾温升高，且尾温升高与模型的疾病状态密切相关**：悬灸治疗 40 分钟后，部分悬灸组 MCAO/R 大鼠出现尾温升高（平均超过 2℃），所占比例为 54.1%。此外，悬灸 15 分钟尾温即开始升高，并且温度峰值持续至悬灸 40 分钟结束。未接受悬灸治疗或悬灸 15 分钟治疗的 MCAO/R 大鼠尾温无变化。悬灸 15 分钟与未接受悬灸治疗的大鼠尾温变化趋势基本相同（见图 1-2-1、图 1-2-2）。

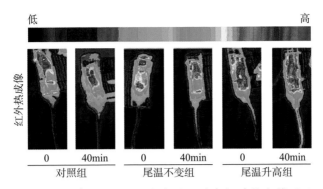

图 1-2-1　艾灸 MCAO/R 大鼠尾温升高红外热成像显示

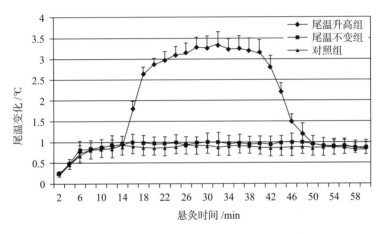

图 1-2-2　艾灸 MCAO/R 大鼠尾温升高时间序列图

（2）产生远部热效应（尾温升高）能提高悬灸疗效：7 天治疗中，悬灸 15 分钟与模型对照组比较，未能改善神经功能缺损评分；悬灸 40 分钟伴有尾温升高组于治疗第 3 天，与模型对照组和悬灸 15 分钟组比较，能明显降低神经功能缺损评分；第 7 天评分时，悬灸 40 分钟伴有尾温升高组（M40-2）与悬灸 40 分钟不伴有尾温升高组（M40-1）、悬灸 15 分钟组（M15）、模型对照组（C）比较，均具有统计学意义，且悬灸 40 分钟不伴有尾温升高组与模型对照组、悬灸 15 分钟组比较，也具有统计学意义。（见表 1-2-3，图 1-2-3）

表 1-2-3 尾温升高与疗效的关系（$\bar{x} \pm s$）

组别	0D	1D（第 1 天）	3D（第 3 天）	7D（第 7 天）
M40-2（悬灸 40min）	12.0 ± 1.5	9.2 ± 1.4	7.1 ± 1.2	4.4 ± 1.0*
M40-1（悬灸 40min）	11.8 ± 1.2	9.8 ± 1.5	8.3 ± 1.6	6.3 ± 1.5
M15（悬灸 15min）	11.0 ± 1.4	9.4 ± 1.5	8.8 ± 1.1	7.5 ± 1.2
C（模型对照组）	12.0 ± 1.5	10.0 ± 1.3	9.6 ± 1.6	7.9 ± 1.4

注：*表示 M40-2 组第 7 天分别与 M40-1 组、M15 组、C 组第 7 天比较，$P<0.01$。

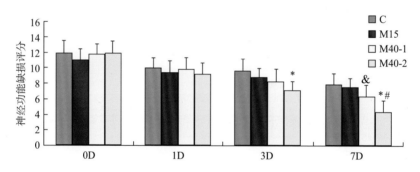

注：*表示 M40-2 组与 C 组比较，$P<0.01$；# 表示 M40-2 组与 M40-1 组比较，$P<$ 0.01；& 表示 M15 组与 C 组比较，$P<0.01$。

图 1-2-3 尾温升高与疗效的关系

以上研究结果表明：

①悬灸时，在 MCAO/R 大鼠模型能产生远部热效应；②产生远部热与疾病状态高度（MCAO/R 大鼠模型）相关；③产生远部热效应能提高悬灸疗效。

上述实验结果与临床热敏现象的特征完全吻合，标志热敏灸动物模型建立成功，同时首次在动物上客观显示了艾灸得气现象，为其生物学机制研究奠定了科学基础。

五、艾灸得气提高疗效的临床证据

得气是针灸获效的基础，而出现热敏灸感是艾灸得气的重要指征。临床实践表明，施灸过程中能否产生艾灸得气，直接影响着灸疗疗效。艾灸相同腧穴治疗疾病时，出现热敏灸感组与未出现热敏灸感组的治疗效果存在明显差异。陈日新等[42]采用神庭、大椎双点温和灸治疗椎动脉型颈椎病患者，每次治疗 50 分钟，每天 1 次，连续治疗 7 天。根据艾灸治疗时有无热敏灸感、出现热敏灸感的次数自然分为热敏灸感组和无热敏灸感组。结果显示，艾灸治疗时有无热敏灸感均有疗效，治疗前后比较均有统计学意义（$P<0.05$），但热敏灸感组在总分项、眩晕项、颈肩痛项明显优于无热敏灸感组（$P<0.05$）。表明悬灸过程中有无艾灸得气现象的出现与疗效密切相关，激发艾灸得气能够提高临床灸疗疗效。

陈日新等[22,43]采用热敏灸治疗膝关节骨性关节炎，依据在艾灸患侧内膝眼、外膝眼二穴过程中有无热感透至膝关节腔内作为艾灸得气的标准，将患者分为热敏灸感组（热感透至膝关节腔内）和普通灸感组（热感未透至膝关节腔内，或仅热感在施灸局部与表面），比较了不同灸感的两组患者临床疗效差异。结果显示，艾灸治疗过程中出现热敏灸感的疗效明显优于普通灸感（总有效率分别为 85.19% 与 58.82%，$P<0.05$），症状总积分及关节消肿程度亦明显优于普通灸感组（$P<0.05$）。以上结果均提示热敏灸感与疗效密切相关，重视热敏灸感是提高疗效的关键。

陈日新与熊俊等[19,44]观察艾灸治疗腰椎间盘突出症急性期不同灸感患者的疗效差异。用艾热探查 131 例腰椎间盘突出症急性期患者大肠俞、阿是穴、委中的灸感，根据患者灸感的不同，分为热敏灸感（6 种特殊的热敏灸感）与温热灸感（仅有局部温热感）。运用倾向评分匹配法对不同灸感患者进行匹配，得到组间协变量均衡的样本，共 30 对，热敏灸感患者为试验组，温热灸感患者为对照组。两组患者均采用艾灸治疗，分别于治疗前、治疗 2 周后、治疗后 6 个月观察两组患者改良日本骨科协会腰痛评分量表（M-JOA）评分及疼痛视觉模拟评分法（VAS）评分。结果显示：治疗 2 周及治疗后 6 个月，两组患者 M-JOA 评分及 VAS 评分均较治疗前显著下降（$P<0.05$ 或 $P<0.01$）。试验组均显著低于对照组（$P<0.05$ 或 $P<0.01$）。结果表明，艾灸治疗腰椎间盘突出症急性期患

者，产生热敏灸感者临床疗效优于温热灸感者，且热敏灸感患者疗效更为稳定。

张伟等[45]比较热敏灸与普通悬灸"关元"穴对原发性痛经（寒湿凝滞型）的疗效差异，探讨了灸感与灸效的相关性。该研究共纳入 180 例合格受试者，经灸感、红外联合探测法探查"关元"穴是否发生热敏化后，二次纳入病例 117 例，分为热敏灸组（灸感法与红外法皆阳性：61 例，均采用热敏灸疗法）和普通悬灸组（灸感法与红外法皆阴性：56 例，采用普通温和灸法）。结果显示：热敏灸组与普通悬灸组比较，对 COX 痛经症状量表（CMSS），经血中前列腺素 $F_{2\alpha}$（$PGF_{2\alpha}$）、前列腺素 E_2（PGE_2）、血管升压素含量的比较皆有非常显著性差异（$P<0.01$）。结果表明：热敏灸"关元"穴治疗原发性痛经疗效明显优于普通悬灸，说明灸感与灸效具有高度相关性。

有研究[46]根据慢性腹泻（脾虚型）患者天枢穴有无热敏灸感分为天枢穴热敏灸感组和非热敏灸感组，观察两组气至病所出现率及其动态过程。结果显示，悬灸时，天枢穴出现热敏灸感组气至病所出现率为 86.7%，未出现热敏灸感组为 22.4%，两组气至病所出现率比较差异有统计学意义（$P<0.01$）。表明艾灸热敏腧穴能高效激发经气，气至病所，这为热敏灸提高灸疗疗效提供了中医理论与临床依据。

上述结果表明，艾灸能像针刺一样激发得气，因此，灸之要，仍然是气至而有效。

第三节 "消敏灸量"新概念

一、消敏灸量的含义

目前常规艾灸每穴施灸时间为 10～15min[1]，远不能满足临床个体化的腧穴充足灸量，艾灸疗效的潜力没有得到发挥。灸量由艾灸强度、艾灸面积、艾灸时间三个因素决定，在前两个因素基本不变的情况下，灸量主要由艾灸时间所决定。陈日新团队通过系统研究灸感 – 灸量 – 灸效的关系，证实了以热敏灸感消失（或消退）为灸时标准，能够达到临床个体化的腧穴充足灸量，显著提高临床灸疗疗效[2]。于是在 2009 年出版的《热敏灸实用读本》专著中正式提出了"消敏灸量"新概念[5]，认为：在施灸时，每穴的施灸时间不应该千人一律，而应以热敏灸感消失（或消退）为度，这才是热敏腧穴的最佳个体化充足灸量，称为"消敏灸量"。达到这个灸量时，穴位的热敏态转化为消敏态（即非热敏态），灸疗疗效的潜力得到充分发挥。消敏灸量新概念的提出，首次解决了中医灸量如何实现个体化与标准化统一的难题，有效指导了临床提高灸疗疗效，为中医标准化提供了新思路。

二、消敏灸量的时效关系证据

陈日新教授等对灸疗过程中灸时与灸感的相关性进行了大样本、多中心临床研究，揭示了灸时－灸感发生发展呈现三个时相变化[5]，即经气激发潜伏期、经气传导期、经气消退期，见图 1-3-1。传统艾灸规定每穴治疗时间为 10～15min，正处在经气激发的潜伏期，灸疗疗效尚未充分发挥；从艾灸开始至经气传导期结束，平均为 40～50min，这主要是经气传导与气至病所期，是灸疗疗效的充分发挥期，达到这个施灸时间，艾灸疗效明显提高；继后是经气消退期，这段时间继续施灸，疗效也无明显增加[16]。经过大量研究发现热敏灸感的持续时间，即从热敏灸感产生到消失的时间，这个参数指标具有以下特征：①与疾病状态高度相关，会随着

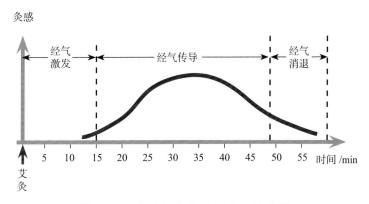

图 1-3-1　灸疗经气激发的时－效曲线

疾病的缓解而缩短；②与疗效高度相关，热敏灸感消失后继续在该穴位施灸，疗效无明显增加，而在热敏灸感消失前就提前结束施灸，疗效的潜力没有充分发挥；③以"热敏灸感消失时间"（即热敏灸感的持续时间）作为个体化施灸时间，疗效最好，这个时间是个体化的，因人、因病、因穴而不同，"消敏灸量"首次实现了施灸时间标准化与个体化的有机统一，突破了长期以来每穴 10～15min 固定灸时的标准，为临床充分发挥灸疗疗效提供了新的量学指导。

动物实验研究同样证实了上述规律。有研究者[39-41]以线栓法大脑中动脉闭塞大鼠模型悬灸 60min 观察其神经保护效应，探索艾灸的时效关系。研究结果表明：悬灸脑缺血模型大鼠的"大椎"穴可以导致部分大鼠的尾温升高。尾温升高的时效关系如图 1-3-2，呈现出明显的潜伏期、上升期、高峰期、下降期时效关系曲线。悬灸 40min 的疗效要优于悬灸 15min 的疗效（此时尾温升高效应还不明显，处在潜伏期），悬灸 40min 并伴有远部热（尾温升高）的疗效明显优于局部热（尾温未升高）的疗效。大鼠尾温升高并不因艾灸的持续存在而继续维持。悬灸 40min 和 60min 疗效无差异，说明当大鼠尾温开始下降时继续施灸对大鼠无明显提高疗效的作用。

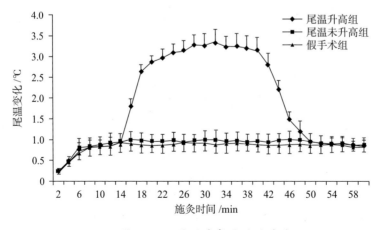

图 1-3-2　尾温升高的时效关系

三、消敏灸量判读的注意事项

"消敏灸量"以施灸过程中热敏灸感的消失为度，但是临床操作中"消敏"过程常常会受到其他因素的影响，需要仔细辨别、区别对待。热敏灸感的产生、消失受环境温度、施灸部位皮肤表面温度、体位的影响。人体在疾病状态下，热敏穴位的开放和热敏灸感的产生需要有一定的环境温度和达到一定的皮肤表面温度。施灸环境温度应在 24~30℃为宜，不宜低于 22℃。如果环境温度过低，不仅患者施灸时容易受寒，而且热敏穴位不容易激发得气。临床研究表明，艾灸得气的最佳激发皮肤温度为 42℃左右，因此我们在探查热敏穴位时常应用回旋灸、雀啄灸、循经往返灸、温和灸、接力灸或其组合手法温热局部气血，提高施灸部位皮肤表面温度。在施灸过程中，需要掸灰，应控制在 10 秒之内，以免皮肤表面温度下降，热敏穴位临时关闭，出现穴位消敏的假象。如果一次治疗内，这种情况反复出现，施灸有效时间减少，会影响施灸效果。如果施灸过程中需要临时暂停，要注意覆盖施灸部位，以免受寒。患者施灸时体位的改变也会影响艾灸得气，通常治疗前会要求患者以舒适的体态，充分暴露施灸部位，肌肉放松。在施灸过程中，患者体位的改变可能造成灸感产生部位肌肉紧张，得气会出现暂时消失，待肌肉放松后得气会再次产生。因此在判别"消敏灸量"时，需要注意环境温度、施灸部位皮肤表面温度、体位等因素，以免误判，影响疗效。临床上，随着施灸时间的延长，穴位热敏灸感变化常常出现以下几个类型：

1. 热敏灸感消失。这表明施灸穴位的此次灸量已饱和，可以结束施灸。

2. 热敏灸感消退或减弱。这表明灸量基本饱和，也可酌情结束此次施灸。

3. 热敏灸感超过 60min 仍然存在。这多见于慢病患者，表明灸量还未饱和，需要多次的灸量补充，但每次施灸也不可时间过长，以免出现疲劳等症状。

4. 一种热敏灸感消失后，另一种灸感出现。这表明灸量还未完全饱和，此时应该继续施灸，直到新的灸感完全消失。例如在腰部穴区施灸时，开始为酸胀感，酸胀感消失后转化为凉感，这种情况应该继续施灸，一直灸到凉感消失。

四、消敏灸量提高疗效的临床证据

（一）艾灸治疗腰椎间盘突出症（急性期）消敏灸量的随机对照试验

由江西中医药大学附属医院牵头，组织 4 家医院采用大样本、多中心、中央随机对照试验方法联合开展了艾灸治疗腰椎间盘突出症（急性期）消敏灸量的随机对照试验研究[47]。各分中心受试对象的随机分配采用中心随机化方法，由中国中医科学院中医临床基础医学研究所统一控制，随机分为试验组（个体化的消敏饱和灸量治疗组）、对照组（传统灸量对照组），分组结果采用"药物临床试验中央随机分配交互式语音操作系统 V1.00（中央随机分配系统）"通过语音电话、网络进行发布。

1. 治疗方案

（1）试验组

1）热敏腧穴的探查：①环境：检测室保持安静，室内温度保持在 24～30℃；②体位：选择舒适、充分暴露病位的体位；③探查工具：江西省中医院生产，规格：直径 22mm×长度 160mm 特制精艾绒艾条；④探查方法：选择俯卧或侧卧体位，充分暴露腰部，用点燃的艾条在患者双侧大肠俞与腰俞构成的三角区域（大肠俞－腰俞－对侧大肠俞区域内），距离皮肤 3cm 左右施行温和灸，当患者感受到艾热发生透热（艾热从施灸部位皮肤表面直接向深部组织穿透）、扩热（以施灸点为中心向周围扩散）、传热（灸热从施灸点开始循某一方向传导）和非热觉中的一种或一种以上感觉时，即为发生腧穴热敏现象，该探查穴点为热敏腧穴。重复上述步骤，直至所有的热敏腧穴被探查出。

2）治疗方法：在上述热敏化强度最强的穴位实施艾条温和悬灸，每天 2 次，每次艾灸时间以热敏灸感消失为度（上限 60min，下限 30min），共治疗 4 天，第 5 天开始每天 1 次，连续治疗 10 次，共治疗 18 次（共 14 天），前 7 天为 1 个疗程，后 7 天为 1 个疗程，第 1 个疗程结束后如痊愈可不进入第 2 个疗程。

（2）对照组：在上述热敏化强度最强的穴位实施艾条温和悬灸，每天 2 次，每次 15min，共治疗 4 天，第 5 天开始每天 1 次，连续治疗 10 次，共治疗 18 次（共 14 天），前 7 天为 1 个疗程，后 7 天为 1 个疗程，第 1 个疗程结束后如痊愈可不进入第 2 个疗程。

2．观察指标、观察周期与时点　采用改良日本骨科协会腰痛评分表（M-JOA）。评分表总分为 30 分，病情程度分级：轻度者总分≤10 分，10＜中度者总分≤20 分，20＜重度者总分≤30 分。改善率＝[（治疗前分值－治疗后分值）/ 治疗前分值]×100%。所选病例均满足治疗前临床症状评分积分值＞10。

目前国内对腰椎间盘突出症尚未制定统一疗效标准，参照国内外文献，认为判定疗效关键在于缓解疼痛，恢复腰部功能，预防及延缓腰椎组织结构改变。结合临床情况，以改良日本骨科协会腰痛评分表为依据拟定以下评判标准：

痊愈：腰部疼痛、下肢放射痛基本消失，腰部功能恢复正常，直腿抬高 70° 以上，改善率≥75%；

显效：腰部疼痛、下肢放射痛明显减轻，腰部活动功能基本正常，50%≤改善率＜75%；

有效：腰部疼痛、下肢放射痛减轻，腰部活动功能部分恢复，30%≤改善率＜50%；

无效：临床症状及腰部功能较治疗前后未改善，改善率＜30%。

观察周期为 14 天，随访观察 6 个月。观察时点分别为治疗前、治疗 1 个疗程后、治疗结束后即刻及治疗结束后 6 个月。

3．研究结果　本临床研究共纳入合格受试者 96 例。其中试验组、对照组分别完成 48 例。治疗完成后脱落共 2 例，占 2.08%。患者的性别、年龄、体重等人口学特征具有可比性（P＞0.05）。腰椎间盘突出症患者中，改良日本骨科协会腰痛评分量表总分、各项因子以及病情严重程度等基线资料均具有可比性（P＞0.05）。

（1）**改良日本骨科协会腰痛评分量表总分**：如表 1-3-1 所示，治疗 7 天，即 1 个疗程时，两组比较有非常显著性差异（P＜0.01）；治疗 14 天，即治疗结束后，两组比较有非常显著性差异（P＜0.01）。随访 6 个月后，两组比较有非常显著性差异（P＜0.01）。结果表明，热敏灸治疗腰椎间盘突出症（急性期），采用个体化消敏灸量优于传统固定灸量。

表 1-3-1　M-JOA 评分量表总分比较（$\bar{x} \pm s$）

观测时点	组别	
	试验组	对照组
治疗前	16.1 ± 4.7	16.5 ± 4.8
治疗 7 天	9.5 ± 3.9 ★◆	11.4 ± 5.0 ★
治疗 14 天	6.6 ± 4.8 ★●	9.0 ± 4.7 ★
随访 6 个月	4.4 ± 3.1 ★●	6.8 ± 3.4 ★

注：★表示与治疗前比较 $P<0.01$，◆表示与对照组比较 $P<0.05$，●表示与对照组比较 $P<0.01$。

（2）治疗结束后两组间临床整体疗效比较：如表 1-3-2 所示，治疗结束后，试验组治愈 18 例、显效 16 例、有效 12 例、无效 1 例，对照组治愈 8 例、显效 8 例、有效 28 例、无效 3 例，两组比较有非常显著性差异（$P<0.01$）。两组愈显率比较，试验组为 72.34%，对照组为 34.04%，具有非常显著性差异（$P<0.01$）。结果表明，热敏灸治疗腰椎间盘突出症（急性期），采用个体化消敏灸量优于传统固定灸量。

表 1-3-2　两组临床整体疗效比较

组别	例数	治愈（治愈率 /%）	显效（显效率 /%）	有效（有效率 /%）	无效（无效率 /%）	愈显数（愈显率 /%）
试验组	47	18（38.30）	16（34.04）	12（25.53）	1（2.13）	34（72.34）
对照组	47	8（17.02）	8（17.02）	28（59.57）	3（6.38）	16（34.04）

4. 研究结论　试验组的 M-JOA 评分、临床整体疗效优于对照组，选取个体化消敏灸量治疗腰椎间盘突出症（急性期）的疗效优于传统固定灸量。

（二）艾灸治疗膝关节骨性关节炎（肿胀型）消敏灸量的随机对照试验

由江西中医药大学附属医院牵头，组织 4 家医院采用大样本、多中心、中央随机对照试验方法联合开展了艾灸治疗膝关节骨性关节炎（肿胀型）消敏灸量的随机对照试验研究[48]。各分中心受试对象的随机分配采用中心随机化方法，由中国中医科学院中医临床基础医学研究所统一控制，随机分为试验组（个体化的消敏饱和灸量治疗组）、对照组（传统灸量对照组），分组结果采用"药物临床试验中央随机分配交互式语音操作系统 V1.00（中央随机分配系统）"通过语音电话、网络进行发布。

1. 治疗方案

（1）试验组

1）热敏腧穴的探查：①环境：检测室保持安静，室内温度保持在 24～30℃；②体位：选择舒适、充分暴露病位的体位；③探查工具：江西省中医院生产，规格：直径 22mm × 长度 160mm 特制精艾绒艾条；④探查方法：选择仰卧体位，充分暴露膝关节，用点燃的艾条在患者膝关节周围（阴陵泉 - 阳陵泉 - 梁丘 - 血海穴组成的区域内），距离皮肤 3cm 左右施行温和灸，当患者感受到艾热发生透热（艾热从施灸部位皮肤表面直接向深部组织穿透）、扩热（以施灸点为中心向周围扩散）、传热（灸热从施灸点开始循某一方向传导）和非热觉中的一种或一种以上感觉时，即为发生腧穴热敏现象，该探查穴点为热敏腧穴。重复上述步骤，直至所有的热敏腧穴被探查出。

2）治疗方法：选择上述热敏化强度最强的穴位实施艾条温和悬灸，每天 2 次，每次施灸时间以该穴热敏灸感消失为度（上限 60min，下限 30min），共治疗 5 天，第 6 天开始每天 1 次，连续治疗 25 次，共治疗 35 次（共 30 天），治疗前、治疗结束后及 6 个月后进行疗效评价。

（2）对照组：选择上述热敏化强度最强的 1 个穴位实施艾条温和悬灸，每天 2 次，每次 15min，共治疗 5 天，第 6 天开始每天 1 次，连续治疗 25 次，共治疗 35 次（共 30 天），治疗前、治疗结束后及 6 个月后进行疗效评价。

两组患者均嘱避风寒，调情志，清淡饮食。在本研究观察期内不允许加用其他治疗本病的相关药物及治疗方法。如患者在治疗期间病情加重，或发生其他病症，或失访，则退出观察组，放弃本治疗方法，改用相应综合治疗。

上述两组患者，由于病情需要，在治疗过程中如有其他用药情况，应如实记录。

2. 观察指标、观察周期与时点 参照《中药新药临床研究指导原则》（2002 年版），按疼痛、活动与疼痛的关系、功能障碍相关的特殊检查分项就其程度进行评分。按下列标准评估膝关节骨性关节炎的轻重程度：轻度<5 分；中度 5～9 分；重度>9 分。本课题所选病例均满足治疗前临床症状评分积分值≥5。

临床控制：症状消失，功能活动正常，临床症状评分减少≥95%；

显效：症状基本消失，关节功能基本正常，能参加正常活动和工作，临床症状评分减少≥70%，<95%；

有效：疼痛基本消失，关节屈伸活动基本正常，参加活动或工作能力有改善，临床症状评分减少≥30%，<70%；

无效：未达到有效标准，临床症状评分减少不足 30%。

观察周期为 30 天，随访观察 6 个月。观察时点分别为治疗前、治疗结束后即刻、治疗结束后 6 个月。

3. 研究结果 本临床研究共纳入合格受试者 72 例。其中试验组、对照组分别完成 36 例。试验完成后失访脱落共 3 例，占 4.17%。患者的性别、年龄、体重等人口学特征具有可比性（$P>0.05$）。膝关节骨性关节炎患者中，膝关节 GPCRND-KOA 评分量表总分、各项因子以及病情严重程度等基线资料均具有可比性（$P>0.05$）。

（1）膝关节 GPCRND-KOA 评分量表总分：如表 1-3-3 所示，治疗 30 天，即治疗结束后，两组积分比较有非常显著性差异（$P<0.01$）。随

表 1-3-3 GPCRND-KOA 评分量表总分比较（$\bar{x}\pm s$）

观测时点	组别	
	试验组	对照组
治疗前	11.22 ± 3.10	10.14 ± 3.00
治疗 30 天	3.44 ± 1.90 ★●	6.13 ± 3.00 ★
随访 6 个月	2.19 ± 1.80 ★●	5.10 ± 2.00 ★

注：★表示与治疗前比较 $P<0.01$，●表示与对照组比较 $P<0.01$。

访 6 个月后，两组积分比较有非常显著性差异（$P<0.01$）。结果表明，选取个体化消敏灸量治疗膝关节骨性关节炎（肿胀型）优于传统固定灸量。

（2）膝关节周径比较：如表 1-3-4 所示，治疗前试验组周径（39.32 ± 3.40）cm，对照组周径（39.01 ± 2.40）cm；治疗 30 天即治疗结束后，试验组周径（36.21 ± 3.40）cm，对照组周径（38.03 ± 2.70）cm，两组比较有显著性差异（$P<0.05$）。随访 6 个月后，试验组周径（35.81 ± 3.60）cm，对照组周径（37.92 ± 2.70）cm，两组比较有显著性差异（$P<0.05$）。结果表明，选取个体化消敏灸量对膝关节骨性关节炎肿胀的改善作用优于传统固定灸量。

表 1-3-4　两组间膝关节周径比较（$\bar{x} \pm s$）

观测时点	组别	
	试验组	对照组
治疗前	39.32 ± 3.40	39.01 ± 2.40
治疗 30 天	36.21 ± 3.40○◆	38.03 ± 2.70
随访 6 个月	35.81 ± 3.60○◆	37.92 ± 2.70○

注：○表示与治疗前比较 $P<0.05$，◆表示与对照组比较 $P<0.05$。

（3）**治疗结束后两组间临床整体疗效比较：**如表 1-3-5 所示，治疗结束后，试验组治愈 9 例、显效 10 例、有效 15 例、无效 2 例，对照组治愈 4 例、显效 6 例、有效 23 例、无效 3 例；两组比较有显著性差异（$P<0.05$）。两组愈显率比较，试验组为 52.78%，对照组为 27.78%，经统计具有显著性差异（$P<0.05$）。结果表明，选取个体化消敏灸量对膝关节骨性关节炎（肿胀期）的临床整体疗效优于传统固定灸量。

表 1-3-5　两组间临床整体疗效比较

组别	例数	治愈（治愈率/%）	显效（显效率/%）	有效（有效率/%）	无效（无效率/%）	愈显数（愈显率/%）
试验组	36	9（25.00）	10（27.78）	15（41.67）	2（5.55）	19（52.78）
对照组	36	4（11.11）	6（16.67）	23（63.89）	3（8.33）	10（27.78）

4．研究结论　试验组的 GPCRND-KOA 评分、关节周径、临床整体疗效优于对照组，选取个体化消敏灸量治疗膝关节骨性关节炎（肿胀期）的疗效优于传统固定灸量。

（三）艾灸治疗慢性前列腺炎消敏灸量的随机对照试验

康明非等[49]比较了热敏灸量与传统灸量治疗慢性前列腺炎的临床疗效差异。热敏灸量组选择天枢 – 中极 – 对侧天枢区域内及肾俞 – 同侧次髎 – 对侧次髎 – 对侧肾俞区域内的热敏腧穴施灸，以热敏灸感消失为度；传统灸量组在上述区域选热敏强度最强的 2 个穴位实施传统悬灸治疗，每次每穴 15min，2 穴共 30min。两组治疗 30 天，于治疗前、后观察各组症状分级量化积分、症状积分指数（NIH-CPSI）及前列腺液中白细胞计数（EPS-WBC）变化。结果显示，与治疗前相比，两组治疗后症状积分、NIH-CPSI 积分、WBC 计数差异均有统计学意义（均 $P < 0.01$）；与传统灸量相比，消敏灸量组症状积分、NIH-CPSI 积分、WBC 计数差异均有统计学意义（均 $P < 0.05$，$P < 0.01$），消敏灸量组愈显率为 45%，与传统灸量组相比，差异均有统计学意义（均 $P < 0.05$）。消敏饱和灸量艾灸治疗慢性前列腺炎临床疗效显著，优于传统灸量组。

（四）艾灸治疗椎动脉型颈椎病消敏灸量的随机对照试验

周小平等[50]将 60 例椎动脉型颈椎病患者随机分为饱和灸量组和常规灸量组，每组 30 例，两组均采用热敏灸治疗，选择热敏灸感最强的 2 个穴位上实施艾条温和悬灸，饱和灸量组艾灸时间以热敏灸感消失为度，常规灸量组每穴灸 15min，两组均每天治疗 2 次，共治疗 4 天，第 5 天起每天 1 次，连续治疗 10 次，共治疗 14 天。结果显示：饱和灸量组治疗后愈显率为 56.7%，6 个月后随访时愈显率为 60.0%，均优于常规灸量组的 26.7% 与 30.0%（$P < 0.01$，$P < 0.05$）；两组患者治疗后及随访时临床症状与功能评分均较治疗前明显升高（均 $P < 0.01$）；饱和灸量组治疗后功能评分为 22.32 ± 4.64，随访时功能评分为 23.01 ± 4.76，常规灸量组治疗后功能评分为 17.43 ± 3.21，随访时功能评分为 18.32 ± 2.13，治疗后及随访时饱和灸量组与常规灸量组比较，临床症状与功能评分升高更明显（$P < 0.01$）。消敏饱和灸量艾灸治疗椎动脉型颈椎病近期及远期疗效均优于传统灸量艾灸治疗。

（五）超饱和灸量研究

郑嵩[51]将60例肩周炎患者随机分为常规灸量组、饱和灸量组（以热敏感觉消失为度）和超饱和灸量组（在热敏感觉消失的基础上增加10min），在治疗前后对肩关节疼痛、功能活动及日常生活活动能力进行对比研究。结果显示：治疗后三组患者疼痛积分、肩关节活动度及日常生活活动评分均有很大的改善，饱和灸量组总有效率为95%，超饱和灸量组总有效率为94.45%，常规热敏灸量组总有效率为84.21%，说明三组不同灸量治疗肩周炎均取得一定的疗效，其中超饱和灸量组与饱和灸量组无显著差异（$P>0.05$），但饱和灸量组明显优于常规热敏灸量组（$P<0.05$），超饱和灸量组亦明显优于常规热敏灸量组（$P<0.05$）。以上研究结果表明，饱和灸量与超饱和灸量疗效明显优于常规灸量，饱和灸量与超饱和灸量疗效无明显差异。

余希婧[52]将90例肌筋膜疼痛综合征患者按照随机数字表随机分为常规灸量组（15min）、饱和灸量组（以热敏感觉消失为度）和超饱和灸量组（在热敏感觉消失的基础上增加15min），每组30例，比较不同热敏灸量治疗肌筋膜疼痛综合征的疗效差异。结果显示：常规灸量组、饱和灸量组、超饱和灸量组三组治疗后愈显率分别为33.3%、80%、73.3%，且饱和灸量组、超饱和灸量组 VAS、PRI、PPI 积分的改善程度优于常规灸量组（均 $P<0.01$）。

李丹[53]在热敏灸治疗颈型颈椎病不同灸量方案的临床疗效观察中得到相同的结论：饱和灸量组与超饱和灸量组疗效明显优于常规热敏灸量组（$P<0.05$），但超饱和灸量组与饱和灸量组疗效无显著差异（$P>0.05$）。以上研究均表明：以热敏感觉消失为度的"消敏灸量"为最佳灸量，临床可以应用"消敏灸量"标准指导灸疗操作。

因此，陈日新团队以灸感的产生与消失规律为基础，提出了"消敏定量"的灸量新标准，此标准是以个体化的热敏灸感消失为度来确定具体的施灸时间，是根据患者机体自身表达出来的需求灸量确定的灸量标准，是最适的个体化充足灸量，是个体化与标准化相结合的示范。

（六）不同灸量的动物实验验证

陈日新等[39-41]通过线栓法制备大鼠脑缺血再灌注损伤模型，证实了热敏现象能在大鼠中出现，并且表现出人体临床相似的特征，表明热敏灸动物模型建立成功，突破了热敏灸机制研究的瓶颈。动物实验结果显示，在悬灸"大椎"穴 15min 左右时大鼠尾温开始升高，40min 后尾温开始降低。伴有大鼠尾温升高的持续悬灸能明显减少大鼠脑梗死面积，降低 MCAO/R 大鼠神经缺损评分。与无尾温升高的 MCAO/R 大鼠相比，伴有尾温升高的 MCAO/R 大鼠环氧合酶 -2（COX-2）及诱导型一氧化氮合酶（iNOS）表达水平的下降尤为明显。伴有尾温升高的 MCAO/R 大鼠胱天蛋白酶 -3（caspase-3）的表达受到抑制。尽管悬灸使大鼠尾温升高明显加强了悬灸的疗效，但悬灸 40min 和 60min 疗效却无差异，表明尾温开始降低后继续施灸对提高悬灸疗效无明显贡献。针对悬灸 40min "大椎"穴减轻大鼠脑缺血损伤的神经保护效应问题，吕志迈[54] 等采用分子生物学技术，研究发现悬灸 40min 组与缺血对照组相比较，再灌注后、再灌注 1 或 3 天后可明显减少梗死面积，再灌注后 3 天可降低神经功能缺损评分，$P < 0.05$，有明显统计学意义。悬灸 40min 组（$P < 0.01$）、悬灸 15min 组（$P < 0.05$）与缺血对照组分别相比，悬灸 40min 组在缺血再灌注 7 天可明显降低缺血大鼠的神经功能缺损评分，传统悬灸 15min 却没有任何神经保护作用。并且悬灸大椎穴 40min 组在降低线栓法大脑中动脉缺血大鼠模型皮质诱导型一氧化氮合成酶、环氧合酶 -2、胱天蛋白酶 -3 的表达、减少脑梗死面积及神经缺损功能评分等方面明显优于悬灸 15min 组。

五、消敏灸量在灸学标准中的示范意义

任何一种治疗方法疗效的产生，剂量都是相当重要的。剂量恰到好处，疗效充分发挥；剂量太小，不起作用或疗效甚微；剂量太大，疗效不增，甚或副作用太大，得不偿失。中医不传之秘在于量，同一种药物，有时用量不同，主治功用就不一样，临床效果就会差别很大，有时甚至会产生相反的效果。同样，灸疗技术的秘诀之一在"灸量"。相同穴位施灸，灸感一样，但是施灸时间不同，获效就会大不一样。中医论治强调个体化、三因制宜；西方医学则认为应该标准化、精准化，灸疗时间个体化与标准化的有机统一值得深入研究与探讨。

古人运用灸法时，对灸疗的用量也是非常重视的。例如《外台秘要》

曰："凡灸有生熟，候人盛衰及老少也。衰老者少灸，盛壮肥实者多灸。"此处"生"是少灸之意，"熟"是多灸之意。说明古人常根据患者的体质、年龄进行灸量调整。《扁鹊心书》曰："大病灸百壮……小病不过三五七壮。"这则是依据疾病的程度确定灸量的记载。明代《医学入门》曰："针灸穴治大同，但头面诸阳之会，胸膈二火之地，不宜多灸，背腹阴虚有火者，亦不宜灸，惟四肢穴最妙，凡上体及当骨处，针入浅而灸宜少，凡下体及肉厚处，针可入深，灸多无害。"这则是根据身体部位的差异给予不同的施灸剂量。这些记载均可说明灸法也是有个体化要求的，但是古代文献记载多为定性描述，没有定量标准。然而现代针灸学教科书中悬灸的标准多为局部有温热感无灼痛为宜，一般每穴 10~15min，至皮肤出现红晕为度。虽然给出了灸量标准，但是没有体现个体化用量。热敏灸"消敏灸量"标准是依据患者自身腧穴状态变化确定的灸量标准，是以个体化的热敏灸感消失为度的施灸时间，这时穴位的热敏状态转化为消敏状态（即非热敏状态）。这是患者腧穴根据自身状态向外界发出的信号，是顺应自然的表现，符合人类本能医学特点，需要时开放，出现热敏灸感，不需要时就会关闭，热敏灸感消失。因此每穴的施灸时间不是固定不变的，而是因人因病因穴而不同，不同热敏穴位施灸时从热敏灸感产生至热敏灸感消失所需要的时间是不同的，时间为 10~200min 不等，这是热敏穴位的最佳个体化施灸剂量，达到这个灸量疗效明显提高。"消敏灸量"标准符合灸时 – 灸感发生发展时相变化规律，在达到消敏灸量的灸疗时间时灸疗疗效充分发挥，此时施灸时间平均为 40min。热敏灸"消敏灸量"标准完美体现了灸疗时间个体化与标准化的有机统一，可以作为临床灸疗的定量标准。

第四节　"辨敏施灸"新概念

一、辨敏施灸的含义

常规艾灸普遍采用的是辨证施灸诊疗模式，即辨证、选穴、施灸。陈日新团队发现腧穴有状态之别后，研究证明了敏化态腧穴对艾灸刺激能产生"小刺激大反应"，于是在 2009 年出版的《热敏灸实用读本》专著中首次提出"辨敏施灸"新概念 [5]，即"辨证、选穴、择敏、施灸"，简称辨敏施灸。陈日新倡导临床操作时不仅重视"辨证选穴"，更强调"择敏施灸"，通过热敏灸感的辨识来确定施灸的选穴，能够显著提高灸疗疗效。继后根据新的临床研究证据，进一步丰富了辨敏施灸的概念内涵 [55]：即辨敏施灸的"择敏"施灸环节不仅包括辨敏选穴，还包括辨敏定量及辨敏判断艾灸适应证等环节。这是辨证施灸的继承和发展，对于构建艾灸理论与技术新体系具有重要价值。

二、辨敏施灸新概念的形成

早在《黄帝内经》中就有"辨敏施针"的相关记载。《灵枢·经筋》强调："以痛为腧。"《素问·缪刺论》说："疾按之，应手如痛，刺之傍三痏，立已。"《灵枢·五邪》列举了辨敏施针的病案："咳动肩背，取之膺中外腧，背三节之傍，以手疾按之，快然乃刺之。"《素问·骨空论》首次论述辨敏同样适用于灸法治疗："切之坚痛如筋者，灸之。"唐代孙思邈的《备急千金要方·灸例》更是明确指出针、灸治疗皆需辨敏："有阿是之法，言人有病痛，即令捏其上，若里当其处，不问孔穴，即得便快成（或）痛处，即云阿是。灸刺皆验，故曰阿是穴也。"上述文献表明，从《黄帝内经》起就一直提倡选取敏感位点作为针灸部位辨敏施术的诊疗原则。

在 20 世纪 80 年代，当时全国针灸临床灸法萎缩，"但见针刺病，不闻艾绒香"。江西中医药大学陈日新团队在临床艾灸过程中陆续发现了一组神奇的灸感现象：透热、扩热、传热、局部不（微）热远部热、表面不（微）热深部热、非热感觉等。当这些现象发生时，灸疗疗效似乎明显提高，然而现代医学不能解释，这就引起了团队的极大兴趣与重视。陈日新教授带领研究团队普查了神经系统、运动系统、消化系统、呼吸系统、生殖系统等近 20 种病症后发现，这些患者在艾灸时都能不同程度地产生上述特殊灸感现象，尤其以寒证、湿证、瘀证、虚证患者居多，急性病和慢性病均可出现，出现率高达 70% 以上，当疾病好转或痊愈后，这种灸感现象消失，而健康人出现率仅 10%。当艾灸出现这些特殊灸感现象后，气至病所率明显提高，表明上述特殊灸感现象的出现具有普遍性，与疾病状态有高度相关性，以及气至病所率的高效性。至此，团队认识了热敏现象出现的基本规律，大家非常振奋，似乎看到了振兴灸法、提高疗效的一道曙光。

然而，产生上述特殊灸感的"位点"与教科书中经穴、奇穴、阿是穴的位置并不重合，并且呈现位置"动态"性、"旁开"的特征。产生特殊灸感的位点是穴位吗？如果是穴位，它不在已知穴位位置上；如果不是穴位，疗效却比已知穴位好。这时现有的穴位理论与临床实践发生了矛盾，引起了陈日新团队的困惑与深深思考。团队意识到这很可能是新的灸学理论与提高灸疗疗效的突破口，于是带着"穴位是什么"的困惑，直溯《黄帝内经》求解。令团队惊讶的是：《黄帝内经》对穴位的论述竟然与在临床灸疗实践中的观察完全一致！他们深感到，中医经典对现代临床的重要指导作用。可以得出结论，艾灸过程中产生特殊灸感的位点不但是穴位，而且是符合《黄帝内经》中穴位原始定义的正宗穴位，是提高灸疗疗效的特异性穴位。

团队抓住"灸位"与"灸量"两个关键技术环节，创立了热敏灸技术：探感定位，辨敏施灸，量因人异、敏消量足。这是一项全新的灸法技术，穴位已不是一个固化的坐标位点，而是一个动态的功能位点；灸时也不是千人一律的 10~15min，而是个体化与标准化结合的灸时标准；灸法已不是以温和灸为主的静灸手法，而是充分应用高效激发得气的动、静灸组合手法；灸感也不是皮肤温热而无灼痛，而是透热、扩热、传热等深部热、远部热；灸效也不是与施灸时间、艾热强度有关，而是与热敏灸感持续时间、强度有关；灸疗适应证也不是用寒热虚实来判断，而是以机体是否开启热敏穴位为指征；辨证施灸已不能满足临床需求了，而是需要辨敏施灸。热敏灸以敏选择穴位、以敏筛选灸法、以敏确定灸量、以敏激发得气、以敏提高疗效、以敏判断适应证，均可以"敏"一线贯穿之。一句话，热敏灸从理论到技术再到疗效，都完全不一样了。至此，辨敏施灸新概念形成了。

三、辨敏施灸与辨证施灸的关系

长期以来灸疗临床多秉承中医辨证论治的思想，采用"辨证、选穴、施灸"的诊疗模式，忽视了穴位状态，缺少择敏的过程，直接影响灸疗疗效的充分发挥。陈日新等在充分认识到腧穴具有状态之别的本质属性后，结合临床施灸经验，提出"辨敏施灸"，即"辨证、选穴、择敏、施灸"的诊疗模式，倡导临床操作时不仅重视"辨证选穴"，更强调"择敏施灸"，显著提高了灸疗疗效[16]。"辨敏施灸"与"辨证施灸"的内涵区别见表1-4-1，优势对比见表1-4-2。

表 1-4-1　辨敏施灸与辨证施灸的要素对比

对比项	辨敏施灸	辨证施灸
辨证	需要辨证	需要辨证
选穴	辨证基础上择敏选穴	辨证选穴
灸量	依敏定量、敏消量足	固定灸时，10 ~ 15min
判断适应证	通过辨敏判断，不拘于寒热虚实	通过辨证判断

表 1-4-2　辨敏取穴与辨证取穴的针灸疗效差异

疾病	辨敏取穴显效率 /%	辨证取穴显效率 /%
过敏性鼻炎	83.34	43.33
原发性痛经	71.67	46.67
慢性前列腺炎	53.57	32.20
膝关节骨性关节炎	80.95	21.05
腰椎间盘突出症	62.32	34.24
神经根型颈椎病	88.21	42.62
肌筋膜疼痛综合征	86.07	24.08
慢性腰肌劳损	51.14	26.27
枕神经痛	85.00	50.00
跟痛症	80.56	40.63

四、辨敏施灸的临床指导作用

（一）探敏定位

腧穴是针灸获效的基础，取穴准确与否直接影响针灸的临床疗效。陈日新教授通过对热敏灸感的系统研究，提出腧穴的精准定位方法是探敏定位，即根据热敏灸感来精准定位。热敏穴位的定位方法是先以传统辨证选穴为基础的经穴部位作为热敏穴位的粗定位，然后在粗定位的区域进行悬灸探查，当悬灸至某一部位出现前述透热、扩热、传热等 10 种热敏灸感中的 1 种或 1 种以上时，此部位就是热敏穴位的准确位置。

（二）辨敏选优

在临床探查热敏穴位过程中，可能出现几个穴位同时发生热敏的情况。陈日新教授认为，不同热敏灸感携带着不同的信息，尽管这些腧穴都表明是热敏腧穴，但有首选与候选、主选与次选之分，需要进一步分析、辨别，可以按照"辨敏选优"原则在所有出现热敏灸感的腧穴中选取最佳的热敏腧穴进行热敏灸操作。按灸感性质来分，以出现非热感觉的热敏穴位为主选热敏穴位，而非热灸感中又以痛感优于酸胀感；按灸感循行路径来分，以出现热敏灸感经过或直达病变部位的热敏穴位为主选热敏穴位；按灸感强度来分，以出现较强的热敏灸感的热敏穴位为首选热敏穴位。

（三）依敏定量

艾灸剂量是决定艾灸疗效的另一个关键环节。陈日新教授等对灸疗过程中灸时与灸感的相关性进行了大样本、多中心临床研究，揭示了灸时－灸感发生发展呈现三个时相变化，即经气激发潜伏期、经气传导期、经气消退期。传统艾灸规定每穴治疗时间为 10～15min，正处在经气激发的潜伏期，灸疗疗效尚未充分发挥；从艾灸开始至经气传导期结束，平均为 40～50min，这主要是经气传导与气至病所期，是灸疗疗效的充分发挥期，达到这个施灸时间，艾灸疗效明显提高；继后是经气消退期，这段时间继续施灸，疗效也无明显增加[1]。因此，艾灸时间应该是"依敏定量"，即"以热敏灸感消失为度"，突破了灸疗临床长期以来每穴 10～15min 固定灸时的固有观念，为临床充分发挥灸疗疗效提供了量学标准。首次实现了灸疗时间标准化与个体化的有机统一。

（四）察敏论灸

艾灸疗法安全有效、操作简便，适应证广泛，但多以寒证、虚证为优势病症。自古以来，对于灸疗是否可以治疗热证，一直争议不断。有研究表明，部分热证使用艾灸疗效极佳，如体表的疔疮疖肿及慢性炎症等[56]。

另一方面，并非所有的寒证、虚证都是灸疗的有效适应证。长期以来，临床上一直缺乏简便、实用的灸疗适应证判断标准，只能是经验推测。灸疗适应证的准确判断能够充分发挥灸疗疗效的潜力。根据腧穴具有热敏化特征及长期的临床实践总结，陈日新教授提出新的、临床实用的灸疗适应证判断标准，即在与病症相关的热敏穴位高发区出现热敏腧穴，该病症就是热敏灸的适应证[5]。热敏腧穴的一个显著特征就是喜热，它是人体对外界热的需求表现，是生物的本能反应，说明人体需要艾热的帮助。自然界从来不做多余的事，生物体也是如此，不足则喜，有余则恶。因此，这条判断标准的建立适应了生物本能的需求，是顺应自然、回归自然的大道至简法则。

五、辨敏施灸的临床潜力

"辨敏施灸"的关键在"敏"，"敏"是指腧穴热敏，热敏的表现就是产生远部热感和深部热感，甚至热至病所，而非局部与表面的热感。陈日新教授在临床实践中系统研究了热敏灸感现象及其临床规律，认为不同的热敏灸感携带着机体不同的生理病理信息，可以反映病情，在临床施灸过程中应重视热敏信息的采集；根据热敏灸感性质、灸感强度可以指导临床灸疗选穴与准确定位；根据热敏灸感的消退与消失，可以指导艾灸确立个体化充足灸量，以"热敏灸感消失为度"作为充足灸疗时间，突破了灸疗临床每穴固定施灸时间的灸量标准，为临床充分发挥灸疗疗效提供了新的量学标准；根据热敏灸感的产生，可以判断灸疗适应证，即在与病症相关的热敏穴位高发区出现热敏腧穴，该病症就是热敏灸的适应证。深入全面认识热敏灸感的产生、变化规律，有利于指导灸疗的规范操作与灸疗疗效的提高。

关于热敏灸感类型在"好中选优"原则中有所体现，但是对于灸感类型的研究还远远不够，对提高临床疗效的作用仍有巨大空间和潜力。例如："好中选优"中按灸感性质来分，以出现非热感觉的热敏穴位为主选热敏穴位，而非热灸感中又以痛感优于酸胀感。然而非热觉的表现非常广泛，包括施灸（悬灸）部位或远离施灸部位产生的酸、胀、压、重、痛、麻、冷等一系列非热感觉，每种非热觉的出现对临床疾病的诊断、热敏腧穴的选择都是具有不同指导意义的。"痛感"的出现常常代表着祛除病邪；

"胀感"多由于患者湿邪内蕴;"酸感"多由于患者正气虚弱等。在热敏灸感产生时常伴随舒适感、身烘热、面红（额汗出）、肢端热、胃肠蠕动反应、皮肤扩散性潮红等灸感反应，这些反应提示了哪些生理病理信息？对艾灸方案的制定有哪些重要意义？这是值得进一步深入研究的。因此，灸感信息蕴藏着人体腧穴的秘密，有待于继续挖掘与认识，在目前"辨敏施灸"基础上的"辨感施灸"规律值得进一步探索。

参考文献

[1] 孙国杰. 针灸学 [M]. 上海：上海科学技术出版社，1997：178.

[2] 陈日新，康明非. 腧穴热敏化艾灸新疗法 [M]. 北京：人民卫生出版社，2006：15.

[3] 陈日新，康明非，陈明人. 岐伯归来——论腧穴"敏化状态说" [J]. 中国针灸，2011，31（2）：134-138.

[4] 陈日新，谢丁一. 再论"腧穴敏化状态说" [J]. 安徽中医药大学学报，2016，35（3）：50-53.

[5] 陈日新，陈明人，康明非. 热敏灸实用读本 [M]. 北京：人民卫生出版社，2009：5.

[6] TIAN N，XI B，SU B Y，et al. Study on infrared radiation characteristic of heat-sensitive acupoints in bronchial asthma [C]. 2011 IEEE International Conference on Bioinoformatics and Biomedicine Workshops，2011.

[7] 田宁，陈日新，谢兵，等. 支气管哮喘患者热敏穴红外辐射特征研究 [J]. 上海针灸杂志，2014，33（2）：174-176.

[8] 陈日新，陈明人，李巧林. 灸感法与红外法检测支气管哮喘（慢性持续期）患者肺俞穴热敏态的对比研究 [J]. 江西中医药，2011，42（1）：12-14.

[9] 陈日新，陈明人，康明非，等. 灸感法与红外法检测腰椎间盘突出症患者腰阳关穴热敏态的对比研究 [J]. 世界针灸杂志，2010，20（2）：21-26.

[10] 李伟，安鑫，陈日新. 腰椎间盘突出症腧穴热敏化红外客观显示研究 [J]. 江西中医学院学报，2010，22（4）：24-26.

[11] CHEN R X，CHEN M R，LI Q L，et al. Assessment of heat-sensitization at Guanyuan (CV 4) in patients with primary dysmenorrhea: A comparative study between moxibustion sensation and infrared thermography[J]. Journal of Acupuncture and Tuina Science，2010，8（3）：163-166.

[12] 周明镜，陈日新，陈明人，等. 灸感法与红外法检测心气虚患者内关穴热敏态的对比研究 [J]. 中国针灸，2010，30（3）：213-216.

[13] 谢丁一，李原浩，陈日新，等. 腰椎间盘突出症患者热敏腧穴温度觉特征研究 [J]. 中华中医药杂志，2017，32（9）：4211-4214.

[14] 谢丁一，谢秀俊，陈日新，等. 神经根型颈椎病患者热敏态腧穴温度觉特征研究 [J]. 安徽中医药大学学报，2017，36（1）：35-39.

[15] XIE D Y，JIANG Y X，CHEN R X，et al. Study on the thermesthesia features of heat-sensitive acupoints in patients with knee osteoarthritis[J]. Journal of Acupuncture and Tuina Science，2016，14（2）：110-114.

[16] 郭义，方剑乔. 实验针灸学 [M]. 北京：中国中医药出版社，2012：239-241.

[17] CHEN M R，CHEN R X，XIONG J，et al. Effectiveness of heat-sensitive moxibustion in the treatment of lumbar disc herniation: study protocol for a randomized controlled trial[J]. Trials，2011，12（1）：226.

[18] CHEN R X，XIONG J，CHI Z H，et al. Heat-sensitive moxibustion for lumbar disc herniation: a meta-analysis of randomized controlled trials[J]. Journal of Traditional Chinese Medicine，2012，32（3）：322-328.

[19] CHEN R X，CHEN M R，XIONG J，et al. Influence of the Deqi sensation by suspended moxibustion stimulation in lumbar disc herniation: study for a multicenter prospective two arms cohort study[J]. Evidence-Based Complementary and Alternative Medicine，2013，2013: 718593.

[20] CHEN R X，CHEN M R，SU T S，et al. A 3-arm, randomized, controlled trial of heat-sensitive moxibustion therapy to determine superior effect among patients with lumbar disc herniation[J]. Evidence-Based Complementary and Alternative Medicine，2014，2014: 154941.

[21] CHEN R X，CHEN M R，KANG M F，et al. The design and protocol of heat-sensitive moxibustion for knee osteoarthritis: a multicenter randomized controlled trial on the rules of selecting moxibustion location[J]. BMC Complementary Medicine and Therapies，2010，10: 32.

[22] CHEN R X，CHEN M R，XIONG J，et al. Comparative effectiveness of the Deqi sensation and non-Deqi by moxibustion stimulation: a multicenter prospective cohort study in the treatment of knee osteoarthritis[J]. Evidence-Based Complementary and Alternative Medicine，2013，2013: 906947.

[23] CHEN R X，CHEN M R，SU T S，et al. Heat-sensitive moxibustion in patients with osteoarthritis of the knee: a three-armed multicentre randomised active control trial[J]. Acupuncture in Medicine，2015，33（4）：262-269.

[24] CHEN R X，CHEN M R，XIONG J，et al. Curative effect of heat-sensitive

moxibustion on chronic persistent asthma: a multicenter randomized controlled trial[J]. Journal of Traditional Chinese Medicine，2013，33（5）：102-109.

[25] CHEN R X，CHEN M R，XIONG J，et al. Comparison of heat-sensitive moxibustion versus fluticasone/salmeterol (seretide) combination in the treatment of chronic persistent asthma: design of a multicenter randomized controlled trial[J]. Trials，2010，11（1）：1-9.

[26] 唐福宇，王继，娄宇明，等. 热敏灸法治疗神经根型颈椎病疗效观察 [J]. 广西中医药，2013，36（4）：32-33.

[27] 李冠豪，曹淑. 热敏灸治疗神经根型颈椎病疗效观察 [J]. 四川中医，2015，33（7）：170-172.

[28] 谢炎烽，阮永队，宁晓军，等. 热敏灸治疗神经根型颈椎病疗效对照研究 [J]. 中国针灸，2010，30（5）：379-382.

[29] 陈日新，康明非. 灸之要，气至而有效 [J]. 中国针灸，2008（1）：44-46.

[30] 陈日新，陈彦奇，谢丁一. 试论艾灸得气 [J]. 中国针灸，2019，39（10）：1111-1114.

[31] 陈日新，谢丁一. 神奇热敏灸 [M]. 北京：人民军医出版社，2013：9.

[32] 董小玉，陈日新，张波，等. 艾灸热敏腧穴产生舒适情感体验的临床观察 [J]. 江西中医药，2011，42（1）：33-35.

[33] 陈日新，吕志迈，谢丁一，等. 热敏灸感条目德尔菲法调查分析 [J]. 中医杂志，2018，59（22）：1915-1919.

[34] 陈日新，吕志迈，谢丁一，等. 热敏灸得气灸感量表的研制与初步评价 [J]. 中国针灸，2018，38（11）：1229-1234.

[35] Liao F F，Zhang C，Bian Z J，et al. Characterizing heat-sensitization responses in suspended moxibustion with high-density EEG[J]. Pain Medicine，2014，15：1272-1281.

[36] 廖斐斐，张潆，边志杰，等. 慢性腰背痛患者艾灸热敏现象的脑电机制初探 [J]. 中国疼痛医学杂志，2013，19（12）：719-726.

[37] WANG J，YI M，ZHANG C，et al. Cortical activities of heat-sensitization responses in suspended moxibustion: an EEG source analysis with sLORETA[J]. Cognitive Neurodynamics，2015，9（6）：581-588.

[38] 黄仙保，李巧林，谢丁一，等. 悬灸不同状态犊鼻穴的脑电功率谱密度特征研究 [J]. 世界中医药，2019，14（8）：1936-1941.

[39] CHEN R X，LV Z M，HUANG D D，et al. Efficacy of suspended moxibustion in stroke rats is associated with a change in tail temperature[J]. Neural Regeneration Research，2013，8（12）：1132-1138.

[40] CHEN R X，LV Z M，CHEN M R，et al. Stroke treatment in rats with tail temperature increase by 40-min moxibustion[J]. Neuroscience Letters，2011，503（2）：131-135.

[41] LV Z M，LIU Z M，HUANG D D，et al. The Characterization of Deqi during Moxibustion in Stroke Rats[J]. Evidence-Based Complementary and Alternative Medicine，2013，2013: 140581.

[42] 陈日新，陈明人，黄建华，等. 热敏灸治疗椎动脉型颈椎病灸感与灸效关系的临床观察 [J]. 江西中医药，2011，42（1）：48-49.

[43] 陈日新，张波，蔡加. 温和灸治疗膝关节骨性关节炎（肿胀型）不同灸感的临床疗效比较研究 [J]. 世界中医药，2013，8（8）：856-858.

[44] 熊俊，耿乐乐，迟振海，等. 艾灸治疗不同灸感腰椎间盘突出症急性期患者60例疗效观察 [J]. 中医杂志，2015，56（21）：1836-1839.

[45] 张伟，李海澜，胡锦玉. 热敏灸"关元"穴治疗原发性痛经的灸感与灸效相关性研究 [J]. 时珍国医国药，2014，25（1）：246-248.

[46] 陈日新，陈明人，付勇，等. 艾灸慢性腹泻（脾虚型）天枢穴气至病所的临床研究 [J]. 江西中医药，2011，42（1）：24-26.

[47] CHEN M R，CHEN R X，XIONG J，et al. Evaluation of different moxibustion doses for lumbar disc herniation: multicentre randomised controlled trial of heat-sensitive moxibustion therapy[J]. Acupuncture in Medicine，2012，30（4）：266-272.

[48] CHEN R X，CHEN M R，XIONG J，et al. Is there difference between the effects of two-dose stimulation for knee osteoarthritis in the treatment of heat-sensitive moxibustion?[J]. Evidence-Based Complementary and Alternative Medicine，2012，2012: 696498.

[49] 康明非，章海凤，付勇，等. 热敏灸治疗慢性前列腺炎不同灸量方案的临床疗效评价 [J]. 时珍国医国药，2015，26（1）：125-127.

[50] 周小平，林华，付勇，等. 热敏灸不同灸量治疗椎动脉型颈椎病：随机对照研究 [J]. 中国针灸，2014，34（5）：461-464.

[51] 郑嵩. 热敏灸治疗肩周炎的量效关系研究 [D]. 南昌：江西中医药大学，2015.

[52] 余希婧. 热敏灸治疗项背部肌筋膜疼痛综合的量效关系研究 [D]. 南昌：江西中医药大学，2015.

[53] 李丹. 热敏灸治疗颈型颈椎病不同灸量方案的临床疗效观察 [D]. 南昌：江西中医药大学，2018.

[54] CHEN R X，LV Z M，CHEN M R，et al. Neuronal apoptosis and inflammatory reaction in rat models of focal cerebral ischemia following 40-minute suspended moxibustion[J]. Neural Regeneration Research，2011（15）：1180-1184.

[55] 安鑫. 陈日新腧穴敏化学术思想及临床经验 [J]. 江西中医药，2011, 42（1）：77-78.

[56] 魏稼. 热证可灸论 [J]. 中医杂志，1980（11）：45-48.

第二章

技术篇

　　影响艾灸疗效的两大关键因素是灸位与灸量。陈日新团队依据"腧穴敏化""灸之要，气至而有效"等理论，创立了热敏灸技术，强调灸位一定要选择热敏穴位，灸量一定要达到消敏饱和灸量，才能够获得古人所描述的"效之信，若风之吹云，明乎若见苍天"的速效、特效。热敏灸位与消敏灸量的判断要依据热敏灸感的辨识，因此，认识掌握热敏灸感是至关重要的。灸感是指施灸时被灸者的自我感觉。悬灸某一部位时通常被灸者在施灸部位产生局部、表面的热感，然而针对热敏穴位施灸，就会产生透热、扩热、传热等非表面、非局部的热敏灸感。不同热敏灸感携带着机体不同的生理病理信息，能指导临床制定灸疗方案。因此，如何找准穴位，如何施足灸量，如何读懂灸感，这些都是热敏灸技术操作的重要环节。本章从热敏灸操作方法、作用与特点、适应病症、操作注意事项及常用穴位热敏灸感五个方面进行介绍。

🔆 第一节　热敏灸操作方法

一、调定灸态

灸态就是艾灸时的状态，调整好灸态是激发得气、获得灸效的前提，包括静、松、匀、守四个方面。

静：静是指环境安静，心神安静。患者和医生都必须保持心神的安定宁静，同时保持环境安静，才能最大限度地激发得气感应。

松：松是指患者肌肉的放松。机体处于自然放松的状态，有利于得气感应的激发。

匀：匀是指患者自然均匀的腹式呼吸。自然均匀的腹式呼吸有利于调整机体自主神经功能，有利于增加机体反应的敏感性。

守：包括两方面，一是指患者应意守灸感处，以体验得气感应；二是指医者必须意守施灸位点以保持施灸热度的稳定性。

二、找准穴位

热敏腧穴是灸疗的特异性穴位，在施灸过程中应通过探感定位确定热敏腧穴的准确位置，并通过好中选优原则选取最佳热敏腧穴治疗，才能达到小刺激、大反应的效果。

（一）探感定位

热敏腧穴的准确位置与传统经穴挂图上的位置不是完全重合的，需要粗定位到细定位二步定位法来探查。

热敏腧穴粗定位：确定疾病状态下相关腧穴发生热敏化的高概率区域。穴位发生热敏化是有规律的，有其高发部位，如：支气管哮喘患者的热敏穴位高发部位在肺俞区域；功能性消化不良患者的热敏穴位高发部位在天枢区域；原发性痛经患者的热敏穴位高发部位在关元区域；过敏性鼻炎患者的热敏穴位高发部位在上印堂区域；面神经麻痹患者的热敏穴位高发部位在翳风区域。高发部位的定位可参照传统经穴的定位方法，如：体表标志法、骨度折量法、指寸法、简便取穴法等。

热敏腧穴细定位：用点燃的艾条，在上述热敏腧穴高发部位上下左右范围内，施以循经、回旋、雀啄、温和组合手法进行悬灸探查，艾热强度以患者局部感觉温热而无灼痛感为宜。上述手法分别具有温热局部气血、加强敏化、激发经气、发动感传等作用。热敏腧穴在艾热刺激下，会产生透热、传热、扩热、局部不（微）热远部热、表面不（微）热深部热、非热觉等灸感，只要出现其中的一种或一种以上灸感就表明该穴位已发生热敏化，即为热敏腧穴。在疾病状态下，热敏腧穴分为速发型和迟发型。速发型热敏腧穴的特征是：热敏灸感敏现速度较迅速，潜伏期较短（平均为10 ~ 15min），在施灸部位皮温达到40 ~ 42℃时，很快产生透热、扩热、传热、局部不（微）热远部热、表面不（微）热深部热及其他非热感觉等热敏灸感。迟发型热敏腧穴的特征是：热敏灸感敏现速度较迟缓，潜伏期较长（平均＞15min），常呈现一过性、短暂的透热、扩热、传热、非热觉等灸感，或施灸局部呈现喜热、耐热等。不同类型的热敏腧穴对艾热刺激的敏感性不同，决定了灸疗操作不同，如果探查为迟发型热敏腧穴，可以通过激发的方法转化为速发型。因此，依据热敏灸感法就能判断热敏腧穴的准确位置。

（二）辨敏施灸

经过探查可能出现多个与病症相关腧穴同时发生热敏的情况，按照"好中选优"原则的顺序选取最佳热敏腧穴施灸。

好中选优三原则：①按灸感性质来分，以出现非热感觉的热敏穴位为首选热敏穴位，而非热灸感中又以痛感优于酸胀感；②按灸感指向来分，以出现热敏灸感经过或直达病变部位的热敏穴位为首选热敏穴位；③按灸感强度来分，以出现较强的热敏灸感的热敏穴位为首选热敏穴位。

如果速发型与迟发型热敏腧穴同时存在，则首选速发型施灸。如果仅有迟发型热敏腧穴，应先对迟发型热敏腧穴进行激发处理，使其热敏反应的潜伏期缩短、热敏灸感强度增强，热敏持续时间延长。迟发型热敏腧穴激发方法因腧穴虚实状态不同而不同：①因机体整体阳气或施灸局部阳气虚衰，以致穴位热敏反应的潜伏期延长，可先行督脉铺灸或温和灸大椎、膏肓、神阙、关元、肾俞、命门、足三里等强壮穴，每次40 ~ 60min，每天1次，促进迟发型热敏穴位转化为速发型热敏穴位；②因穴位局部寒湿

痰瘀等阴邪导致局部形成水肿、条索状结节、块状筋结、筋膜粘连、肌肉
痉挛、瘀血阻络的迟发型热敏穴位，可先选用熨灸、筋膜松解术、刺络拔
罐、刺络放血、麦粒灸、针刀等手段疏通经络，减轻施灸局部经气运行
阻力，然后采用雀啄灸、循经往返灸等动灸手法加强敏化，每次 40min，
每天 1 次，以温通局部经络，促进迟发型热敏穴位转化为速发型热敏
穴位。

三、用对手法

（一）热敏灸常用探查手法

采用适宜的探查手法是快速有效激发热敏腧穴产生得气的必要条件。
热敏灸常用探查手法有回旋灸、雀啄灸、循经往返灸、温和灸。探查热敏
腧穴时，可以采用 4 种手法中任何一种，也可采用 4 种手法的组合，灸至
皮肤潮红为度。

回旋灸：用点燃的艾条，与施灸部位皮肤保持一定距离，均匀地往复
旋转施灸，以施灸部位皮肤温热潮红为度。回旋灸有利于温热施灸部位的
气血，主要用于胸腹背腰部穴位（图 2-1-1）。

雀啄灸：用点燃的艾条，对准施灸部位一上一下地活动施灸，如鸟雀
啄食一样，以施灸部位皮肤温热潮红为度。雀啄灸有利于施灸部位进一步
加强敏化，从而为局部的经气激发奠定基础（图 2-1-2）。

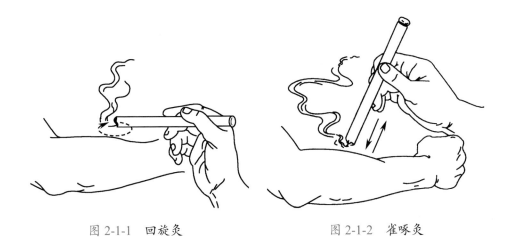

图 2-1-1　回旋灸　　　　　　　　　　图 2-1-2　雀啄灸

循经往返灸：用点燃的艾条在患者体表，距离皮肤 3cm 左右，匀速地沿经脉往返移动施灸，以施灸路线温热潮红为度。循经往返灸有利于温通经络，激发得气（图 2-1-3）。

温和灸：用点燃的艾条，对准施灸部位，距离皮肤 3cm 左右处施灸，使患者局部感觉温热而无灼痛感，以施灸部位皮肤温热潮红为度。温和灸有利于施灸部位进一步激发经气，发动感传（图 2-1-4）。

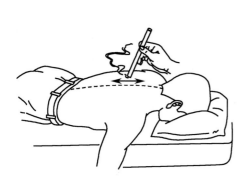 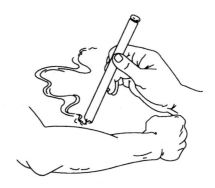

图 2-1-3　循经往返灸　　　　图 2-1-4　温和灸

（二）热敏灸常用治疗手法

热敏灸治疗过程中，可以采用单点灸、双点灸、接力灸、循经往返灸等手法施灸。

单点灸：针对单个热敏腧穴施灸。将点燃的艾条对准选择的一个热敏穴位，在距离皮肤 3cm 左右处施行手法，可选择回旋灸、雀啄灸、温和灸等单个手法或其组合手法施灸（图 2-1-5）。

双点灸：同时对两个热敏腧穴进行施灸，可选择回旋灸、雀啄灸、温和灸等单个手法或其组合手法施灸。双点灸主要用于左右对称的同名穴位或同一经脉的两个穴位（图 2-1-6）。

接力灸：如果经气传导不理想，在上述单点灸基础上，可以在经气传导路线上远离施灸穴位的端点再加一单点灸，这样可以延长经气传导的距离（图 2-1-7）。

循经往返灸：此手法既可用于探查穴位，又是治疗的常用手法。用点燃的艾条在距离患者体表皮肤 3cm 左右处，沿经脉往返匀速移动施灸。此法适用于正气不足，得气较弱的患者（图 2-1-8）。

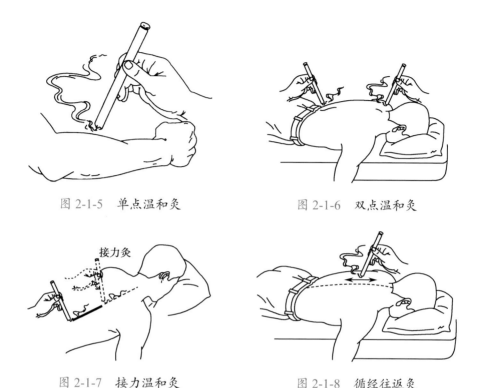

图 2-1-5 单点温和灸   图 2-1-6 双点温和灸

图 2-1-7 接力温和灸   图 2-1-8 循经往返灸

四、施足灸量

施足灸量是产生得气、提高疗效的关键要素之一，正如古人所说："凡灸诸病，必火足气到，始能求愈。"艾灸剂量由艾灸强度、艾灸面积、艾灸时间三个因素决定，在前两个因素基本不变的情况下，艾灸剂量主要由艾灸时间所决定。热敏灸研究表明，每穴的施灸时间不是固定不变的，是因人因病因穴不同而不同。不同热敏腧穴热敏灸感产生至消失所需要的时间可为 10～200min。热敏灸治疗每穴每次的施灸剂量标准是"敏消量足"，即以施灸过程中热敏灸感的消失（或消退）为度，这是热敏腧穴的最佳个体化饱和灸量。达到这个灸量，疗效明显提高，腧穴由热敏状态转化为消敏状态（即静息态）。热敏灸疗程灸量是指与某疾病相关的热敏腧穴均被灸至消敏，只要存在与疾病相关的热敏腧穴，就需要进行疗程施灸。慢病患者由于自身阳虚等特点，必须持之以恒地坚持半年到数年的科学、规范的常灸，才能够获得满意的艾灸疗效。

热敏灸的操作技术关键可用十六字来概括：探感定位、辨敏施灸、量因人异、敏消量足。前两句是有关施灸部位的操作技术关键，后两句是有关施灸剂量的操作技术关键，整个操作流程见图2-1-9：

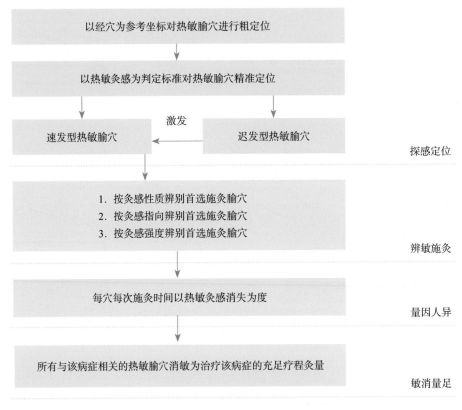

图 2-1-9　热敏灸操作流程图

🎐 第二节　热敏灸作用与特点

一、治疗作用

热敏灸是传统悬灸传承与创新的一项新灸法，它的最大特点是高效激发得气、气至病所，因此具有以下治疗作用：温补阳气、温化寒湿、温经通络、温养心神。

（一）温补阳气

热敏灸温补阳气的作用就是可使阳气不足的机体得到阳气的补充。《素问·生气通天论篇》曰："阳气者，若天与日，失其所，则折寿而不彰。"阳气是机体生命活动产生的源动力，有一份阳气就有一份生机。阳气不足，脏腑功能衰退，卫外功能减弱，阴邪重生，固扶阳气是防治疾病的根本。艾叶性属纯阳，艾火温热属阳，两阳相加，补火助阳，温阳益气。《本草从新》说："艾叶苦辛，生温熟热，纯阳之性，能回垂绝之元阳。"热敏灸通过热敏穴位，小刺激激发大反应，扶助人体阳气。临床上阳气不足所致的胃寒、宫寒、脾失健运、神倦乏力、肢端凉等，通过热敏灸治疗，有显著的效果。

（二）温化寒湿

热敏灸温化寒湿的作用就是可使体内寒湿之邪得以祛除。寒邪收引，湿性黏滞重浊、缠绵难除，寒湿属阴邪，易损伤阳气，阻遏气机，聚湿成饮成痰，湿久郁热，湿遏热伏。《本草从新》说："艾叶苦辛，生温熟热，纯阳之性……逐寒湿，暖子宫。"热敏灸芳香化湿、温脾除湿、温中散寒、温化痰饮、温透郁热。临床中反复证明，一些湿阻中焦的患者舌苔厚腻，食欲不佳，大便黏腻不成形，如果艾灸中脘、水分等穴激发得气，经过2~3次治疗，患者舌苔明显变薄，食欲改善，大便成形。因此，寒湿为病均可用热敏灸治疗。

（三）温经通络

热敏灸温经通络的作用就是可使瘀阻的经络得以温通。《灵枢·经脉》篇强调："经脉者，所以能决死生，处百病，调虚实，不可不通。"说明经络通畅对于人体健康起着极其重要的作用。气血遇寒，或久病入络，可导致血运不畅，经络痹阻。《本草从新》说艾灸能"透诸经而除百病"，热敏灸激发得气，透热、扩热、传热，温经散寒，温阳益气，气行则血行，血得温则行，血行则瘀散。临床上气虚血瘀所致的心脑血管疾病及寒湿痹阻所致的颈肩腰腿痛均可以用热敏灸治疗。

（四）温养心神

热敏灸温养心神的作用就是可使患者身心舒畅，负性情绪得到舒缓。《黄帝内经》云："得神者昌，失神者亡。"说明"神"关系到人的生老病死。焦虑、抑郁、失眠、精神萎靡、情绪低落或烦躁不安等情志异常，均是心神失养的表现，而心神异常又会加重脏腑功能紊乱，导致疾病加重或病程延长。针灸疗法非常重视治神，强调"凡刺之法，必先本于神"，又说"用针之要，无忘其神"。热敏灸得气时产生的一身烘热、一身轻松、心情舒畅，体现了温养心神的作用，能够减轻患者负性情绪，增强抗病机能，调节紊乱的生理生化功能，促进疾病康复，这是热敏灸的独特优势。临床上情绪低落、郁郁寡欢及许多心身紧张性疾病均可用热敏灸治疗。

二、效应特点

热敏灸的热刺激可以通过激发体内固有的调节系统功能，使失调、紊乱的生理生化功能恢复正常，这与针灸作用原理类同，具有以下特点：

（一）双向调节

双向调节特点是指热敏灸能产生兴奋或抑制双重效应。用适宜的艾灸刺激作用于热敏穴位，其效应总是促进偏离的功能朝着正常态转化，使紊乱的功能恢复正常。在身体功能状态低下时，热敏灸可使之增强；功能状态亢进时又可使之降低，而对正常生理功能无明显影响。如艾灸天枢穴，既可治疗功能性便秘又能治疗功能性腹泻；艾灸内关穴，既能治疗心动过速又能治疗心动过缓等。热敏灸的双向调节特点，是其无不良反应的根本原因。

（二）整体调节

整体调节特点包括两方面含义：一是指热敏灸可在不同水平上同时对多个器官、系统功能产生影响；二是指热敏灸对某一器官功能的调节作用，是通过该器官所属系统甚至全身各系统功能的综合调节而实现的。用适宜的艾灸刺激作用于热敏穴位，通过调整交感神经和迷走神经张力，从而调节胃肠动力与胃酸分泌、保护胃肠黏膜等，达到治疗胃肠功能紊乱的效果。热敏灸对身体各系统、各器官功能均能发挥多环节、多水平、多途径的综合调节作用。整体调节特点是热敏灸具有广泛适应证的治疗学基础。

（三）品质调节

品质调节特点是指热敏灸具有增强体内各调节系统调节能力的作用，以维持身体各功能态的稳定。热敏灸的这一品质调节作用揭示了热敏灸对偏离正常状态的紊乱功能呈现双向调节效应，而对正常态生理功能无明显影响。在临床上的表现是对疾病产生治疗作用（双向调节作用），而对正常状态呈现防病保健作用，使得身体对继后受到的干扰因素（致病因素）引起的功能紊乱显著减少。如经常艾灸足三里穴可以增强身体的免疫力，减少感冒次数，提高身体的防病能力就是艾灸品质调节作用的具体体现。热敏灸的品质调节作用是其防病保健作用的内在原理，具有重要的意义，是一块待开垦的新领域。

（四）自限调节

自限性调节特点包括两方面含义：一是指热敏灸的调节能力与针刺疗法一样，是有限度的，只能在生理调节范围内发挥作用；二是指热敏灸的调节能力必须依赖于有关组织结构的完整与潜在的功能储备。热敏灸发挥作用的原理是通过激发机体的调节系统功能，使失调、紊乱的状态恢复正常，这就决定了热敏灸作用具有以上的自限性。与针刺麻醉中的镇痛不全一样，这是针刺镇痛的固有"本性"。又如对某些器官功能衰竭或组织结构已发生不可逆损害者，热敏灸对相应脏腑的调节就难以奏效。了解热敏灸调节的自限性，有利于我们正确认识热敏灸的适应范围与合理应用，从而提高临床疗效。

三、热敏灸与传统悬灸比较

热敏灸与传统悬灸都是对准穴位"悬空"而灸的艾灸疗法，但是两种方法适应证判别、灸位定位、灸感要求、灸法选择、灸量定量的标准不同（表2-2-1）。热敏灸激发得气，气至病所，实现古人"气至而有效"的要求，因此热敏灸的疗效较传统悬灸疗法有显著提高。

（一）适应证判别标准不同

热敏灸适应证判别标准：在与病症相关的热敏穴位高发区出现热敏腧穴，该病症就是热敏灸的适应证，不限于热证、寒证、虚证、实证、表证、里证。传统悬灸没有明确适应证判别标准，一般以寒证、虚证为主。

（二）灸位标准不同

热敏灸是选择热敏腧穴施灸，容易激发得气，产生"小刺激大反应"。而传统悬灸由于未认识到腧穴有敏化状态与静息状态之别，不要求辨别与选择热敏腧穴施灸，因此激发得气的效率很低。

（三）灸感标准不同

灸感即施灸时患者的自我感觉。对于艾灸疗法，艾热作用于体表，自然产生热感。热敏灸强调施灸过程中产生透热、传热、扩热、非热觉、喜热、身烘热、面红（或额汗出）、肢端热、胃肠蠕动反应、皮肤扩散性潮红等10种热敏灸感，气至病所，而传统悬灸仅要求有局部和表面的热感。

（四）灸法标准不同

灸法是指灸疗过程中的操作手法。热敏灸的最大特点是高效激发得气、气至病所从而提高疗效。由于热敏穴位有阻性穴位与容性穴位的不同，因此热敏灸在施灸过程中的操作手法均是动静手法的组合。因为动灸手法（如回旋灸、雀啄灸、循经往返灸）容易激发容性穴位的得气，静灸手法（温和灸）容易激发阻性穴位的得气。传统悬灸未认识穴位有阻性穴位与容性穴位的不同，因此未重视动静手法的有序组合，气至病所率较低。

（五）灸量标准不同

灸量是指每次艾灸的有效作用剂量。在进行热敏灸时，每穴每次的施灸时间不是固定不变的，而是因人因病因穴而不同，以个体化的热敏灸感消失为度。这是患病机体自身表达出来的需求灸量，是最适宜的个体化充足灸量即饱和消敏灸量。传统悬灸的灸量每次每穴一般10~15min，或以局部皮肤潮红为度，往往达不到治疗个体化的饱和灸量。

表 2-2-1　**热敏灸与传统悬灸的比较**

对比项	热敏灸	传统悬灸
适应证判别标准	与病症相关的热敏穴位高发区出现热敏腧穴，该病症就是热敏灸的适应证	寒证、虚证为主
灸位标准	要求选择热敏穴位	不要求选择热敏穴位
灸感标准	透热、传热、扩热、非热觉、喜热、身烘热、面红（或额汗出）、肢端热、胃肠蠕动反应、皮肤扩散性潮红等 10 种热敏灸感	局部和表面的热感
灸法标准	要求动、静灸手法有序结合	不要求动、静灸手法有序结合
灸量标准	施灸时间不是固定不变的，而是因人因病因穴而不同，一般以热敏灸感消失为度	悬灸每次每穴均为 10～15min，或者以局部皮肤潮红为度

第三节　热敏灸适应病症

　　热敏腧穴的出现是人体在疾病状态下对外界发出的需求信号，表明此时机体需要借助外界的热量，帮助机体调动自身抗病潜力。热敏灸具有温补阳气、温化寒湿、温经通络、温养心神等作用，因此，临床上凡是出现热敏腧穴的病症，无论热证、寒证、虚证、实证、表证、里证，均是热敏灸的适应病症。

（一）寒湿病症

　　寒邪收引，湿性凝滞，寒湿为邪，经络闭阻，热敏灸温经通络、祛湿散寒，能够治疗寒湿郁表、寒痹经脉引起的各种表证、里证，有"以阳制阴"之意，可收事半功倍之效。

（二）阳虚病症

艾为纯阳之品，可温通经络；艾火温热，可直达经络，补虚起陷。对于阳虚为主的病症，热敏灸具有大补阳气、升阳举陷之功。

（三）血瘀病症

寒邪凝涩，血运不畅成瘀，或气滞血瘀、血虚成瘀等，阻滞经络。热敏灸能温经通阳，温运气血，气行则血行，血行则瘀散。对于血瘀病症，热敏灸具有活血通络之功。

（四）气阴虚证

金元四大家之一朱震亨认为热证用灸，乃"从治"之意，之所以用于阴虚证的治疗，是因灸有补阳之功效，而"阳生则阴长"也。气虚、阴虚者，用灸法以热补气，使脾胃气盛，运化正常，则气阴得补，此为"以阳化阴"之意，故气阴虚为主的病证亦可用灸。

（五）郁热病症

历代有不少医家提出热证禁灸的问题，如汉代张机指出热证灸治可引起不良后果，并告诫人们无论是阳盛的热证或是阴虚的热证，均不可用灸法。清代医家王士雄还提出了"灸可攻阴"之说，把灸法用于热证视为畏途。近代也有艾灸教材把热证定为禁灸之列，有些人甚至认为"用之则犹如火上添油，热势更炽"。然而，通考《黄帝内经》全文，并无"发热不能用灸"的条文与字句，却有"热病二十九灸"之说。《素问·六元正纪大论》认为"火郁发之"，灸法可以使血脉通畅，血流加速，腠理宣通，从而达到"火郁发之"、散热退热与驱邪外出的目的。明代龚居中在其《痰火点雪》一书中，更是明确指出灸法用于寒热虚实诸症，无往不宜。因此，热敏灸并非"以火济火"，而恰恰是"热能行热"。故郁热之证，亦可灸之。

经过多年临床研究与经验总结，我们发现，热敏灸尤其适合下述病症：

（1）**脊柱关节痛症**：如颈椎病、腰椎间盘突出症、膝关节骨性关节炎。

（2）**过敏性病症**：如过敏性鼻炎、荨麻疹、支气管哮喘。

（3）**胃肠功能性病症**：如非溃疡性消化不良、功能性肠病。

（4）**男性前列腺病症**：如慢性前列腺炎、前列腺肥大、性功能障碍。

（5）**女性宫寒性病症**：如原发性痛经、卵泡发育不良、卵巢功能早衰。

（6）**皮肤病症**：如湿疹、神经性皮炎、带状疱疹。

（7）**正气虚湿气盛病症**：如亚健康、慢性病、肿瘤放化疗后的阳虚气虚诸症。

第四节 热敏灸操作注意事项

（一）施灸前

施灸前应详细告知被灸者施灸操作过程及 10 种热敏灸感，特别是对首次接受热敏灸者。被灸者应以平静信任的心态进行治疗，消除对艾灸的紧张感。并告知被灸者在施灸过程中，应注意灸感的交流，以便施灸者及时调整施灸方案。对于需要常灸的患者应详细告知患者常灸操作方法与要求，坚定患者持之以恒的常灸信心。

（二）施灸中

1. **施灸艾条** 应选择艾绒纯净，艾条包裹松紧适宜，施灸时热力温和、不刚烈的艾条，有利于激发热敏灸感，促进气至病所，同时避免艾火掉落烫伤皮肤或烧坏衣物。施灸结束后，须将燃着的艾条熄灭，以防复燃。

2. **施灸环境** 施灸时环境温度应保持在 24～30℃为宜，不宜过低（低于 22℃），以免受寒。艾灸治疗室应通风良好，或设有排烟、消烟装置，避免艾烟浓度过高，对人体产生不良影响。

3. **施灸体位** 选择合适、舒适的体位，充分暴露施灸部位，保持肌肉放松。

4. **施灸皮温** 施灸皮温应在 40～42℃之间，温度过高易发生灼伤，温度过低不易激发热敏灸感。施灸过程中，掸灰时间最好不超过 10 秒，以免皮肤表面温度下降，影响热敏灸感的稳定性。

5．施灸时间　施灸时严格掌握"消敏灸量"标准，每穴每次施灸时间以热敏灸感消失为度，热敏灸感消失后不宜继续施灸。

6．不宜施灸部位　孕妇的腹部和腰骶部慎灸，以免发生流产；感觉障碍、皮肤溃疡处慎灸，以免灼伤。

7．不宜施灸状态　过饥、过饱、过劳、过悲、酒醉等状态禁灸，以免晕灸；精神紧张、抑郁、亢奋等状态不宜施灸。

8．不宜施灸对象　婴幼儿、灸感表达障碍者，要慎灸，以免灼伤。

9．不宜施灸病症　昏迷、脑出血急性期、大量吐（咯）血者不宜施灸，以免延误其他治疗。

（三）施灸后

施灸后 2 小时内均应注意保暖，以免受寒。

纠偏反应与处理方法：热敏灸在调整人体紊乱功能的过程中，正气祛邪，疏通经络，少数人可能会有一些不适反应，这是打破病理稳态过程中的伴发反应，要正确认识，正确辨别，正确引导，避免误把正常认为不正常。纠偏反应常有以下几种：①对于少数气血不畅患者，可能灸后出现短暂的嗳气、肛门排气、病痛局部疼痛加重或短暂的失眠。这种情况一般不需特殊处理。②对于少数痰湿内蕴患者，可能灸后出现短暂的咳痰变多，或排稀便、黏便。这种情况一般不需特殊处理。③对于少数素体郁热患者，可能灸后出现短暂的皮肤发痒、局部湿疹、大小便灼热等反应。一般停灸 2～3 次，上述症状消失后可继续施灸。④对于少数素体较虚患者，可能灸后短暂的失眠或疲乏无力，发困欲睡。可嘱患者多休息或喝小米温粥，以温养胃气。⑤对于少数慢病患者，可能灸后有时出现正邪相搏引起的短暂性症状加重反应。应向患者及时宣教有关知识，消除紧张心理。⑥如果没有灸准热敏穴位或热敏灸感消失后继续施灸，可能会有上火现象，如口干、咽干等。一般停灸 3～5 次，上述症状消失后可继续施灸。

第五节 常用穴位与热敏灸感

一、头项部

（一）阳白

【归经】属足少阳胆经。

【穴位定位】在前额部，当瞳孔直上，眉上 1 寸处。

【主治病症】面神经麻痹，夜盲，眶上神经痛，偏头痛，眩晕，视物模糊，目痛，眼睑下垂。

【热敏灸感】

面瘫：常出现热感深透颅内，或热感扩散至整个额部，或自觉局部有紧、压、酸、胀感等非热觉反应，临床常配合翳风穴单点灸、颊车穴单点灸、合谷穴单点灸。

偏头痛：常出现热感深透颅内，或热感扩散至整个额部，或自觉局部有紧、压、酸、胀感等非热觉反应，临床常配合太阳穴双点灸、风池穴双点灸、外关穴单点灸。

三叉神经痛：常可出现热感扩散至整个额部，或自觉局部有紧、压、酸、胀感等非热觉反应，临床常配合承泣穴单点灸、风池穴双点灸。

（二）下关

【归经】属足阳明胃经。

【穴位定位】在面部耳前方，当颧弓与下颌切迹所形成的凹陷中，张口时隆起处。

【主治病症】耳聋，耳鸣，聤耳；牙痛，口噤，口眼㖞斜，面痛，三叉神经痛，面神经麻痹，下颌疼痛，牙关紧闭，张嘴困难，颞颌关节炎。

【热敏灸感】

耳聋耳鸣：常出现热感渗透或热感扩散至一侧面颊的灸感反应，临床常配合外关穴单点灸或合谷穴单点灸。

牙痛：常出现热感渗透牙龈或局部出现酸胀等非热觉的灸感反应，临床常配合合谷穴单点灸。

（三）颊车

【归经】属足阳明胃经。

【穴位定位】位于面颊部，下颌角前上方约 1 横指，当咀嚼时咬肌隆起、放松时按之凹陷处。

【主治病症】牙痛，颊肿，下颌关节紊乱，口噤不语，三叉神经痛。

【热敏灸感】

牙痛：常出现热感渗透牙龈或局部出现酸胀等非热觉的灸感反应，临床常配合合谷穴单点灸。

下颌关节紊乱：常出现热感渗透下颌关节内，或关节内出现酸胀的非热觉灸感反应，临床常配合合谷穴单点灸。

面瘫：常出现热感渗透深部或热感扩散整个面颊的灸感反应，临床常配合翳风穴单点灸、合谷穴单点灸。

（四）迎香

【归经】属手阳明大肠经。

【穴位定位】在鼻翼外缘中点旁开约 0.5 寸，当鼻唇沟中。

【主治病症】嗅觉减退，面神经麻痹或痉挛，胆道蛔虫。

【热敏灸感】

鼻部疾病（如鼻塞、不闻香臭、鼻衄、鼻渊）：常出现热感扩散或热感渗透深部组织的灸感反应，临床常配合印堂穴组成三点灸，灸至热敏灸感消失。

口眼㖞斜：常可出现热感扩散的灸感反应，临床常配合翳风穴单点灸、合谷穴单点灸。

（五）通天

【归经】属足太阳膀胱经。

【穴位定位】在头部，当前发际正中直上 4 寸，旁开 1.5 寸。

【主治病症】头痛，眩晕，鼻塞，鼻衄，鼻渊。

【热敏灸感】

头痛：常出现热感深透颅内，或热感扩散，临床常配合太阳穴双点灸、风池穴双点灸、合谷穴单点灸。

过敏性鼻炎：常出现热感深透颅内，或热感扩散，临床常配合印堂穴单点灸、迎香穴双点灸、合谷穴单点灸。

（六）百会

【归经】属督脉。

【穴位定位】在头部，当前发际正中直上 5 寸，两耳连线的中点处，或以两眉头中间向上 1 横指起，直到后发际正中点。

【主治病症】头重脚轻，痔疮，高血压，低血压，宿醉，目眩，失眠，焦躁等。

【热敏灸感】

失眠：常出现热感深透颅内，或出现灸感向前额或向后项沿督脉传导，临床常配合心俞穴双点灸、至阳穴单点灸、涌泉穴双点灸。

缺血性中风：常出现热感透至颅内，或热感向四周扩散，或热感向前额或后项沿督脉传导的灸感，临床常配合风池穴双点灸、手三里穴双点灸、阳陵泉穴双点灸。

头痛：常出现热感透至颅内，或热感沿督脉前行至额部后行至颈项部，临床常配合太阳穴双点灸、合谷穴双点灸、风府穴单点灸。

腹泻：常出现热感透至颅内，或热感扩散至头顶部，临床常配合天枢穴双点灸、次髎穴双点灸、足三里穴双点灸。

胃下垂：常出现热感透至颅内，或热感向前额或后项沿督脉传导灸感，临床常配合中脘穴单点灸、神阙穴单点灸、足三里穴双点灸。

（七）上印堂

【归经】经外奇穴。

【穴位定位】在额部，当两眉头中间上 1 寸。

【主治病症】头痛，项强，鼻炎，眩晕，目赤，目痛，癫狂痫。

【热敏灸感】

过敏性鼻炎：常出现收紧感、麻木感、酸胀感、重压感等非热觉反应，或出现热感扩散至前额部，或出现热流沿鼻梁下行至鼻根部，临床常配合迎香穴双点灸，神阙、关元穴双点灸，肾俞穴双点灸，肺俞穴双点灸。

头痛：常出现收紧感、麻木感、酸胀感、重压感等非热觉反应，或出现热感扩散至前额部，临床常配合太阳穴双点灸、百会穴单点灸、风池穴双点灸。

（八）风池

【归经】属足少阳胆经。

【穴位定位】风池在后头项部，当头枕骨下，平风府穴（入后发际正中上 1 寸），斜方肌上端和胸锁乳突肌之间凹陷中。

【主治病症】头痛，眩晕，目赤肿痛，鼻渊，耳鸣，面瘫，颈项强痛，癫痫，中风，热病，疟疾，瘿气，神经症，高血压，失眠，肩膀酸痛，足跟痛，电光性眼炎，视网膜动脉阻塞，面肌痉挛，荨麻疹。

【热敏灸感】

头痛、偏头痛、眩晕：常出现热感渗透深部，或热感扩散至头后部及颈项部，或出现热感上传头顶部或下传至项背部，部分可出现穴位处酸胀反应，临床常配合百会穴单点灸、太阳穴双点灸、外关穴单点灸、太冲穴双点灸。

感冒、鼻塞、过敏性鼻炎：常出现热感渗透深部，或热感扩散至头后部及颈项部，临床常配合印堂穴单点灸、肺俞穴双点灸。

三叉神经痛、面肌痉挛：常可出现热感渗透深部，或热感扩散至头后部及颈项部，临床常配合阳白穴单点灸、四白穴单点灸、合谷穴单点灸。

枕神经痛：常出现热感渗透深部，或热感扩散至头后部及颈项部，或出现热感上传头顶部或下传至项背部，部分可出现穴位处酸胀反应，临床常配合百会穴单点灸、阿是穴单点灸。

颈椎病：常出现热感渗透深部，或热感上传头顶部下传至项背部，临床常配合大椎穴组成三点灸、颈项部阿是穴单点灸、列缺穴单点灸。

（九）翳风

【归经】属手少阳三焦经。

【穴位定位】位于耳垂后方，当乳突与下颌角之间的凹陷中。

【主治病症】面瘫，面肌痉挛，口眼㖞斜；疖腮，颊肿，瘰疬。

【热敏灸感】

面瘫：常出现热感深透且扩散至患侧面部，或出现穴位处酸痛、酸胀等非热觉反应，临床常配合颊车穴单点灸、风池穴双点灸。

耳鸣、耳聋：常出现热感深透且扩散至患侧耳部及面颊，临床常配合听宫穴单点灸、外关穴单点灸。

（十）太阳

【归经】经外奇穴。

【穴位定位】在颞部（前额两侧），当眉梢和外眼角的中点向后的凹陷处，大约 0.5 寸。

【主治病症】头痛，偏头痛，视疲劳，牙痛等疾病。

【热敏灸感】

感冒：常出现热感扩散至整个颞部，或出现热感渗透颅内，临床常配合上印堂单点灸，大椎、风池穴三点灸。

头痛：常出现热感扩散至整个颞部，或出现热感渗透颅内，或出现局部酸胀、皮肤收紧感、重压感等非热觉反应，临床常配合上印堂穴单点灸，百会穴单点灸，风池、大椎穴三点灸。

二、胸腹部

（一）中府

【归经】属手太阴肺经。

【穴位定位】位于胸部，前正中线旁开 6 寸，平第 1 肋间隙处。

【主治病症】胸胁胀痛，咳嗽气喘。

【热敏灸感】

感冒咳嗽：常出现热感透至胸腔并传至上肢，或热感扩散胸前的灸感，临床上常配合风池穴双点灸、肺俞穴双点灸。

气喘：常出现热感渗透至胸腔并传至上肢的灸感，临床常配合大椎、至阳、命门穴循经往返灸和接力灸，肺俞穴双点灸及神阙穴单点灸。

慢性支气管炎：常出现热感渗透至胸腔并传至上肢的灸感，临床常配合大椎、至阳、命门穴循经往返灸和接力灸，肺俞穴双点灸及脾俞穴双点灸。

肩周炎：常出现热感渗透至肩关节深部，或出现施灸局部酸胀痛的灸感反应，临床常配合局部压痛点单点灸、膏肓穴和肩井穴患侧单点灸，常出现热感深透或酸胀感。

（二）天枢

【归经】属足阳明胃经。

【穴位定位】位于腹部，脐中旁开2寸。

【主治病症】急性胃肠炎，小儿腹泻，痢疾，便秘，胆囊炎，肝炎，痛经，子宫内膜炎，异常子宫出血，肾炎等。

【热敏灸感】

腹痛腹胀：自觉热感深透至腹腔，或沿带脉向两侧腰部及背部传导，或出现表面不热而腹腔深部感觉热感扩散，临床常配合双侧足三里穴单点灸、神阙穴单点灸。

便秘、腹泻、痢疾：自觉热感深透至腹腔，或扩散至整个腹部，沿带脉向两侧腰部及背部传导，或出现表面不热而腹腔深部感觉热感扩散，临床常配合阴陵泉穴单点灸、双侧足三里穴单点灸。

月经不调、痛经：自觉热感深透至腹腔，或沿带脉向两侧腰部及背部传导，临床常配合阴陵泉穴单点灸、三阴交穴单点灸、合谷穴单点灸。

妇科炎症：自觉热感深透至腹腔，或扩散至整个腹部，或沿带脉向两侧腰部及背部传导，临床常配合阴陵泉穴单点灸、足三里穴单点灸、太冲穴单点灸。

（三）中脘

【归经】属任脉。

【穴位定位】仰卧位，前正中线之脐上4寸。取穴时于前正中线上，取肚脐与胸骨下缘之中点。

【主治病症】胃痛，腹痛，腹胀，呕逆，反胃，食不化；肠鸣，泄泻，便秘，便血，胁下坚痛；喘息不止，失眠，脏躁，癫痫，尸厥；胃炎，胃溃疡，胃扩张，子宫脱垂，荨麻疹，食物中毒。

【热敏灸感】

消化性溃疡：常出现热感透至腹腔内，或热感扩散至整个上腹部，或出现胃肠蠕动反应，临床常配合双点温和灸天枢、胃俞、阴陵泉等穴。

功能性消化不良：常出现热感透至腹腔内，或出现胃脘部发热现象，或出现胃肠蠕动反应，临床常配合关元、肝俞、膈俞、上巨虚等穴双点灸。

（四）关元

【归经】属任脉。

【穴位定位】在下腹部，前正中线，当脐中下 3 寸。

【主治病症】中风、腹痛、痢疾、脱肛、疝气、遗尿、小便不利、遗精、早泄、阳痿、月经不调、阴部瘙痒、消渴、眩晕、神经衰弱、细菌性痢疾、胃肠炎、肠道蛔虫症、肝炎、肾炎、尿路感染、盆腔炎、睾丸炎。

【热敏灸感】

慢性前列腺炎：可出现热感深透至腹腔，或出现腹腔内发热现象，或出现热感沿带脉传导至腰骶部，临床常配合关元、中极穴双点灸，肾俞穴双点灸，命门、次髎穴三点灸。

阳痿：可出现热感深透至腹腔，或出现腹腔内发热现象，临床常配合关元、气冲穴三点灸，肾俞穴双点灸，腰阳关穴单点灸，三阴交穴双点灸。

盆腔炎：可出现热感深透至腹腔，或出现腹腔内发热现象，或出现热感呈带状向两侧腰际传导甚至到达腰骶部，临床常配合关元、天枢穴三点灸，肾俞穴双点灸，次髎穴双点灸，三阴交穴双点灸。

原发性痛经：可出现热感深透至腹腔，或出现热感扩散至整个腹部，临床常配合关元、子宫穴三点灸或关元、天枢穴三点灸。

保健：可出现热感渗透腹腔，或出现热感扩散至整个腹腔，或出现腹腔深部发热感觉，或出现热感呈带状向两侧腰际传导，临床常配合腰阳关穴单点灸、足三里穴双点灸。

（五）子宫

【归经】经外奇穴。

【穴位定位】在下腹部，当脐中下 4 寸，中极旁开 3 寸。

【主治病症】月经不调，带下，痛经，产后恶露不下，阴挺，产后子宫神经痛、尿频、尿急。

【热敏灸感】

原发性痛经：常出现热感透至腹腔，或热感扩散至整个腹部，临床常配合关元、子宫穴三点灸，腰阳关穴单点灸。

盆腔炎：常出现热流深透整个下腹部，或出现热感扩散如巴掌大小，或出现热感呈带状向两侧腰际传导，临床常配合关元、子宫穴三点灸，次髎穴双点灸。

（六）神阙

【归经】属任脉。

【穴位定位】位于肚脐正中。

【主治病症】腹痛，泄泻，脱肛，水肿，虚脱。

【热敏灸感】

支气管哮喘：可出现热流逐渐扩散至整个腹部，或有热流如水柱向腹腔深部灌注灸感，临床常配合大椎、至阳、命门循经往返灸，中府穴双点灸、肺俞穴双点灸。

过敏性鼻炎：可出现热感深透至腹腔灸感，临床常配合上印堂穴单点灸、通天穴双点灸、风池穴双点灸、肺俞穴双点灸。

荨麻疹：可出现热感深透至腹腔灸感，临床常配合肺俞穴双点灸、至阳穴单点灸、曲池穴双点灸、血海穴双点灸、三阴交穴双点灸。

失眠：可出现热感深透至腹腔，或出现腹腔深部发热的灸感反应，临床常配合百会穴单点灸、心俞穴双点灸、至阳穴单点灸、涌泉穴双点灸。

面瘫：可出现热感深透至腹腔，或热感呈带状沿两侧扩散至腰部，临床常配合单点灸阳白、下关、颊车等穴，双点灸足三里穴。

腹胀、腹泻、便秘：可出现热感深透至腹腔，或热感呈带状沿两侧扩散至腰部，或出现腹腔深部发热的灸感反应，临床常配合天枢穴双点灸、次髎穴双点灸、足三里穴双点灸。

保健：可出现热感深透腹腔，或出现热感扩散至整个腹腔，或出现腹腔深部发热感觉，或出现热感呈带状向两侧腰际传导，临床常配合腰阳关穴单点灸、足三里穴双点灸。

（七）膻中

【归经】属任脉。

【穴位定位】位于胸部，当前正中线上，平第4肋间，两乳头连线的中点。

【主治病症】咳嗽，气喘，咯唾脓血，胸痹心痛，心悸，心烦，产妇少乳，噎膈，臌胀。

【热敏灸感】

胸闷、心痛：可出现热感扩散至胸部，或出现热流沿任脉上下循行，可配合心俞穴双点灸、内关穴双点灸。

三、腰背部

（一）肩井

【归经】属足少阳胆经。

【穴位定位】在大椎穴与肩峰连线中点，肩部最高处。取穴时一般采用正坐、俯伏或者俯卧的姿势，此穴位于人体的肩上，前直乳中，当大椎与肩峰端连线的中点，即乳头正上方与肩线交接处。在后颈根最高突起下凹陷与肩外侧骨突连线的中点，按压有痛感。

【主治病症】肩膀酸痛，头酸痛，头重脚轻，视疲劳，耳鸣，高血压，落枕，肩背痹痛，手臂不举，颈项强痛，乳痈，中风，瘰疬，难产，诸虚百损。

【热敏灸感】

肩周炎：常出现热感透向深部并向四周扩散，或出现重压、酸胀、酸痛感，或热感经肩部沿上肢外侧向下传导，部分感传可直接到腕部，如感传不显著者，可采用接力灸方法，取一支点燃的艾条分别放置于肩髃、臂臑、曲池、手三里、外关穴进行温和灸，依次接力使感传到达手背部，最后将两支艾条分别固定于肩井穴和手三里穴进行温和灸。

（二）大椎

【归经】属督脉。

【穴位定位】在后正中线上，第 7 颈椎棘突下凹陷中。

【主治病症】热病，疟疾，咳嗽，喘逆，骨蒸潮热，项强，肩背痛，腰脊强，角弓反张，小儿惊风，癫狂痫，五劳虚损，七伤乏力，中暑，霍乱，呕吐，黄疸，风疹。

【热敏灸感】

颈椎病：常出现热感透向深部，或自觉肩部有重压、酸胀、酸痛感，或热感上传至颈项部，临床常配合颈部阿是穴单点灸，风池、大椎穴三点灸。

（三）至阳

【归经】属督脉。

【穴位定位】在背部，当后正中线上，第7胸椎棘突下凹陷中。

【主治病症】胸胁胀痛，脊强，腰背疼痛，黄疸，胆囊炎，胆道蛔虫病，胃肠炎，肋间神经痛。

【热敏灸感】

胸胁胀满：常出现热感扩散至胸背部，或热感沿督脉上行至大椎、下行至腰骶部，感传不显著者，可采用接力灸方法，用另一点燃艾条，沿督脉依次在大椎、至阳、命门穴循经往返灸和接力灸，使灸感接力上行下循，常可配合膻中穴单点灸、日月穴单点灸。

支气管哮喘：常出现热感沿督脉上行，可达风府，部分感传不显著者，可采用接力灸方法，用另一点燃艾条，沿督脉依次在大椎、至阳、命门穴循经往返灸和接力灸，使灸感接力上行下循，临床常配合肺俞穴双点灸，中府穴双点灸，神阙、关元穴双点灸。

腰背疼痛：常出现热感扩散至胸背部，或热感沿督脉上行至大椎、下行至腰骶部，感传不显著者，可采用接力灸方法，用另一点燃艾条，沿督脉依次在大椎、至阳、命门穴循经往返灸和接力灸，使灸感接力循行，常可配合阿是穴单点灸，肾俞、腰阳关穴三点灸。

阳虚病证：常出现热感沿督脉上行可达风府、下行至腰骶部，部分感传不显著者，可采用接力灸方法引导，临床常配合神阙、关元穴双点灸，腰阳关穴单点灸，足三里穴双点灸。

（四）肺俞

【归经】属足太阳膀胱经。

【穴位定位】在背部，当第3胸椎棘突下，旁开1.5寸。

【主治病症】咳嗽，气喘，咯血，鼻塞，骨蒸潮热，盗汗，皮肤瘙痒，瘾疹。

【热敏灸感】

感冒、咳嗽：常出现热感渗透胸腔，或腋下热，或热感沿手臂内侧下行至肘、腕，或热感扩散至肩胛区，临床常配合大椎穴单点灸、风池穴双点灸。

慢性支气管炎、支气管哮喘：常出现热感渗透胸腔，或热感沿手臂内侧下行至肘、腕，临床常配合中府穴单点灸、肾俞穴双点灸。

过敏性鼻炎：常出现热感渗透胸腔，或热感沿手臂内侧下行至肘、腕，或热感扩散至肩胛区，临床常配合印堂穴单点灸、风池穴双点灸、肾俞穴双点灸，灸至热敏灸感消失。

颈椎病：常可出现热感上行至风府、风池穴，或热感沿手臂内侧下行至肘、腕，临床常配合颈部阿是穴单点灸，风池穴双点灸。

荨麻疹：常出现热感透至胸腔，或热感沿手臂内侧下行传导，临床常配合肾俞穴双点灸、至阳穴单点灸、足三里穴单点灸、神阙穴单点灸。

（五）脾俞

【归经】属足太阳膀胱经。

【穴位定位】在背部，第 11 胸椎棘突下，旁开 1.5 寸。

【主治病症】腹胀、腹泻、呕吐、痢疾、便血等脾胃肠腑病症。

【热敏灸感】

慢性支气管炎：常出现热感透至深部，或热感扩散至整个腰背部，临床常配合中府穴单点灸、肺俞穴双点灸。

腹胀、消化不良：常出现热感深透至腹腔，或热感扩散至背腰部，或出现胃脘部发热现象，或出现胃肠间歇性蠕动，临床上常配合足三里穴双点灸、中脘穴单点灸、神阙穴单点灸。

（六）胃俞

【归经】属足太阳膀胱经。

【穴位定位】位于背部，当第 12 胸椎棘突下，旁开 1.5 寸。

【主治病症】消化系统疾病，如胃溃疡、胃炎、胃痉挛、呕吐、恶心等。

【热敏灸感】

腹胀、胃脘痛、消化不良：常可出现热感深透至腹腔，或热感扩散至背腰部，或出现胃脘部发热现象，或出现胃肠间歇性蠕动，临床上常配合足三里穴双点灸、中脘穴单点灸、神阙穴单点灸。

（七）命门

【归经】属督脉。

【穴位定位】位于腰部，当后正中线上，第 2 腰椎棘突下凹陷中。

【主治病症】虚损腰痛，脊强反折，遗尿，尿频，泄泻，遗精，白浊，阳痿，早泄，赤白带下，胎屡堕，五劳七伤，头晕耳鸣，癫痫，惊恐，手足逆冷。

【热敏灸感】

腰痛：常出现热感渗透深部，或热感扩散至腰骶部，或热感呈带状向两侧腰际传导，或出现热感呈带状向一侧或两侧臀部、下肢部传导，如感传不显著者，可采用接力灸方法，取另一点燃艾条依次艾灸环跳、承扶、委中、承山穴，使灸感依次接力下行至踝部，最后艾灸腰阳关、委中穴，临床常配合腰部阿是穴单点灸、肾俞穴双点灸。

阳痿、早泄：常出现热感渗透深部，或热感呈带状向两侧腰际传导，或出现下腹部腹腔内发热感觉，或出现下腹部及双侧腹股沟处发热反应，临床常配合肾俞穴双点灸、神阙中极穴双点灸、三阴交穴双点灸。

腹胀、腹泻：常出现热感渗透深部，或热感呈带状向两侧腰际传导，或出现下腹部腹腔内发热感觉，临床常可配合天枢、神阙穴三点灸，足三里穴双点灸。

慢性支气管炎，支气管哮喘：常出现热感沿督脉上行，可达风府，部分感传不显著者，可采用接力灸方法，用另一点燃艾条，沿督脉依次在大椎、至阳、命门穴循经往返灸和接力灸，使灸感接力上行至颈项部，临床常配合肺俞穴双点灸，中府穴双点灸，神阙关元穴双点灸，大椎、至阳、腰阳关穴三点灸。

肾阳虚病症：常出现热感渗透深部，或热感沿督脉上行，可达风府，部分感传不显著者，可采用接力灸方法，用另一点燃艾条，沿督脉依次上行，使灸感接力上行至颈项部，临床常配合神阙、关元穴双点灸，至阳穴单点灸，足三里穴双点灸。

（八）肾俞

【归经】属足太阳膀胱经。

【穴位定位】在背部，第 2 腰椎棘突下，旁开 1.5 寸。

【主治病症】遗尿，遗精，阳痿，月经不调，白带，水肿，耳鸣，耳聋，腰痛。

【热敏灸感】

阳痿、早泄：常出现热感深透至腹腔，或热感扩散至腰骶部，或热感向两侧腰部传导，或出现腹部神阙关元穴发热现象，临床常配合神阙关元穴双点灸、三阴交穴双点灸、足三里穴双点灸。

慢性前列腺炎：常出现热感深透至腹腔，或热感扩散至腰骶部，或热感向两侧腰部传导，或出现腹部神阙关元穴发热现象，或出现两侧腹股沟发热现象，临床常配合关元中极穴双点灸、三阴交穴双点灸、血海穴双点灸。

肾虚病症：常出现热感深透至腹腔，或热感扩散至腰骶部，或热感向两侧腰部传导，或出现热感沿足太阳膀胱经上下传导，或出现腹腔内发热现象，临床常配合神阙、关元穴双点灸，三阴交穴双点灸，足三里穴双点灸。

（九）腰阳关

【归经】属督脉。

【穴位定位】在腰部，当后正中线上，第4腰椎棘突下凹陷中。

【主治病症】腰骶疼痛，下肢痿痹，月经不调、赤白带下等妇科病症，遗精、阳痿等男科病症。

【热敏灸感】

腰痛：常出现热感渗透深部，或热感扩散至腰骶部，或热感呈带状向两侧腰际传导，或出现热感呈带状向一侧或两侧臀部、下肢部传导，如感传不显著者，可采用接力灸方法，取另一点燃艾条依次艾灸环跳、承扶、委中、承山穴，使灸感依次接力下行至踝部，最后艾灸腰阳关、委中穴，灸至热敏灸感消失。或出现局部酸胀、酸痛等非热觉反应。临床常配合腰部阿是穴的单点灸、肾俞穴双点灸。

妇科病症：常出现热感渗透深部，或热感扩散至腰骶部，或热感呈带状向两侧腰际传导，或出现下腹部腹腔内发热感觉，或出现下腹部及双侧腹股沟处发热反应，临床常配合次髎穴双点灸、天枢穴双点灸。

阳痿、早泄：常出现热感渗透深部，或热感呈带状向两侧腰际传导，或出现下腹部腹腔内发热感觉，或出现下腹部及双侧腹股沟处发热反应，临床常配合肾俞穴双点灸、神阙中极穴双点灸、三阴交穴双点灸。

腹胀、腹泻：常出现热感渗透深部，或热感呈带状向两侧腰际传导，或出现下腹部腹腔内发热感觉，临床常可配合天枢、神阙穴三点灸，足三里穴双点灸。

（十）大肠俞

【归经】属足太阳膀胱经。

【穴位定位】位于腰部，当第4腰椎棘突下，旁开1.5寸。

【主治病症】腹胀，泄泻，便秘，腰痛，坐骨神经痛。

【热敏灸感】

腰痛：常出现热感渗透深部甚至腹腔，或热感向四周扩散至腰骶部，或热感下行经臀部向下肢传导，或出现热感呈带状向两侧腰部传导，或局部出现酸胀、酸痛非热觉反应，临床常配合肾俞穴双点灸、委中穴单点灸。

腹泻、便秘：常出现热感渗透深部甚至腹腔，或热感向四周扩散至腰骶部，或出现热感呈带状向两侧腰部传导，或出现肠蠕动等非热觉反应，或出现下腹部腹腔内发热现象，临床常配合天枢穴双点灸、足三里穴双点灸。

（十一）次髎

【归经】属足太阳膀胱经。

【穴位定位】在骶部，当髂后上棘内下方，适对第2骶后孔处。

【主治病症】疝气，月经不调，痛经，带下，小便不利，遗精，腰痛，下肢痿痹。

【热敏灸感】

妇科病症：常出现热感深透至腹腔，或热感扩散至腰骶部，或热感呈带状向两侧腰部传导甚至到达腹部，或出现下腹部腹腔内发热现象，临床常配合天枢关元穴三点灸、三阴交穴双点灸。

腹胀、腹泻、便秘：常出现热感深透至腹腔，或热感扩散至腰骶部，或热感呈带状向两侧腰部传导甚至到达腹部，或出现下腹部腹腔内发热现象，或出现肠蠕动现象，临床常配合天枢穴两点或三点灸、足三里穴双点灸。

腰痛：常出现热感渗透深部甚至腹腔，或热感向四周扩散至腰骶部，或热感下行经臀部向下肢传导，或出现热感呈带状向两侧腰部传导，或局部出现酸胀、酸痛非热觉反应，临床常配合肾俞穴双点灸、委中穴单点灸。

四、上肢部

（一）肩贞

【归经】属手太阳小肠经。

【穴位定位】位于人体的肩关节后下方，臂内收时，腋后纹头直上1寸。

【主治病症】肩周炎，瘰疬瘿气，目疾，肩胛疼痛，腋下痛等。

【热敏灸感】

肩周炎：常出现热感渗透肩关节内，或热感沿上臂内侧下行，或热感上行至肩、颈项部，或艾灸局部甚至关节腔内出现酸胀、酸痛等非热觉灸感，临床常配合臑俞、肩髃穴双点灸，臂臑穴单点灸。临床也可采用隔姜灸，常出现肩关节内酸胀酸痛等非热觉灸感，或出现热感沿上臂内侧下行，一般可灸5~7壮。

乳腺增生：可出现热透深部，或热流沿上臂内侧下行传导，临床常配合足三里穴单点灸、中府穴单点灸、乳根穴单点灸。

（二）曲池

【归经】属手阳明大肠经。

【穴位定位】屈肘，在肘横纹桡侧端凹陷处。取法：①屈肘成直角，当肘弯横纹尽头处；②屈肘，于肘横纹外侧端与肱骨外上髁连线的中点处。

【主治病症】咽喉肿痛，牙痛，目赤痛，瘰疬，瘾疹，热病，上肢不遂，手臂肿痛，腹痛吐泻，高血压，癫狂。

【热敏灸感】

热病：常出现热感沿前臂前缘下传至手，或沿上臂前缘上行至肩部，临床常配合大椎穴单点灸、风池穴双点灸。

头面五官疾病：常出现热感沿上臂前缘上行至肩部，经过接力灸，热感可上行至患处。临床常配合合谷穴单点灸、局部压痛点单点灸。

瘾疹：常出现灸感沿前臂前缘下传至手，临床常配合合谷穴单点灸、风门穴双点灸、足三里穴双点灸。

腹部疾病：常出现热感渗透深部组织，并沿前臂前缘下传至手，临床常配合中脘天枢三点灸、次髎穴双点灸、足三里穴双点灸。

上肢不遂、手臂肿痛：常出现局部酸胀痛的反应或热感渗透深部组织，临床常配合局部压痛点单点灸。

（三）内关

【归经】属手厥阴心包经。

【穴位定位】在前臂掌侧，当曲泽与大陵的连线上，腕横纹上 2 寸，掌长肌腱与桡侧腕屈肌腱之间。

【主治病症】心痛，心悸，胸闷气急，呃逆，胃痛，失眠，孕吐，晕车，手臂疼痛，头痛，胸胁痛，上腹痛，心绞痛，月经痛，腹泻，精神异常等。

【热敏灸感】

胃痛：常出现热感沿手厥阴心包经上行传导，或出现胃蠕动现象，临床常配合中脘穴单点灸、足三里穴双点灸。

呃逆：常出现热感沿手厥阴心包经上行传导，临床常配合膈俞穴双点灸、足三里穴双点灸。

失眠：常出现热感渗透，或热感沿手厥阴心包经上行传导，临床常配合神阙穴单点灸、心俞穴单点灸、足三里穴双点灸。

五、下肢部

（一）膝眼

【归经】经外奇穴。

【穴位定位】屈膝，在髌韧带两侧凹陷处，在内侧的称内膝眼，在外侧的称外膝眼（即犊鼻穴）。

【主治病症】腿膝痛，痿痹不仁。

【热敏灸感】

膝关节骨性关节炎：常出现热流渗透膝关节腔内，或出现热感扩散至整个膝关节，或出现酸胀、酸痛等非热觉反应，临床常配合梁丘、血海穴双点灸，阳陵泉、阴陵泉穴双点灸。

（二）血海

【归经】属足太阴脾经。

【穴位定位】位于髌骨底内侧缘上2寸，当股四头肌内侧头的隆起处。简便取法是：患者屈膝，医者以左手掌心按于患者右膝髌骨上缘，二至五指向上伸直对着大腿，拇指约45°角斜置，拇指尖下是穴。对侧取法仿此。揉按此穴有酸胀之感。

【主治病症】月经不调，经闭，崩漏，膝股内侧痛，瘾疹，湿疹，丹毒。

【热敏灸感】

膝关节骨性关节炎：常出现热感渗透深部，或热感扩散至膝关节内侧面，或膝关节内出现酸胀、酸痛等非热觉反应，临床常配合内外膝眼双点灸、阳陵泉穴单点灸、梁丘穴单点灸。

月经不调、痛经：常出现热感渗透深部，或热感沿大腿向上传导，部分感传可直接到达下腹部，如感传仍不能上至下腹部者，再取一支点燃的艾条放置于感传所达部位的近心端点，进行接力灸，使感传到达下腹部，最后将两支艾条分别固定于血海和下腹部进行温和灸，临床常配合三阴交穴单点灸、天枢穴双点灸。

荨麻疹：常出现热感渗透深部，或热感沿大腿向上传导，部分感传可直接到达腹部，临床常配合三阴交穴单点灸、神阙穴或关元穴单点灸、风门穴或肺俞穴双点灸。

慢性前列腺炎、阳痿：常可出现热感渗透深部，或热感沿大腿向上传导至下腹部，部分感传不能上至下腹部者，采用接力灸方法，使感传到达下腹部，最后将两支艾条分别固定于血海和下腹部进行温和灸，临床常配合三阴交穴单点灸、关元穴单点灸。

（三）梁丘

【归经】属足阳明胃经。

【穴位定位】在大腿前面，当髂前上棘与髌底外侧端的连线上，髌底上2寸。简易取穴法：伸展膝盖用力时，膝盖外侧筋肉凸出处的凹陷；或从膝盖骨右端，约3个手指左右的上方也是该穴。

【主治病症】膝关节肿痛，下肢不遂，急性胃痛，腹泻，乳痈。

【热敏灸感】

膝关节骨性关节炎：自觉热感透至膝关节内并扩散至整个膝关节，临床常配合阴陵泉穴双点温和灸。

肠易激综合征：常出现热感沿足阳明经上行至腹部，临床常配合足三里穴单点灸。

（四）上巨虚

【归经】属足阳明胃经。

【穴位定位】在小腿前外侧，当犊鼻下6寸，距胫骨前缘1横指（中指）。

【主治病症】阑尾炎，胃肠炎，泄泻，痢疾，疝气，便秘，消化不良；脑血管病后遗症，下肢麻痹或痉挛，膝关节肿痛。

【热敏灸感】

腹泻、便秘：常出现热感渗透局部深部，或出现热感沿足阳明经传导，部分感传可直接到达腹部，如感传不能上至腹部者，再取一支点燃的艾条放置于感传所达部位的近心端点，进行接力灸，使感传到达腹部，最后将两支艾条分别固定于上巨虚和腹部进行温和灸，临床常配合足三里穴单点灸、天枢穴双点灸。

（五）犊鼻

【归经】属足阳明胃经。

【穴位定位】屈膝，在髌骨下缘，髌韧带（髌骨与胫骨之间大筋）两侧有凹陷，其外侧凹陷中取穴。

【主治病症】风湿、类风湿关节炎，膝关节骨性关节炎，外伤等各种膝关节痛患者，犊鼻穴为常用腧穴。膝部神经痛或麻木，下肢瘫痪，犊鼻穴常为辅助用穴。

【热敏灸感】

膝关节骨性关节炎：常出现热感渗透至膝关节腔内，或艾灸局部出现酸胀甚至疼痛等非热觉反应，临床常配合梁丘穴单点灸、内膝眼单点灸、局部阿是穴单点灸。

（六）丰隆

【归经】属足阳明胃经。

【穴位定位】小腿前外侧，当外踝尖上 8 寸，条口穴外，距胫骨前缘 2 横指（中指）。

【主治病症】气逆，喉痹卒喑，狂癫，足不收，胫枯，胸腹痛，呕吐，便秘，脚气，厥头痛，眩晕等。

【热敏灸感】

下肢痿痹、下肢不遂：常出现热感深透，或热感向上或向下沿足阳明胃经传导，临床常配合足三里穴单点灸、阴陵泉穴单点灸。

痰饮病症：常出现热感深透，或热感向上沿足阳明胃经上行至腹部，临床常配合足三里穴单点灸、合谷穴单点灸、中脘穴单点灸。

（七）足三里

【归经】属足阳明胃经。

【穴位定位】正坐屈膝，在小腿前外侧，当犊鼻下 3 寸，距胫骨前缘 1 横指。

【主治病症】胃痛，呕吐，噎膈，腹胀，泄泻，消化不良，痢疾，便秘，肠痛，下肢痹痛，膝痛，失眠，心悸，头晕，乳痈。

【热敏灸感】

胃肠疾病，如胃痛、呕吐、噎膈、腹胀、腹泻、肠鸣、便秘、痢疾等：常出现热感渗透，或热感沿足阳明胃经上行至腹部、下行至足背，如感传仍不能上至腹部者，再取一支点燃的艾条放置于感传所达部位的近心端点，进行接力灸使感传到达腹部，最后将两支艾条分别固定于足三里与腹部进行温和灸，临床常配合阴陵泉穴单点灸、中脘天枢穴三点灸。

下肢痿痹，下肢不遂：常出现热感渗透，或热感沿足阳明胃经上行至腹部、下行至足背，临床常配合丰隆穴单点灸、承山穴单点灸。

面瘫：艾灸此穴，有部分灸感感传可直接到达腹部，如感传不能上至腹部者，再取一支点燃的艾条放置于感传所达部位的近心端点，进行接力灸使感传到达腹部，最后将两支艾条分别固定于足三里与腹部进行温和灸，临床常配合合谷穴单点灸、翳风穴单点灸。

补益正气，养生保健：艾灸此穴，有部分灸感感传可直接到达腹部，如感传不能上至腹部者，再取一支点燃的艾条放置于感传所达部位的近心端点，进行接力灸，使感传到达腹部，最后将两支艾条分别固定于足三里与腹部进行温和灸，临床常配合神阙关元穴双点灸。

（八）阳陵泉

【归经】属足少阳胆经。

【穴位定位】位于小腿外侧当腓骨头前下方凹陷处。

【主治病症】肩周炎，膝关节炎，风湿性关节炎，类风湿关节炎，偏瘫，坐骨神经痛，扭挫伤，胆囊炎，胆绞痛，胆结石。

【热敏灸感】

膝关节骨性关节炎：常出现热感透至膝关节内并扩散至整个膝关节，或穴位处出现酸胀、酸痛等非热觉反应，临床常配合内外膝眼双点灸、局部阿是穴单点灸。

偏头痛：常出现热感沿躯体侧面上行甚至传导至头，部分感传不显著者，采用接力灸方法，依次接力使感传到达头面部，最后将两支艾条分别固定于阳陵泉和头面部进行温和灸，临床常配合太阳穴单点灸、风池穴双点灸、太冲穴单点灸。

腰椎间盘突出症：常出现腰骶部发热现象，或热感沿下肢外侧上行至腰骶部，或下行至外踝及足背部，部分感传不显著者，可采用接力灸的方法进行感传引导，使热感感传直达病所，临床常配合肾俞穴腰阳关穴三点灸、委中穴单点灸。

胸胁胀痛：常出现热感沿躯体侧面上行甚至传导至胸胁部，部分感传不显著者，可采用接力灸方法，将热感感传引导至胸胁部，临床常可配合日月穴单点灸、肝俞穴双点灸。

（九）阴陵泉

【归经】属足太阴脾经。

【穴位定位】在小腿内侧，当胫骨内侧髁后下方凹陷处。

【主治病症】急慢性肠炎，细菌性痢疾，尿潴留，尿失禁，尿路感染，阴道炎，膝关节及周围软组织疾患。

【热敏灸感】

膝关节骨性关节炎：常出现热感渗透深部，或热感扩散至膝关节内侧面，或膝关节内出现酸胀、酸痛等非热觉反应，临床常配合内外膝眼双点灸、阳陵泉穴单点灸，血海、梁丘穴双点灸。

腹胀、腹泻：常出现热感渗透深部，或热感沿足太阴脾经上行，部分感传可直接到达腹部，如感传不能上至腹部者，再取一支点燃的艾条进行接力灸，依次接力使感传到达腹部，最后将两支艾条分别固定于阴陵泉和腹部进行温和灸，临床常配合足三里穴单点灸、天枢穴双点灸。

消化性溃疡：常出现热感渗透深部，或热感沿足太阴脾经上行，再取一支点燃的艾条采用接力灸法，依次接力使感传到达腹部，最后将两支艾条分别固定于阴陵泉和腹部进行温和灸，临床常配合足三里穴单点灸、中脘天枢穴三点灸，灸至热敏灸感消失。慢性消化性溃疡，也可采用麦粒灸法，艾灸时可出现热感渗透深部，或热感沿足太阴脾经上行至大腿内侧，一般可灸 7～10 壮。

盆腔炎症：常出现热感渗透深部，或热感沿足太阴脾经上行，采用接力灸法，使热感传至下腹部，最后将两支艾条分别固定于阴陵泉和腹部进行温和灸，临床常配合三阴交穴单点灸、子宫穴双点灸、神阙穴单点灸、次髎穴双点灸，灸至热敏灸感消失。慢性盆腔炎症经久难愈者，也可采用麦粒灸法，艾灸时可出现热感渗透深部，或热感沿足太阴脾经上行至大腿内侧，一般可灸 7～10 壮。

慢性前列腺炎：自觉热感沿大腿向上传导，部分感传可直接到达下腹部，如感传仍不能上至下腹部者，再取一支点燃的艾条放置于感传所达部位的近心端点，进行接力灸，依次接力使感传到达下腹部，最后将两支艾条分别固定于阴陵泉和下腹部进行温和灸，灸至热敏灸感消失。也可采用麦粒灸法，艾灸时可出现热感渗透深部，或热感沿足太阴脾经上行至大腿内侧，一般可灸 7～10 壮。

（十）三阴交

【归经】属足太阴脾经。

【穴位定位】位于小腿内侧，当足内踝尖上 3 寸，约 4 横指宽，按压有一骨头为胫骨，胫骨后缘靠近骨边凹陷处。

【主治病症】妇科病如月经不调、痛经、崩漏、带下、不孕、难产、阴挺；男科病如疝气、遗精、阳痿、早泄；消化系统病如腹胀腹痛、肠鸣泄泻、便秘。

【热敏灸感】

腹胀、腹泻：常可出现热感渗透深部，或热感沿足太阴脾经上行，部分感传可直接到达腹部，如感传不能上至腹部者，再取一支点燃的艾条进行接力灸，依次接力使感传到达腹部，最后将两支艾条分别固定于三阴交和腹部进行温和灸，临床常配合足三里穴单点灸、天枢穴双点灸。

妇产科病症：常可出现热感沿足太阴脾经上行至腹部，如感传不能上至腹部者，再取一支点燃的艾条进行接力灸，依次接力使感传到达腹部，最后将两支艾条分别固定于三阴交和腹部进行温和灸，临床常配合足三里穴单点灸、神阙穴单点灸、子宫穴双点灸及次髎穴双点灸，灸至热敏灸感消失。也可采用麦粒灸法，艾灸时可出现热感渗透深部，或热感沿足太阴脾经上行至小腿内侧，一般可灸7~10壮。

失眠：常可出现热感渗透深部，或出现热感沿足太阴脾经上行至腹部，如感传不能上至腹部者，可采用接力灸方法，依次接力使感传到达腹部，最后将两支艾条分别固定于三阴交和腹部进行温和灸，临床常配合足三里穴单点灸、神阙穴单点灸、内关穴单点灸，灸至热敏灸感消失。也可采用麦粒灸法，艾灸时可出现热感渗透深部，或热感沿足太阴脾经上行至小腿内侧，一般可灸7~10壮。

荨麻疹：常可出现热感深透，或向上或向下沿足太阴脾经传导，临床常配合肺俞穴双点灸、腰阳关穴肾俞穴三点灸，灸至热敏灸感消失。慢性荨麻疹患者，也可采用麦粒灸法，艾灸时可出现热感渗透深部，或热感沿足太阴脾经上行至小腿内侧，一般可灸7~10壮。

保健：常可出现表面不热或微热而深部热感强烈，或热流向上传导至腹部，如感传不显著者，再采用接力灸法，依次接力使感传到达腹部，最后将两支艾条分别固定于三阴交和腹部进行温和灸，临床常配合足三里穴单点灸，神阙穴单点灸，腰阳关穴、肾俞穴三点灸。

（十一）公孙

【归经】属足太阴脾经。

【穴位定位】位于足内侧缘，当第1跖骨基底的前下方，赤白肉际处。

【主治病症】胃痛，呕吐，腹胀，腹痛，泄泻，痢疾，心痛，胸闷。

【热敏灸感】

腹痛、腹泻：常出现热感沿足太阴脾经上行传导，部分感传可直接到达腹部，如感传不能上至腹部者，再取一支点燃的艾条放置于感传所达部位的近心端点，进行接力灸，使感传到达腹部，最后将两支艾条分别固定于公孙穴和腹部进行温和灸，临床常配合神阙、天枢穴三点灸，灸至热敏灸感消失。也可采用麦粒灸法，艾灸时可出现热感渗透深部，或热感沿足太阴脾经上行至小腿内侧，一般可灸 7 ~ 10 壮。

失眠：常出现热感渗透深部，或热感沿足太阴脾经上行传导，临床常采用接力灸，使感传到达腹部，最后将两支艾条分别固定于公孙穴和神阙穴进行温和灸，临床常配合太阳穴双点灸，脾俞、心俞穴四点灸，灸至热敏灸感消失。也可采用麦粒灸法，艾灸时可出现热感渗透深部，或热感沿足太阴脾经上行至小腿内侧，一般可灸 7 ~ 10 壮。

（十二）委中

【归经】属足太阳膀胱经。

【穴位定位】腘横纹中点，当股二头肌腱与半腱肌肌腱的中间。

【主治病症】腰背痛、下肢痿痹等腰及下肢病症；腹痛，急性吐泻；小便不利，遗尿，丹毒。

【热敏灸感】

腰腿痛：常可出现热感透向深部并向四周扩散，或热感沿足太阳膀胱经下行至足部（部分感传不能传至足跟部者，再取一支点燃的艾条依次放置于合阳、承筋、承山、昆仑穴进行温和灸，依次接力使感传到达足部，最后将两支艾条分别固定于委中穴和昆仑穴），或热感沿足太阳膀胱经上行至腰骶部（部分感传不能传至腰骶部者，再取一支点燃的艾条依次放置于殷门、承扶、环跳、腰阳关穴进行温和灸，依次接力使感传到达腰骶部，最后将两支艾条分别固定于委中穴和腰阳关穴），或出现腰骶部发热现象，临床常配合昆仑穴单点灸，腰阳关、肾俞穴三点灸。

（十三）太冲

【归经】属足厥阴肝经。

【穴位定位】在足背上，第 1、2 跖骨间隙后方的凹陷处。

【主治病症】头晕头痛，目赤肿痛，面瘫，耳鸣耳聋，咽喉肿痛，月经不调，崩漏，疝气，遗尿；小儿惊风，中风，原发性高血压，胁痛，下肢痿痹。

【热敏灸感】

面瘫：常出现热感渗透至足底，或热感沿足背上行经踝关节前部至小腿前侧，临床常可配合翳风穴单点灸、颊车穴单点灸、合谷穴单点灸。

胸胁胀痛：常出现热感沿足背上行经踝关节前部至小腿前侧，少部分患者可出现热感上传至胸胁，部分患者经过接力灸的方法也可使热感上行至胸胁部，临床常配合日月穴章门穴双点灸，阳陵泉穴单点灸。

眩晕、耳鸣：常出现热感沿足背上行经踝关节前部至小腿前侧，少部分患者经过接力灸的方法可出现热感上传至头面部，临床常配合合谷穴单点灸、风池穴双点灸、阳陵泉穴单点灸。

第三章

治疗篇

第一节 上呼吸道感染

上呼吸道感染是一种常见的由多种病毒引起的呼吸道传染病。中医学认为，本病是六淫之邪、时行疫毒侵袭人体，邪犯肺卫，以致卫表不和，肺失宣肃为病。由于感邪之不同、体质强弱不一，证候可表现为风寒、风热及夹湿、夹暑、夹燥、夹虚的不同。感冒全年均可发病，冬季多感风寒，春季多感风热，夏季多夹暑湿，秋季多兼燥邪，但以风寒感冒多见。如果病情较重，在一个时期内广泛流行，称为"时行感冒"。

【临床表现】

主要症状有鼻塞、流涕、喷嚏、咳嗽、咽干、声音嘶哑等，严重者有发热、轻度畏寒、全身酸痛、头痛等。

【灸法治则】

本病以祛风、解表、散寒为基本治疗原则。根据督脉主一身阳气理论，表寒重症的灸疗以温督通阳、解表散寒为主。

【治疗方案】

（一）探感选穴，准确定位

1. 高发穴区 热敏穴位高发区一般多位于上印堂、太阳、风池、风府、大椎、至阳、腰阳关等穴区，对这些部位进行热敏探查常能发现热敏腧穴。

2. 探查手法 在本病热敏穴位高发区，按下述步骤分别依序进行回旋、雀啄、往返、温和灸四步操作。

回旋灸 $\xrightarrow[\text{2分钟}]{\text{温热局部气血}}$ 雀啄灸 $\xrightarrow[\text{1分钟}]{\text{加强敏化}}$ 往返灸 $\xrightarrow[\text{1分钟}]{\text{激发经气}}$ 温和灸 $\xrightarrow[\text{2分钟}]{\text{发动传感}}$ 出现热敏灸感 $\rightarrow$ 确定热敏穴位

3. 热敏灸感 灸上印堂穴，灸感多为紧压感、扩热；灸太阳穴，灸感多为扩热；灸风池、风府、大椎、至阳、腰阳关穴，灸感多为透热、扩热、传热。

（二）循序激发，辨敏施灸

按照以下顺序，择优选穴施灸：

上印堂穴单点灸→太阳穴双点灸→大椎、风池穴双点灸→风府、大椎、至阳、腰阳关穴循经往返和接力灸。

上述热敏穴区不是每位患者全都出现，没有出现穴位热敏的就不做相应操作。

1. 上印堂穴单点灸　上印堂穴位于印堂穴上 1 寸，具有解表、疏利头目、通鼻窍之功效，适用于流鼻涕、打喷嚏、鼻塞、前额紧痛的风寒感冒。患者可觉热感或紧压重感扩散至整个前额，灸至热敏灸感消失（图 3-1-1）。

2. 太阳穴双点灸　适用于流鼻涕、打喷嚏、鼻塞、前额紧痛的风寒感冒。患者可感觉热感扩散至两侧颞部，灸至热敏灸感消失（图 3-1-2）。

3. 大椎、风池穴双点灸　大椎、风池穴分别为督脉与足少阳胆经穴位，具有疏风散寒、通鼻窍、退热等功效，适用于头项强痛的风寒感冒。患者可觉热感透至深部并扩散至整个头项背部，灸至热敏灸感消失（图 3-1-3）。

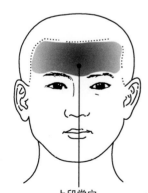

上印堂穴
定位：在额部，当两眉头之中间为
　　　印堂穴，在印堂穴上 1 寸
功效：解表，疏利头目，通鼻窍

图 3-1-1　上印堂穴单点灸

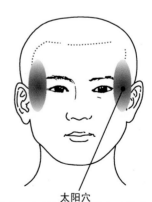

太阳穴
定位：在颞部，当眉梢与目外眦
　　　之间，向后约一横指的凹陷处
功效：解表退热，清利头目

图 3-1-2　太阳穴双点灸

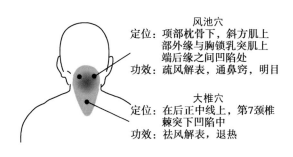

风池穴
定位：项部枕骨下，斜方肌上部外缘与胸锁乳突肌上端后缘之间凹陷处
功效：疏风解表，通鼻窍，明目

大椎穴
定位：在后正中线上，第7颈椎棘突下凹陷中
功效：祛风解表，退热

图 3-1-3　大椎、风池穴双点灸

4. 风府、大椎、至阳、腰阳关穴循经往返灸和接力灸　风府、大椎、至阳、腰阳关穴俱为督脉穴位，具有振奋督脉阳气，祛寒、疏风、解表、通络之功效。适用于恶风、恶寒发热、全身乏力的风寒感冒。患者可感觉到热感沿头项背腰部督脉传导，灸至热敏灸感消失（图 3-1-4）。

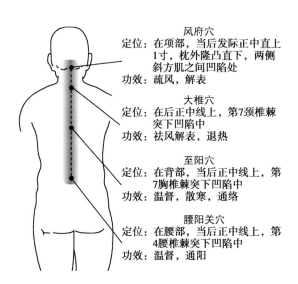

风府穴
定位：在项部，当后发际正中直上1寸，枕外隆凸直下，两侧斜方肌之间凹陷处
功效：疏风，解表

大椎穴
定位：在后正中线上，第7颈椎棘突下凹陷中
功效：祛风解表，退热

至阳穴
定位：在背部，当后正中线上，第7胸椎棘突下凹陷中
功效：温督，散寒，通络

腰阳关穴
定位：在腰部，当后正中线上，第4腰椎棘突下凹陷中
功效：温督，通阳

图 3-1-4　风府、大椎、至阳、腰阳关穴循经往返灸和接力灸

（三）量因人异，敏消量足

每次每穴的施灸时间以热敏灸感消失为度，每天 2 次，直至症状消失。一般 1~2 天即可痊愈。风寒表证较重的患者，应重灸督脉，灸至汗出为佳。

（四）灸后防护，巩固疗效

1. 风寒感冒，可以在艾灸前喝点姜糖水，助力驱散寒气。
2. 艾灸后 2 小时内，要注意避风寒。
3. 易感冒患者平时可做保健灸，比如灸足三里、关元穴。

【验案举例】

张先生，27 岁，因天气变化未及时添加衣物，今晨起出现鼻塞，流清涕，打喷嚏，头痛，伴全身乏力酸痛，体温 37.7℃，诊断为感冒。在大椎、右风池、上印堂穴区探及有明显透热、传热等灸感。选取上印堂穴区行单点灸，即感热流如"水注"向深部灌注并向鼻根部传导，并觉前额"酸胀压迫感"，灸感持续大约 15 分钟后感鼻腔渐通，同时上印堂穴区皮肤有灼热感，即停灸。改灸大椎、右风池穴，自觉有热感扩散至整个颈项部，5 分钟后向头顶部传导，10 分钟后整个头颅均有温热感，灸感持续约 30 分钟后渐回缩并感施灸点皮肤灼热，停止热敏灸，完成 1 次治疗。治疗后感鼻塞、头痛明显减轻，体温 36.8℃。嘱回家后避风寒，注意保暖。次日复诊，患者痊愈。

⚖ 第二节　慢性支气管炎

慢性支气管炎是指气管、支气管黏膜及其周围组织的慢性非特异性炎症，长期吸烟、烟雾、粉尘、空气污染或气温突变均可诱发本病，体质虚弱者、老年人患病率较高。本病属于中医学"咳嗽""喘证""痰饮"等范畴。中医学认为，本病多由外邪侵袭肺系，或脏腑功能失调，内邪干肺，引起肺失宣肃，肺气上逆所致。疾病的发展和转归与肺、脾、肾三脏关系密切。

【临床表现】

以慢性咳嗽、咳痰、喘息或气急为主要临床表现，痰液多为白色泡沫状，合并有感染的可见黄色或黄绿色脓痰，每年持续 3 个月或以上，连续发作 2 年或更长时间。

【灸法治则】

本病以宣肺止咳、降气化痰为基本治疗原则。根据肺主气、司呼吸、主宣发肃降，脾主运化水湿，肾主纳气等理论，选择相关穴位探感定位，辨敏施灸。

【治疗方案】

（一）探感选穴，准确定位

1. **高发穴区** 热敏穴位高发区一般多位于大椎、至阳、命门、中府、肺俞、脾俞、肾俞等穴区，对这些部位进行穴位热敏探查常能发现热敏穴位。

2. **探查手法** 在本病热敏穴位高发区，按下述步骤分别依序进行回旋、雀啄、往返、温和灸四步操作。

回旋灸 $\xrightarrow[\text{2分钟}]{\text{温热局部气血}}$ 雀啄灸 $\xrightarrow[\text{1分钟}]{\text{加强敏化}}$ 往返灸 $\xrightarrow[\text{1分钟}]{\text{激发经气}}$ 温和灸 $\xrightarrow[\text{2分钟}]{\text{发动传感}}$ 出现热敏灸感 $\rightarrow$ 确定热敏穴位

3. **热敏灸感** 灸大椎、至阳、命门穴，灸感多为透热、扩热、传热；灸肺俞、中府穴，灸感多为透热、传热；灸脾俞、肾俞穴，灸感多为透热、传热。

（二）循序激发，辨敏施灸

按照以下顺序，择优选穴施灸：

大椎、至阳、命门穴循经往返灸和接力灸→中府穴双点灸→肺俞穴双点灸→脾俞穴双点灸→肾俞穴双点灸。

上述热敏穴区不是每位患者全都出现，没有出现穴位热敏的就不做相应操作。

1. **大椎、至阳、命门穴循经往返灸和接力灸** 大椎、至阳、命门皆为督脉要穴，督脉主一身阳气。三穴合用，温督通阳，既有元阳资纳，又有肺卫阳气布散，使得上下内外皆相通达。患者可自觉热感沿头项背腰部督脉传导，灸至热敏灸感消失（图3-2-1）。

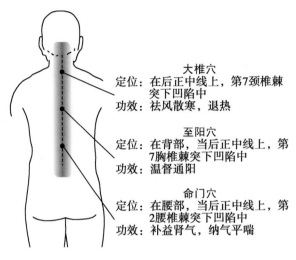

大椎穴
定位：在后正中线上，第7颈椎棘突下凹陷中
功效：祛风散寒，退热

至阳穴
定位：在背部，当后正中线上，第7胸椎棘突下凹陷中
功效：温督通阳

命门穴
定位：在腰部，当后正中线上，第2腰椎棘突下凹陷中
功效：补益肾气，纳气平喘

图 3-2-1　大椎、至阳、命门穴循经往返灸和接力灸

2．中府穴双点灸　中府是肺经募穴，手足太阴经的交会穴，具有宣利肺气、止咳平喘、化痰的功效。患者可自觉热感透至胸腔并传至上肢，灸至热敏灸感消失（图3-2-2）。

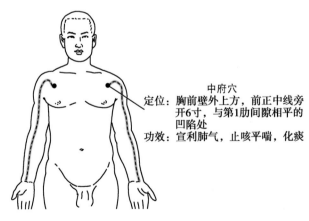

中府穴
定位：胸前壁外上方，前正中线旁开6寸，与第1肋间隙相平的凹陷处
功效：宣利肺气，止咳平喘，化痰

图 3-2-2　中府穴双点灸

3．肺俞穴双点灸　肺俞是肺气输注于背部的部位，可治本脏之疾，具有补肺气、化痰止咳的功效。患者常可觉热感透至胸腔并向颈项传导，灸至热敏灸感消失（图3-2-3）。

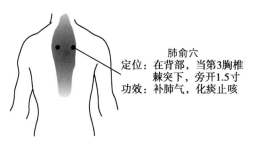

肺俞穴
定位：在背部，当第3胸椎
棘突下，旁开1.5寸
功效：补肺气，化痰止咳

图 3-2-3 肺俞穴双点灸

4. **脾俞穴双点灸** 脾俞是脾气输注于背部的部位，可治本脏之疾，具有补脾益气、化痰止咳的功效。患者常可觉热感透至深部或扩散至整个腰背部，灸至热敏灸感消失（图 3-2-4）。

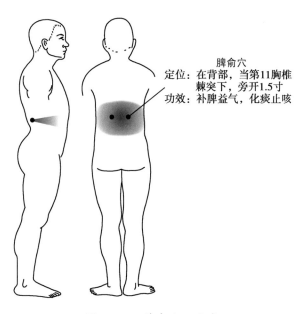

脾俞穴
定位：在背部，当第11胸椎
棘突下，旁开1.5寸
功效：补脾益气，化痰止咳

图 3-2-4 脾俞穴双点灸

5. **肾俞穴双点灸** 肾俞是肾气血在背部的输注部位，具有纳气平喘的功效。患者可自觉热感透至深部并扩散至腰背部且向下腹部传导，灸至热敏感消失（图 3-2-5）。

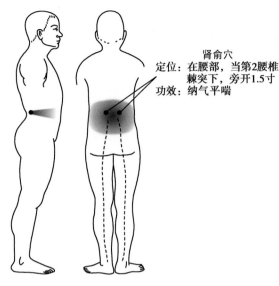

肾俞穴
定位：在腰部，当第2腰椎棘突下，旁开1.5寸
功效：纳气平喘

图 3-2-5　肾俞穴双点灸

（三）量因人异，敏消量足

选取上述 1～2 组穴位，每天 1 次，每次每穴的施灸时间以热敏灸感消失为度，疗程灸量以与病症相关热敏腧穴消敏为度。一般 10 次为 1 个疗程，疗程间休息 2～5 天，共 2～3 个疗程。

（四）灸后防护，巩固疗效

1. 热敏灸治疗本病有一定疗效，病情重者，应采取综合治疗。由其他心肺疾病引起的咳嗽，应积极治疗原发病。

2. 应避风寒，清淡饮食，限烟酒，避免接触粉尘、烟雾和刺激性物质，以防复发。

【验案举例】

刘先生，50 岁，6 年前无明显诱因反复出现发热、咳嗽、咳痰。今又不慎感受风寒，咳嗽、咳白痰，来我科求诊。胸部正侧位 X 线片示有慢性支气管炎改变。随即在大椎穴、至阳穴探及穴位热敏。嘱俯卧位，于大椎穴、至阳穴区施循经往返灸 10 分钟，感热流呈片状扩散，故在至阳穴、大椎穴双点灸，感热流继向腰背部传导，并感热流徐徐入里且深透至前胸，灸感持续约 20 分钟后，热流渐回缩至至阳穴并感皮肤灼热，乃停灸。继灸大椎穴，仍有扩热、传热现象，灸感持续约 10 分钟后热流渐回缩至大椎穴且皮肤灼热，乃停灸，完成 1 次治疗。次日复诊时，于双脾俞穴探及穴位热敏，施双点灸，即有扩热、透热现象，5 分钟后热流汇合成片，整个腰部温热舒适，灸感持续约 20 分钟后回缩至双脾俞穴并感皮肤灼热，乃停灸，完成 1 次治疗。按上述方法探敏治疗 30 次后，患者咳嗽、咳痰症状消失，半年后随访未有复发。

第三节　支气管哮喘

支气管哮喘是一种以慢性气道炎症和气道高反应性为特征的异质性疾病。接触变应原，冷空气，物理、化学性刺激等可诱发本病，患者多有过敏史或家族遗传史。本病属于中医的"哮病""喘证"范畴，因肺、脾、肾三脏功能不足，水湿内聚为痰饮，遇外邪引动而发，痰随气升，气因痰阻，相互搏结，阻于气道，肺失宣肃而出现咳喘痰鸣，甚则不能平卧，胸闷，咳痰不爽等症。

【临床表现】

症状为反复发作性喘息、呼吸困难、胸闷或咳嗽，常在夜间或清晨发作或加剧，多数患者可自行缓解或经治疗后缓解。发作时双肺在呼气过程可听到散在或弥漫性的哮鸣音，呼气时间延长。

【灸法治则】

本病以宣肺定喘为基本治疗原则。根据肺主皮毛、主宣发肃降，为水之上源，脾主运化水湿，肾主纳气等理论，选择相关穴位探感定位，辨敏施灸。

【治疗方案】

（一）探感选穴，准确定位

1. 高发穴区　热敏穴位高发区一般多位于大椎、至阳、命门、肺俞、肾俞、神阙等穴区，对这些部位进行穴位热敏探查常能发现热敏穴位。

2. 探查手法　在本病热敏穴位高发区，按下述步骤分别依序进行回旋、雀啄、往返、温和灸四步操作。

回旋灸 $\xrightarrow[\text{2分钟}]{\text{温热局部气血}}$ 雀啄灸 $\xrightarrow[\text{1分钟}]{\text{加强敏化}}$ 往返灸 $\xrightarrow[\text{1分钟}]{\text{激发经气}}$ 温和灸 $\xrightarrow[\text{2分钟}]{\text{发动传感}}$ 出现热敏灸感 $\rightarrow$ 确定热敏穴位

3. 热敏灸感　灸大椎、至阳、命门穴，灸感多为透热、扩热、传热；灸肺俞穴，灸感多为透热、传热；灸肾俞穴，灸感多为透热、传热；灸神阙穴，灸感多为透热。

（二）循序激发，辨敏施灸

按照以下顺序，择优选穴施灸：

大椎、至阳、命门穴循经往返灸和接力灸→肺俞穴双点灸→肾俞穴双点灸→神阙穴单点灸。

上述热敏穴区不是每位患者全都出现，没有出现穴位热敏的就不做相应操作。

1. 大椎、至阳、命门穴循经往返灸和接力灸　振奋督脉阳气。大椎、至阳、命门皆为督脉要穴，督脉主一身阳气；三穴合用，温督通阳，既有元阳资纳，又有肺卫阳气布散，从而上下内外皆相通达。患者可自觉热感沿头项背腰部督脉传导，灸至热敏灸感消失（图 3-3-1）。

2. 肺俞穴双点灸　肺俞是肺气输注于背部的部位，可治本脏之疾，具有补肺气、化痰止咳的功效。患者可自觉热感透至胸腔或扩散至整个背部并向上肢传导，灸至热敏灸感消失（图 3-3-2）。

3. 肾俞穴双点灸　肾俞是肾气血在背部的输注部位，具有纳气平喘的功效。患者可自觉热感透至深部并扩散至腰背部且向下腹部传导，灸至热敏灸感消失（图 3-3-3）。

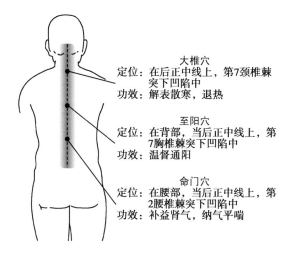

大椎穴
定位：在后正中线上，第7颈椎棘
突下凹陷中
功效：解表散寒，退热

至阳穴
定位：在背部，当后正中线上，第
7胸椎棘突下凹陷中
功效：温督通阳

命门穴
定位：在腰部，当后正中线上，第
2腰椎棘突下凹陷中
功效：补益肾气，纳气平喘

图 3-3-1 大椎、至阳、命门穴循经往返灸和接力灸

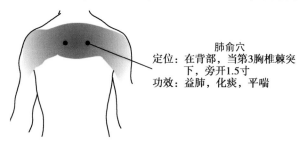

肺俞穴
定位：在背部，当第3胸椎棘突
下，旁开1.5寸
功效：益肺，化痰，平喘

图 3-3-2 肺俞穴双点灸

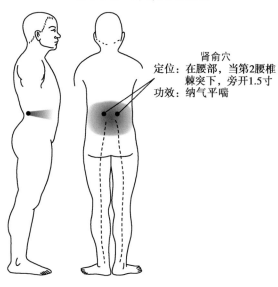

肾俞穴
定位：在腰部，当第2腰椎
棘突下，旁开1.5寸
功效：纳气平喘

图 3-3-3 肾俞穴双点灸

111

4．神阙穴单点灸　　神阙为任脉禁针宜灸要穴，具有大补元气、益肾、纳气平喘的功效。患者可自觉热感透至腹腔，灸至热敏灸感消失（图 3-3-4）。

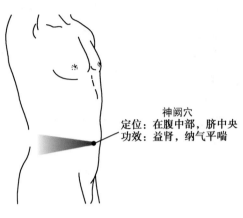

神阙穴
定位：在腹中部，脐中央
功效：益肾，纳气平喘

图 3-3-4　神阙穴单点灸

（三）量因人异，敏消量足

每次选取上述 1～2 组穴位，每天 1 次，每次每穴的施灸时间以热敏灸感消失为度。10 次为 1 个疗程，疗程间休息 2～5 天，共 2～3 个疗程。

（四）灸后防护，巩固疗效

1．热敏灸治疗哮喘缓解期和慢性持续期均有满意疗效。如由其他心肺疾病等引起喘息、胸闷、咳嗽症状，要积极治疗原发病。

2．饮食宜清淡，忌油腻，避风寒，有明确过敏史的患者应避免接触致敏原。

3．发时治标，平时治本。急性发作期以控制症状为主，应攻邪治标，祛痰利气。缓解期应培补正气，采用补肺、健脾、益肾三法。

4．因患本病者多有过敏史或家族史，所以应注意对致敏原的预防。

【验案举例】

高女士，43 岁，2 年前受寒后出现胸闷、气憋，呼吸困难，无法平卧休息，经治疗症状缓解。但该症每逢冬春季节天气变化时发作，诊断为支气管哮喘。今来我科诊治。经查左肺俞、至阳、命门穴三穴出现穴位热敏。于左肺俞穴处施温和灸，即感热流深透远传，约 5 分钟后，感左腋部温热舒适，约 20 分钟后，热感沿上臂内侧下行，到肘尖附近停止。30 分钟后，热流渐回缩至左肺俞穴且感皮肤灼热，遂停灸。改灸至阳穴、命门穴区，先给予循经往返灸 5 分钟，热流沿后背正中向上传导，遂在至阳穴、命门穴双点灸。数分钟后，感热流徐徐入里，渐深透至前胸，顿感整个前胸温热，灸感持续约 30 分钟后热流渐回缩至至阳穴，并感皮肤灼热，乃停灸。此时命门穴仍有透热现象，续灸 10 分钟后灸感消失，且感皮肤灼热，遂停灸，完成 1 次热敏灸治疗。次日复诊，神阙穴探及穴位热敏，于该穴施温和灸，感热流逐渐扩散，5 分钟后感觉到热感透至腹腔，灸感持续约 35 分钟后透、扩现象消失并感皮肤灼热，乃停灸，完成 1 次热敏灸治疗。按上述方法连续探敏治疗 30 次，发作性胸闷、气憋未见发作。6 个月后随访未见发作。

第四节　消化性溃疡

消化性溃疡是指胃肠黏膜发生的炎性缺损，包括胃和十二指肠溃疡，通常与胃液的胃酸和消化作用有关，病变穿透黏膜肌层或达更深层次。多由饮食无规律，进食生、冷、硬和刺激性食物，精神紧张诱发或加重。本病属中医"胃痛"范畴，认为与感受外邪、饮食不节、情志不遂、素体虚弱等有关，多因中焦气滞不畅、脾胃升降功能失调发病，病位在胃，与肝、脾关系密切。

【临床表现】

临床上以慢性、周期性、节律性发作的上腹部疼痛为主要表现，常兼有嗳气、反酸、恶心、呕吐、上腹胀、腹泻或便秘等症。

【灸法治则】

本病以理气、和胃止痛为基本治疗原则。根据肝主疏泄，脾主升、胃主降，脾主运化水湿等理论，选择相关穴位探感定位、辨敏施灸。

【治疗方案】

(一) 探感选穴, 准确定位

1. 高发穴区　热敏穴位高发区一般多位于中脘、天枢、脾俞、胃俞、阴陵泉等穴区。对这些部位进行穴位热敏探查常能发现热敏穴位。

2. 探查手法　在本病热敏穴位高发区, 按下述步骤分别依序进行回旋、雀啄、往返、温和灸四步操作。

回旋灸 $\xrightarrow[\text{2分钟}]{\text{温热局部气血}}$ 雀啄灸 $\xrightarrow[\text{1分钟}]{\text{加强敏化}}$ 往返灸 $\xrightarrow[\text{1分钟}]{\text{激发经气}}$ 温和灸 $\xrightarrow[\text{2分钟}]{\text{发动传感}}$ 出现热敏灸感 $\rightarrow$ 确定热敏穴位

3. 热敏灸感　灸中脘、天枢穴, 灸感多为透热、扩热; 灸脾俞、胃俞穴时, 灸感多为透热、扩热; 灸阴陵泉穴时, 灸感多为传热、透热。

(二) 循序激发, 辨敏施灸

按照以下顺序, 择优选穴施灸:

中脘穴单点灸→天枢穴双点灸→脾俞穴双点灸→胃俞穴双点灸→阴陵泉双点灸。

上述热敏穴区不是每位患者全都出现, 没有出现穴位热敏的就不做相应操作。

1. 中脘穴单点灸　中脘位于任脉, 胃募穴, 具有健脾和胃、消食导滞的功效。患者可自觉热感透至腹腔内或扩散至整个上腹部, 灸至热敏灸感消失 (图 3-4-1)。

2. 天枢穴双点灸　天枢是调理胃肠疾病的要穴, 能够化瘀止痛、理气消滞。患者可自觉热感透至腹腔或沿两侧扩散至腰部, 灸至热敏灸感消失 (图 3-4-1)。

3. 脾俞穴双点灸　脾俞是脾气输注于背部的部位, 可治本脏之疾, 具有补脾益气、化痰止咳的功效。患者常可觉热感透至深部或扩散至整个腰背部, 灸至热敏灸感消失 (图 3-4-2)。

4. 胃俞穴双点灸　胃俞是胃腑之气在背部的输注部位, 灸之可健脾和胃。患者可自觉热感透至深部或扩散至整个背腰部, 灸至热敏灸感消失

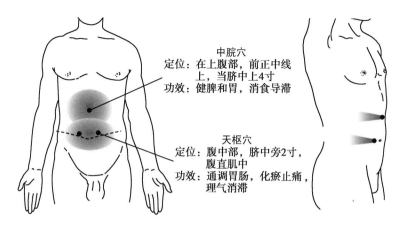

中脘穴
定位：在上腹部，前正中线
上，当脐中上4寸
功效：健脾和胃，消食导滞

天枢穴
定位：腹中部，脐中旁2寸，
腹直肌中
功效：通调胃肠，化瘀止痛，
理气消滞

图 3-4-1　中脘穴单点灸、天枢穴双点灸

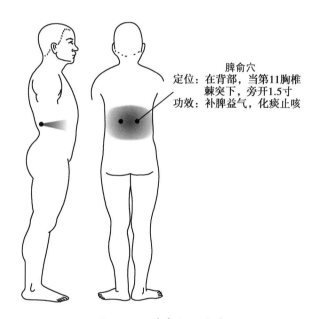

脾俞穴
定位：在背部，当第11胸椎
棘突下，旁开1.5寸
功效：补脾益气，化痰止咳

图 3-4-2　脾俞穴双点灸

（图3-4-3）。

5．阴陵泉穴双点灸　阴陵泉属于脾经的合穴，具有运中焦、健脾胃、化湿滞的功效。部分患者可自觉热感直接传到腹部；如感传仍不能上至腹部，则再取一支点燃的艾条悬于感传所达部位的近心端点，进行温和灸，依次接力使感传到达腹部，最后将两支艾条分别固定于阴陵泉和腹部进行温和灸，灸至热敏灸感消失（图3-4-4）。

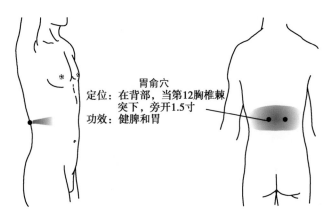

图 3-4-3　胃俞穴双点灸

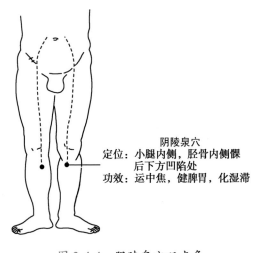

图 3-4-4　阴陵泉穴双点灸

（三）量因人异，敏消量足

每次选取上述 1～2 组穴位，每天 1 次，每次每穴的施灸时间以热敏灸感消失为度。10 次为 1 个疗程，疗程间休息 2～5 天，共 2～3 个疗程。

（四）灸后防护，巩固疗效

1. 热敏灸能加强胃动力、促进胃排空，调节胃酸分泌，增强胃黏膜修复功能，有利于胃溃疡的愈合，对治疗此病有较好的效果。在治疗过程中，如果腹痛加重，或出现黑便，应及时到医院就诊，以免延误病情。

2. 平时应注意胃部保暖，调情志，限烟酒，忌食生、冷、硬和刺激性食物。

【验案举例】

曾先生，48 岁，8 年前因饮食不规律、酗酒出现上腹部疼痛不适，伴有嗳气吞酸，常于餐后出现，持续 1~2 小时，后去医院做相关检查，胃镜示胃溃疡，大便潜血阳性。采用西医常规治疗，症状减轻，每当饮食不规律后又即发作，反复至今。现患者上腹部疼痛 1 日入我院，伴食欲不振、嗳气等症状。对中脘穴实施单点灸，出现上腹部片状热，3 分钟后，热流往里渗透，10 分钟后，整个上腹部里面皆热，且胃部感一股热流，20 分钟后，患者肠蠕动增强，突有食欲想进食，25 分钟后灸感逐渐消失。继续换灸天枢穴，先以脐部为中心行回旋灸 3 分钟，后发现在天枢穴出现强烈透热现象，患者顿时感觉整个少腹有一股热流往里渗透，且患者感觉艾灸局部不热。30 分钟后，透热现象逐渐减弱消失，停灸，完成 1 次治疗。按上述方法治疗 25 次后，患者食欲恢复正常，体重增加 4kg，腹部疼痛不适消失。嘱患者规律进食，且清淡饮食，少吸烟酗酒，1 年后随访未复发。

第五节　功能性消化不良

消化不良为一组临床症状群，其以上腹部疼痛或烧灼感、餐后上腹部饱胀和早饱为主症，还可伴有食欲不振、嗳气、恶心或呕吐等症状，分为器质性消化不良及功能性消化不良。功能性消化不良是指具有以上消化不良症状，但其临床表现不能完全用器质性、系统性或代谢性疾病等来解释。中医学认为本病病位在胃，涉及肝、脾两脏，多因饮食不节，损伤脾胃；或忧思恼怒，损伤肝脾；或中气不足，外邪内侵等，使脾失健运，胃失和降，导致中焦气机阻滞，脾胃升降失常，胃肠功能紊乱而发病。

【临床表现】

表现为慢性复发性或持续性上腹部疼痛、烧灼感、饱胀、早饱、嗳气、食欲不振、恶心呕吐等症状，内镜检查未发现胃及十二指肠溃疡、糜烂、肿瘤等器质性病变。

【灸法治则】

本病以健脾和胃、疏肝理气为治疗原则。根据脾主升清、胃主降浊、肝主疏泄、三焦通畅气机等理论，选择相关穴位探感定位、辨敏施灸。

【治疗方案】

（一）探感选穴，准确定位

1．高发穴区　热敏穴位高发区一般多位于天枢、中脘、下脘、关元、肝俞、膈俞、胃俞、上巨虚等穴区。对这些部位进行穴位热敏探查常能发现热敏穴位。

2．探查手法　在本病热敏穴位高发区，按下述步骤分别依序进行回旋、雀啄、往返、温和灸四步操作。

$$回旋灸 \xrightarrow[2分钟]{温热局部气血} 雀啄灸 \xrightarrow[1分钟]{加强敏化} 往返灸 \xrightarrow[1分钟]{激发经气} 温和灸 \xrightarrow[2分钟]{发动传感} 出现热敏灸感 \rightarrow 确定热敏穴位$$

3．热敏灸感　灸天枢穴，灸感多为透热、扩热；灸中脘、下脘、关元穴，灸感多为透热；灸肝俞、膈俞、胃俞穴，灸感多为透热、扩热；灸上巨虚穴，灸感多为传热。

（二）循序激发，辨敏施灸

按照以下顺序，择优选穴施灸：

天枢穴双点灸→中脘、关元穴双点灸→下脘穴单点灸→肝俞穴双点灸→膈俞穴双点灸→胃俞穴双点灸→上巨虚穴双点灸。

上述热敏穴区不是每位患者全都出现，没有出现穴位热敏的就不做相应操作。

1. **天枢穴双点灸**　天枢是调理胃肠疾病的要穴，能够调理胃肠、理气消滞。患者可自觉热感深透至腹腔或沿两侧扩散至腰部，灸至热敏灸感消失（图 3-5-1）。

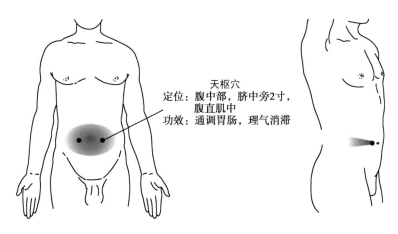

天枢穴
定位：腹中部，脐中旁2寸，腹直肌中
功效：通调胃肠，理气消滞

图 3-5-1　天枢穴双点灸

2. **中脘、关元穴双点灸**　中脘位于任脉，胃募穴，具有健脾和胃、消食导滞的功效。关元亦居任脉，是任脉与足三阴经的交会穴，具有温补元阳、健脾益胃的功效。患者可自觉热感透至腹腔内，灸至热敏灸感消失（图 3-5-2）。

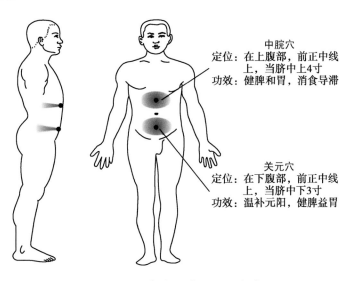

中脘穴
定位：在上腹部，前正中线上，当脐中上4寸
功效：健脾和胃，消食导滞

关元穴
定位：在下腹部，前正中线上，当脐中下3寸
功效：温补元阳，健脾益胃

图 3-5-2　中脘、关元穴双点灸

3．下脘穴单点灸　下脘位于任脉，具有健脾和胃、消食导滞的功效。患者可自觉热感透至腹腔内，灸至热敏灸感消失（图3-5-3）。

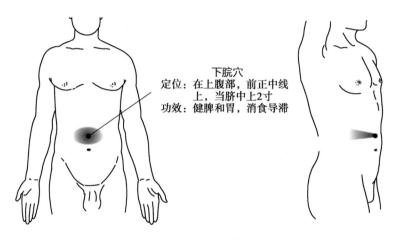

下脘穴
定位：在上腹部，前正中线上，当脐中上2寸
功效：健脾和胃，消食导滞

图 3-5-3　下脘穴单点灸

4．肝俞穴双点灸　肝俞是肝脏之气在背部的输注部位，灸之可疏肝、理气、和胃。患者可自觉热感深透至腹腔或扩散至背腰部，灸至热敏灸感消失（图3-5-4）。

5．膈俞穴双点灸　膈俞乃血会，具有调理气血、利膈的功效。患者可自觉热感深透至腹腔或扩散至背腰部或沿两侧扩散至胸部，灸至热敏灸感消失（图3-5-4）。

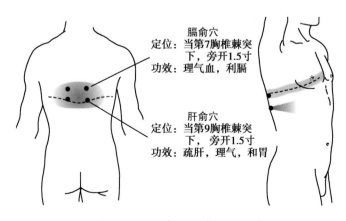

膈俞穴
定位：当第7胸椎棘突下，旁开1.5寸
功效：理气血，利膈

肝俞穴
定位：当第9胸椎棘突下，旁开1.5寸
功效：疏肝，理气，和胃

图 3-5-4　肝俞、膈俞穴双点灸

6. **胃俞穴双点灸** 胃俞是胃腑之气在背部的输注部位，灸之可健脾、和胃。患者可自觉热感透至深部或扩散至整个背腰部，灸至热敏灸感消失（图 3-5-5）。

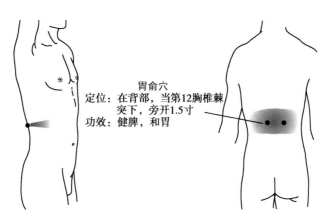

胃俞穴

定位：在背部，当第12胸椎棘突下，旁开1.5寸

功效：健脾，和胃

图 3-5-5 胃俞穴双点灸

7. **上巨虚穴双点灸** 上巨虚在胃经，大肠的下合穴，能调理脾胃、宽肠下气。患者可自觉热感深透，或向上或向下沿足阳明胃经传导，灸至热敏灸感消失（图 3-5-6）。

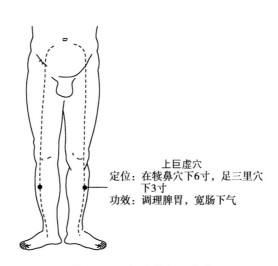

上巨虚穴

定位：在犊鼻穴下6寸，足三里穴下3寸

功效：调理脾胃，宽肠下气

图 3-5-6 上巨虚穴双点灸

（三）量因人异，敏消量足

每次选取上述 1~2 组穴位，每天 1 次，每次每穴的施灸时间以热敏灸感消失为度。10 次为 1 个疗程，疗程间休息 2~5 天，共 2~3 个疗程。

（四）灸后防护，巩固疗效

1. 热敏灸能温胃散寒，增强胃动力，促进胃排空，疗效可靠，无任何不良反应。

2. 加强体育锻炼，调畅情志，保持良好的饮食习惯，避免进食肥甘厚腻及刺激性食物。

【验案举例】

李女士，50 岁，5 年前因饱餐后感上腹部胀满不适、嗳气，自服健胃消食片，症状消除，但经常反复发作，并伴有食欲不佳、精神不振、乏力等。到当地医院就诊，各项检查指标均正常，确诊为功能性消化不良。现来我科就诊，经探查，于双胃俞、下脘、双天枢穴探及穴位热敏。于双侧胃俞实施双点灸，数分钟后感热流扩散并汇合在一起，10 分钟后热流由腰背部逐渐渗透至上腹部，感热流涌动，整个上腹部温热、舒适，灸感持续约 15 分钟后逐渐减弱消失，并感双侧胃俞灼热，乃停灸。改灸下脘及双侧天枢穴，数分钟后感热流如水柱向腹腔深部灌注，并向下腹涌动，整个下腹部感到滚烫，自觉下腹温度明显高于施灸点，灸感持续约 30 分钟下腹热流回缩至天枢穴并感皮肤灼热，停灸。按上述方法治疗 15 次，上述症状基本消失，并嘱咐患者规律饮食，勿暴饮暴食，随访 6 个月未复发。

第六节　肠易激综合征

肠易激综合征系指一种以腹痛伴排便习惯改变为特征而无器质性病变的常见功能性肠病。病变有关部位包括结肠、小肠、胃、食管等整个消化道。中医学将本病归属于"泄泻""腹痛""便秘"与"郁病"等范畴，多由于感受外邪、饮食所伤、情志失常而致脾虚肝郁、肝脾不和、脾失健运、大肠传导失司而发病，病位在肠。

【临床表现】

以腹痛、腹胀、腹泻或便秘为主，伴有神经症；一般情况良好，无消瘦及发热，系统体检仅发现腹部压痛；多次（至少3次）粪常规及培养均阴性，粪潜血试验阴性。

【灸法治则】

本病以疏肝健脾为基本治疗原则。根据肝主疏泄、脾主运化、大小肠皆属于胃等理论，选择相关穴位探感定位、辨敏施灸。

【治疗方案】

（一）探感选穴，准确定位

1. 高发穴区　热敏穴位高发区一般多位于关元、天枢、大肠俞、命门、足三里等穴区，对这些部位进行穴位热敏探查常能发现热敏穴位。

2. 探查手法　在本病热敏穴位高发区，按下述步骤分别依序进行回旋、雀啄、往返、温和灸四步操作。

$$回旋灸 \xrightarrow[2分钟]{温热局部气血} 雀啄灸 \xrightarrow[1分钟]{加强敏化} 往返灸 \xrightarrow[1分钟]{激发经气} 温和灸 \xrightarrow[2分钟]{发动传感} 出现热敏灸感 \rightarrow 确定热敏穴位$$

3. 热敏灸感　灸关元、天枢穴，灸感多为透热、扩热；灸大肠俞、命门穴，灸感多为透热、扩热；灸足三里穴，灸感多为传热。

（二）循序激发，辨敏施灸

按照以下顺序，择优选穴施灸：

关元、天枢穴温和灸→大肠俞、命门穴温和灸→足三里穴温和灸。

上述热敏穴区不是每位患者全都出现，没有出现穴位热敏的就不做相应操作。

1. 关元、天枢穴温和灸 关元、天枢穴合用具有通调肠胃、理气消滞的功效。患者可自觉热感深透至腹腔或沿两侧扩散至腰部，灸至热敏灸感消失（图 3-6-1）。

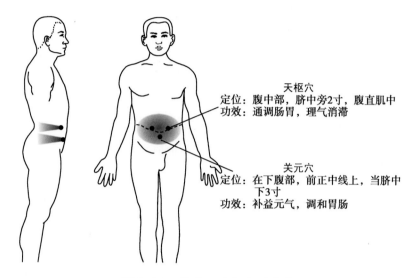

天枢穴
定位：腹中部，脐中旁2寸，腹直肌中
功效：通调肠胃，理气消滞

关元穴
定位：在下腹部，前正中线上，当脐中下3寸
功效：补益元气，调和胃肠

图 3-6-1 关元、天枢穴温和灸

2. 大肠俞、命门穴温和灸 大肠俞、命门穴合用具有补肾通腑、调理胃肠的功效。患者可自觉热感深透至腹腔或扩散至腰骶部或向下肢传导，灸至热敏灸感消失（图 3-6-2）。

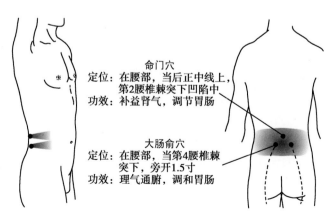

命门穴
定位：在腰部，当后正中线上，第2腰椎棘突下凹陷中
功效：补益肾气，调节胃肠

大肠俞穴
定位：在腰部，当第4腰椎棘突下，旁开1.5寸
功效：理气通腑，调和胃肠

图 3-6-2 大肠俞、命门穴温和灸

3. 足三里穴温和灸　足三里乃足阳明胃经的合穴，具有调理脾胃、宽肠理气的功效。部分患者的感传可直接到达腹部；如感传仍不能上至腹部者，再取一支点燃的艾条悬灸感传所达部位的近心端点，进行接力灸使感传到达腹部，最后将两支艾条分别固定于足三里与腹部进行温和灸，灸至热敏灸感消失（图 3-6-3）。

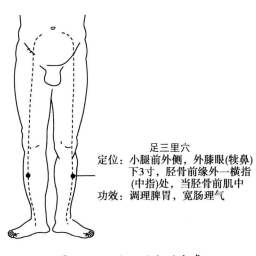

足三里穴
定位：小腿前外侧，外膝眼(犊鼻)下3寸，胫骨前缘外一横指(中指)处，当胫骨前肌中
功效：调理脾胃，宽肠理气

图 3-6-3　足三里穴温和灸

（三）量因人异，敏消量足

每次选取上述 1 ~ 2 组穴位，每天 1 次，10 次为 1 个疗程，疗程间休息 2 ~ 5 天，共 2 ~ 3 个疗程。

（四）灸后防护，巩固疗效

1. 热敏灸对肠易激综合征疗效肯定，临床可作为首选疗法。
2. 加强锻炼，增强体质，保持情绪舒畅，睡眠充足，少食多餐，避免刺激性食物和过冷过热的饮食，限烟酒，避风寒。

【验案举例】

叶先生，28 岁，腹痛腹泻反复发作 3 年，多于排便后缓解。近日因精神紧张或饮食油腻后症状加重，痛则欲泻，泻后痛减，大便每日 3 ~ 5 次，不夹血及黏液，肠镜及实验室检查未见异常，诊断为肠易激综合征。

经探查，在双天枢穴探及穴位热敏，即行双点灸，数分钟后热感渗透入腹腔，并向两侧扩散，整个腹部感温热舒适，灸感约持续 40 分钟后，热流渐向双天枢回缩，乃停止，遂完成 1 次灸疗。次日复诊，于关元穴探及穴位热敏，施温和灸，立感热感深透至腹腔，持续 20 分钟左右热流渐回缩至关元，并感皮肤灼热，乃停灸，完成 1 次热敏灸治疗。按上述方法探敏治疗 25 次，腹部无疼痛，便软色黄并成形，日 1 行。半年后随访未见复发。

第七节 功能性便秘

功能性便秘是由于肠动力不足引起的排便次数减少、粪便干硬和排便困难。其发生可能与心理因素、先天性异常、炎症刺激、滥用泻药及长期有意识抑制排便，或与支配肛门内外括约肌的神经功能异常有关。本病属中医学"便秘"范畴，多由大肠有热，或气滞、寒凝、阴阳气血亏虚，使大肠传导功能失常所致。若肠胃有病，或燥热内结，或气机郁滞，或气虚传送无力，或血虚肠道失润，以及阴寒凝结等，均能导致便秘。常与肺、脾、肾有关。

【临床表现】

每周排便少于 3 次，排便困难，每次排便时间长，粪便干结如羊粪且数量少，排便后仍有粪便未排尽的感觉，可有下腹疼痛、食欲减退、疲乏无力、头晕、烦躁、焦虑、失眠等症状。

【灸法治则】

本病以通调肠腑、通便为基本治疗原则。根据大肠主传导、以通为顺，肺与大肠相表里，肾主水，脾主运化，大、小肠皆属于胃等理论，选择相关穴位探感定位、辨敏施灸。

【治疗方案】

（一）探感选穴，准确定位

1. **高发穴区**　热敏穴位高发区一般多位于天枢、大肠俞、次髎、上巨虚等穴区。对这些部位进行穴位热敏探查常能发现热敏穴位。

2. **探查手法**　在本病热敏穴位高发区，按下述步骤分别依序进行回旋、雀啄、往返、温和灸四步操作。

回旋灸 —温热局部气血／2分钟→ 雀啄灸 —加强敏化／1分钟→ 往返灸 —激发经气／1分钟→ 温和灸 —发动传感／2分钟→ 出现热敏灸感 → 确定热敏穴位

3. **热敏灸感**　灸天枢穴，灸感多为透热、扩热；灸大肠俞穴，灸感多为透热、扩热；灸次髎穴，灸感多为透热、扩热、传热；灸上巨虚穴，灸感多为传热。

（二）循序激发，辨敏施灸

按照以下顺序，择优选穴施灸：

天枢穴双点灸→大肠俞穴双点灸→次髎穴双点灸→上巨虚穴双点灸。

上述热敏穴区不是每位患者全都出现，没有出现穴位热敏的就不做相应操作。

1. **天枢穴双点灸**　天枢是大肠募穴，具有疏调胃肠、理气消滞的功效。患者可自觉热感深透至腹腔或沿两侧扩散至腰部，灸至热敏灸感消失（图3-7-1）。

2. **大肠俞穴双点灸**　大肠俞是大肠的背俞穴，具有理气通腑、调和胃肠的功效。自觉热感深透至腹腔或向两侧扩散沿带脉传至腹部，灸至热敏灸感消失（图3-7-2）。

3. **次髎穴双点灸**　次髎具有利尿通便、调理下焦的功效。患者可自觉热感深透至腹腔或扩散至腰骶部或向下肢传导，灸至热敏灸感消失（图3-7-3）。

4. **上巨虚穴双点灸**　上巨虚是大肠的下合穴，具有调理脾胃、宽肠导气的功效。部分患者的感传可直接到达腹部；如感传仍不能上至腹部

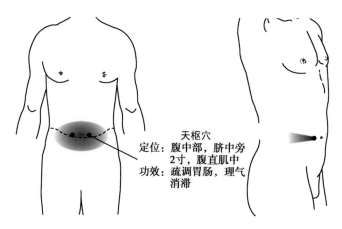

天枢穴
定位：腹中部，脐中旁
2寸，腹直肌中
功效：疏调胃肠，理气
消滞

图 3-7-1　天枢穴双点灸

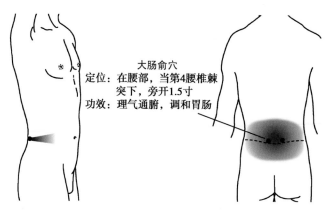

大肠俞穴
定位：在腰部，当第4腰椎棘
突下，旁开1.5寸
功效：理气通腑，调和胃肠

图 3-7-2　大肠俞穴双点灸

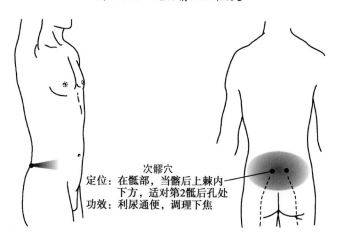

次髎穴
定位：在骶部，当髂后上棘内
下方，适对第2骶后孔处
功效：利尿通便，调理下焦

图 3-7-3　次髎穴双点灸

者，再取一支点燃的艾条悬灸感传所达部位的近心端点，进行接力灸，使感传到达腹部，最后将两支艾条分别固定于上巨虚和腹部进行温和灸，灸至热敏灸感消失（图 3-7-4）

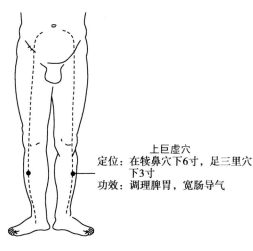

上巨虚穴
定位：在犊鼻穴下6寸，足三里穴
下3寸
功效：调理脾胃，宽肠导气

图 3-7-4　上巨虚穴双点灸

（三）量因人异，敏消量足

每次选取上述 1 ~ 2 组穴位，每天 1 次，每次每穴的施灸时间以热敏灸感消失为度。10 次为 1 个疗程，疗程间休息 2 ~ 5 天，共 2 ~ 3 个疗程。

（四）灸后防护，巩固疗效

1. 热敏灸具有调整肠道动力的作用，治疗功能性便秘疗效确切。
2. 养成定期排便的好习惯，适当进行体育锻炼，以增强肠道蠕动，促进排便。养成良好的饮食习惯，多吃蔬菜、水果，少吃辛辣食物。

【验案举例】

陈先生，61 岁，7 年前开始出现排便困难，始每 3 ~ 4 天排便 1 次，后渐加重，每 5 ~ 7 天大便 1 次，伴头晕、乏力。曾自服中、西泻药，症状可缓解。就诊时于双天枢穴探及穴位热敏，即施双点灸，数分钟后感热流如"水注"向腹腔深部灌注，并向下腹涌动，立感整个下腹滚烫，自觉下腹温度明显高于施灸点皮温，该灸感持续约 35 分钟后热流渐回缩至双天枢穴，2 分钟后感皮肤灼热乃停灸，完成 1 次热敏灸治疗。治疗当晚即排便 1 次，按上述方法治疗 10 次，每 2~3 天自行解大便 1 次，大便通畅，已无头晕、乏力等症状。嘱睡前自灸天枢穴，每穴半小时，每日 1 次，连续 7 天以巩固疗效。3 个月后随访，未见复发。

第八节　原发性痛经

原发性痛经主要表现为从月经初潮开始，行经前后或月经期出现下腹疼痛、坠胀，伴腰酸或其他不适症状，如头痛、乏力、头晕、恶心、呕吐、腹泻、腹胀、腰腿痛等，但生殖器官无器质性病变。本病中医称"痛经"或"经行腹痛"，多为气血运行不畅所致。常由于经期受寒饮冷，坐卧湿地，寒湿伤于下焦，客于胞宫，经血为寒湿所凝，运行不畅而作痛；或肝郁气滞，血行受阻，冲任运行不畅，经血滞于胞宫，不通则痛；或禀赋虚弱，肝肾不足，孕育过多，精血亏损，行经之后血海空虚，胞脉失于滋养故经后作痛。

【临床表现】

以行经前后或月经期下腹疼痛、坠胀不适、腰骶酸重为主要临床表现，可伴头痛、乏力、头晕、恶心、呕吐、腹泻、腹胀等症状；辅助检查如 B 超、宫腔镜等均未发现器质性病变。

【灸法治则】

本病以温经散寒、通络止痛为治疗原则。但根据急则治标原则，痛经当以缓急止痛为先。根据肝主疏泄、喜条达、藏血而司血海，肾主生殖及前后二阴等理论，选择相关穴位探感定位、辨敏施灸。

【治疗方案】

（一）探感选穴，准确定位

1. **高发穴区** 热敏穴位高发区一般多位于关元、子宫、次髎、三阴交等穴区，对这些部位进行穴位热敏探查常能发现热敏穴位。

2. **探查手法** 在本病热敏穴位高发区，按下述步骤分别依序进行回旋、雀啄、往返、温和灸四步操作。

回旋灸 →（温热局部气血 2分钟）→ 雀啄灸 →（加强敏化 1分钟）→ 往返灸 →（激发经气 1分钟）→ 温和灸 →（发动传感 2分钟）→ 出现热敏灸感 → 确定热敏穴位

3. **热敏灸感** 灸关元、子宫穴，灸感多为透热、扩热；灸次髎穴，灸感多为透热、扩热、传热；灸三阴交穴，灸感多为传热。

（二）循序激发，辨敏施灸

按照以下顺序，择优选穴施灸：

关元、子宫穴温和灸→次髎穴双点灸→三阴交穴双点灸。

上述热敏穴区不是每位患者全都出现，没有出现穴位热敏的就不做相应操作。

1. **关元、子宫穴温和灸** 关元位居任脉，是任脉和足三阴经的交会穴，具有温补元阳、暖胞宫、散寒止痛的功效。子宫亦是调理胞宫的要穴，能调经止痛。患者可自觉热感透至腹腔并扩散至整个腹部，灸至热敏灸感消失（图3-8-1）。

2. **次髎穴双点灸** 次髎是治疗泌尿生殖系统病症的要穴，具有调经止痛的功效。患者可自觉热感深透至腹腔或扩散至腰骶部或向下肢传导，灸至热敏灸感消失（图3-8-2）。

3. **三阴交穴双点灸** 三阴交为足三阴之交会穴，妇科常用要穴，具有调血通经、祛瘀止痛的功效。部分患者的感传可直接到达腹部；如感传仍不能上至腹部，再取一支点燃的艾条悬灸感传所达部位的近心端，进行温和灸，依次接力使感传到达腹部，最后将两支艾条分别固定于三阴交和腹部进行温和灸，灸至热敏灸感消失（图3-8-3）。

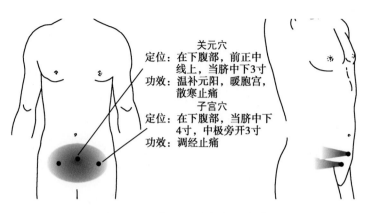

关元穴
定位：在下腹部，前正中
　　　线上，当脐中下3寸
功效：温补元阳，暖胞宫，
　　　散寒止痛
子宫穴
定位：在下腹部，当脐中下
　　　4寸，中极旁开3寸
功效：调经止痛

图 3-8-1　关元、子宫穴温和灸

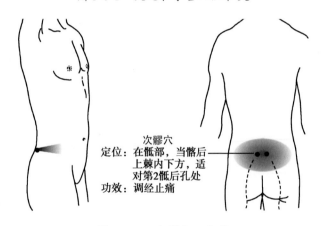

次髎穴
定位：在骶部，当髂后
　　　上棘内下方，适
　　　对第2骶后孔处
功效：调经止痛

图 3-8-2　次髎穴双点灸

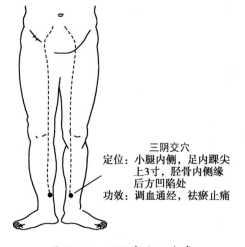

三阴交穴
定位：小腿内侧，足内踝尖
　　　上3寸，胫骨内侧缘
　　　后方凹陷处
功效：调血通经，祛瘀止痛

图 3-8-3　三阴交穴双点灸

（三）量因人异，敏消量足

每次选取上述 2 组穴位，每天 1 次，自月经临来前 3 天开始，每次每穴的施灸时间以热敏灸感消失为度。连续 5 天为 1 个疗程，共 3 个月经周期。

（四）灸后防护，巩固疗效

1. 热敏灸具有温肾暖宫、活血化瘀的功效，治疗原发性痛经疗效确切。月经前后和行经期应注意保暖，避免受凉，忌劳累。
2. 注意精神调养，解除心理焦虑，使情绪舒畅。

【验案举例】

张女士，24 岁，未婚。自诉 13 岁初潮，每次临行经之时下腹胀痛难忍，甚痛至床上翻滚，曾口服中成药物治疗（具体用药不详）。此次求诊时下腹胀满疼痛已 1 小时余，伴腰膝酸软，难以忍受，见其面色苍白，全身冷汗淋漓，立刻给予热敏灸治疗，经探查，其关元穴及双侧次髎穴有明显的喜热、透热现象。先于关元穴区行热敏灸治疗，约 2 分钟，患者即感整个下腹部温热舒适，热流直渗入腹腔，15 分钟后自诉疼痛感明显减轻，灸感持续约 45 分钟，热感由腹腔回缩至皮肤表面，遂停灸关元穴。改灸次髎穴，于次髎穴施行双点灸，约 10 分钟，患者自觉腰背部片状温热感，腹腔内亦感温暖舒适，继灸 20 分钟，次髎穴区皮肤感灼热乃停灸。此 1 次治疗后患者腹痛已减之八九，仅微觉胀满。次日复诊诉月经量色正常，无任何不适。嘱患者每于行经前 3 天左右自灸关元穴，每日 1 次，每次约灸半小时，连续 5 天，坚持 3 个月经周期，以防复发。半年后随访，未复发。

第九节 盆腔炎症

盆腔炎症指女性生殖道及其周围组织的炎症，主要包括子宫内膜炎、输卵管炎、输卵管卵巢脓肿、盆腔腹膜炎等，分为急性和慢性两类。中医学认为本病属于"带下病""癥瘕"等范畴，认为由脾虚湿盛，或食膏粱厚味，酿生湿热，或肝郁化火，蕴生肝热脾湿，湿热下注而致；或因久居湿地、房事不洁、六淫湿热之邪直犯少腹而成；或素体阳虚，寒湿内盛，或寒湿邪气直犯少腹、胞宫而致；或素性抑郁，气机不畅，或手术器械损伤胞宫脉络，瘀血阻滞，气滞血瘀而致本病。总之本病主要由于湿热邪毒、寒湿之邪或瘀血留于少腹胞宫，影响冲任而发病。

【临床表现】

急性盆腔炎常见下腹痛、发热、阴道分泌物增多，腹痛为持续性；而慢性盆腔炎常见下腹部坠胀、疼痛及腰骶部酸痛，多在劳累、性交后及月经前后加剧。若病情严重可有寒战、高热、头痛、食欲缺乏及不同程度的月经失调，表现为经量增多，不规则阴道出血或痛经等，白带色、质异常。

【灸法治则】

本病以清热利湿、活血化瘀为基本治疗原则。根据肾主生殖、肝主疏泄、脾主运化水湿、冲任主月事、带脉主带下等理论，选择相关穴位探感定位、辨敏施灸。

【治疗方案】

（一）探感选穴，准确定位

1. 高发穴区　热敏穴位高发区一般多位于腰阳关、次髎、关元、子宫、归来、三阴交、阴陵泉等穴区，对这些部位进行穴位热敏探查常能发现热敏穴位。

2. 探查手法　在本病热敏穴位高发区，按下述步骤分别依序进行回旋、雀啄、往返、温和灸四步操作。

回旋灸 $\xrightarrow[\text{2分钟}]{\text{温热局部气血}}$ 雀啄灸 $\xrightarrow[\text{1分钟}]{\text{加强敏化}}$ 往返灸 $\xrightarrow[\text{1分钟}]{\text{激发经气}}$ 温和灸 $\xrightarrow[\text{2分钟}]{\text{发动传感}}$ 出现热敏灸感 $\longrightarrow$ 确定热敏穴位

3. 热敏灸感　灸腰阳关、次髎穴，灸感多为透热、扩热、传热；灸关元、子宫穴，灸感多为透热、扩热；灸归来穴，灸感多为透热、扩热；灸三阴交穴，灸感多为传热；灸阴陵泉穴，灸感多为传热、透热。

（二）循序激发，辨敏施灸

按照以下顺序，择优选穴施灸：

腰阳关、次髎穴温和灸→关元、子宫穴温和灸→归来穴双点灸→三阴交穴双点灸→阴陵泉穴双点灸。

上述热敏穴区不是每位患者全都出现，没有出现穴位热敏的就不做相应操作。

1. **腰阳关、次髎穴温和灸** 腰阳关位于督脉，具有补肾调经、散寒止痛的功效；次髎位于足太阳膀胱经，具有理气、调经的功效。患者可自觉热感深透至腹腔或扩散至腰骶部或向下肢传导，灸至热敏灸感消失（图 3-9-1）。

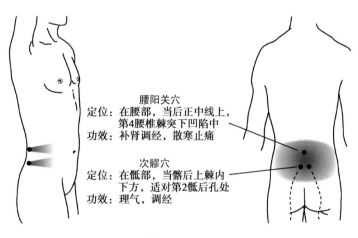

图 3-9-1 腰阳关、次髎穴温和灸

2. **关元、子宫穴温和灸** 关元、子宫穴位于下焦，合用具有温补元阳、调经止痛的功效。患者可自觉热感向深部穿透至腹腔，灸至热敏灸感消失（图 3-9-2）。

3. **归来穴双点灸** 归来穴属足阳明胃经，具有益气活血、祛瘀止痛的功效，患者可自觉热感向深部穿透至腹腔，灸至热敏灸感消失（图 3-9-3）。

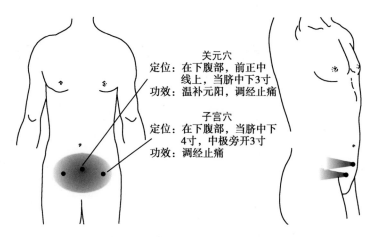

关元穴
定位：在下腹部，前正中
线上，当脐中下3寸
功效：温补元阳，调经止痛

子宫穴
定位：在下腹部，当脐中下
4寸，中极旁开3寸
功效：调经止痛

图 3-9-2　关元、子宫穴温和灸

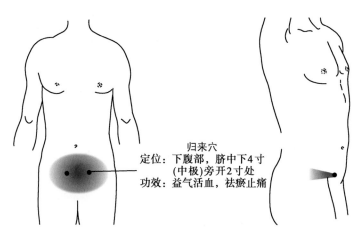

归来穴
定位：下腹部，脐中下4寸
(中极)旁开2寸处
功效：益气活血，祛瘀止痛

图 3-9-3　归来穴双点灸

4. 三阴交穴双点灸　三阴交乃足三阴经的交会穴，具有调血补阴、祛瘀止痛的功效。部分患者的感传可直接到达腹部；如感传仍不能上至腹部者，再取一支点燃的艾条悬灸感传所达部位的近心端点，进行温和灸，依次接力使感传到达腹部，最后将两支艾条分别固定于三阴交和腹部进行温和灸，灸至热敏灸感消失（图 3-9-4）。

5. 阴陵泉穴双点灸　阴陵泉是足太阴脾经的合穴，具有健脾、化湿、调经的功效。部分患者的感传可直接到达腹部；如感传仍不能上至腹部者，再取一支点燃的艾条悬灸感传所达部位的近心端点，进行温和灸，依次接力使感传到达腹部，最后将两支艾条分别固定于阴陵泉和腹部进行温和灸，灸至热敏灸感消失（图 3-9-5）。

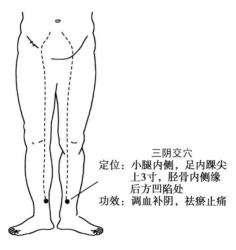

三阴交穴
定位：小腿内侧，足内踝尖
　　　上3寸，胫骨内侧缘
　　　后方凹陷处
功效：调血补阴，祛瘀止痛

图 3-9-4　三阴交穴双点灸

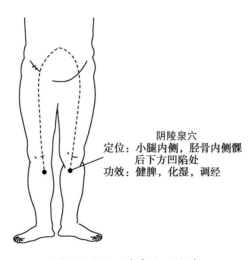

阴陵泉穴
定位：小腿内侧，胫骨内侧髁
　　　后下方凹陷处
功效：健脾，化湿，调经

图 3-9-5　阴陵泉穴双点灸

（三）量因人异，敏消量足

每次选取上述 2 组穴位，每天 1 次，每次每穴的施灸时间以热敏灸感消失为度。连续 10 天为 1 个疗程，共 3 ~ 5 个疗程。

（四）灸后防护，巩固疗效

1. 热敏灸具有改善循环、化湿通络的作用，治疗慢性盆腔炎有较好效果。月经前后和行经期应注意保暖，忌劳累。

2. 注意性生活卫生，做好经期、流产后、产褥期的卫生保健。

【验案举例】

黄女士，38岁。2年前因过度劳累出现下腹部疼痛，白带增多，诊断为急性盆腔炎。经治疗上述症状消失，但劳累及月经前后常感下腹坠胀、疼痛，月经量增多，虽经治疗疗效不佳。现感下腹坠胀、隐隐作痛，并感腰骶部酸痛。双次髎、腰阳关探查出现传热现象。遂温和灸双次髎、腰阳关三穴以清热利湿、活血化瘀。在次髎、腰阳关行温和灸，数分钟后热流汇合成片，10分钟后呈片状沿右侧腰部传至小腹，感整个小腹酸胀舒适，灸感持续约20分钟后渐回缩至腰阳关，并感皮肤灼热，乃停灸腰阳关穴。继灸次髎穴仍有透热现象，5分钟后，施灸点皮肤灼热，遂停灸，完成1次热敏灸治疗。次日复诊，诉下腹坠胀、疼痛稍有减轻。按上述方法每月治疗7~8次，连续4个月经周期，共30次。治疗后患者已无下腹疼痛，妇科检查未见异常。6个月后随访，未见复发。

第十节　勃起功能障碍

勃起功能障碍，又称阳痿，是指在有性欲要求时，阴茎不能勃起或勃起不坚，或者虽然有勃起且有一定程度的硬度，但不能保持性交的足够时间，因而妨碍性交或不能完成性交。引起勃起功能障碍的原因很多，一是精神方面的因素，如夫妻间感情冷漠或因某些原因产生紧张心情导致勃起功能障碍。二是生理方面的原因，如阴茎勃起中枢发生异常。一些重要器官如肝、肾、心、肺患严重疾病时，尤其是长期患病，也可能会影响到性生理的精神控制。中医认为因房劳纵欲过度，久犯手淫，以致精气虚损，命门火衰，引起阳事不举；或思虑忧郁，伤及心脾，惊恐伤肾，使气血不足、宗筋失养而导致阳痿；亦有湿热下注，宗筋受灼而弛纵者。

【临床表现】

在性生活时阴茎不能勃起、勃而不坚或坚而不持久，不能进行正常性生活；常伴有神倦乏力，腰膝酸软，畏寒肢冷，耳鸣等症状；夜间或清晨常有自发性勃起，排除器质性病变或药物所致的阳痿。

【灸法治则】

本病以补益肾气为基本治疗原则。根据肾主生殖、肝主疏泄等理论，选择相关穴位探感定位、辨敏施灸。

【治疗方案】

（一）探感选穴，准确定位

1. 高发穴区　热敏穴位高发区一般多位于关元、气冲、肾俞、腰阳关、血海等穴区，对这些部位进行穴位热敏探查常能发现热敏穴位。

2. 探查手法　在本病热敏穴位高发区，按下述步骤分别依序进行回旋、雀啄、往返、温和灸四步操作。

回旋灸 $\xrightarrow[\text{2分钟}]{\text{温热局部气血}}$ 雀啄灸 $\xrightarrow[\text{1分钟}]{\text{加强敏化}}$ 往返灸 $\xrightarrow[\text{1分钟}]{\text{激发经气}}$ 温和灸 $\xrightarrow[\text{2分钟}]{\text{发动传感}}$ 出现热敏灸感 $\rightarrow$ 确定热敏穴位

3. 热敏灸感　灸关元、气冲穴时，灸感多为透热、传热；灸肾俞、腰阳关穴时，灸感多为透热、扩热、传热；灸血海穴时，灸感多为传热、透热。

（二）循序激发，辨敏施灸

按照以下顺序，择优选穴施灸：

关元、气冲穴温和灸→肾俞穴双点灸→腰阳关穴单点灸→血海穴双点灸。

上述热敏穴区不是每位患者全都出现，没有出现穴位热敏的就不做相应操作。

1. **关元、气冲穴温和灸**　关元、气冲均为调理下焦的要穴，合用具有温补元气、舒筋和血的功效。患者可自觉热感深透至腹腔或传至阴茎根部，灸至热敏灸感消失（图3-10-1）。

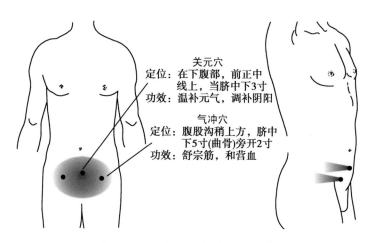

关元穴
定位：在下腹部，前正中线上，当脐中下3寸
功效：温补元气，调补阴阳

气冲穴
定位：腹股沟稍上方，脐中下5寸(曲骨)旁开2寸
功效：舒宗筋，和营血

图3-10-1　关元、气冲穴温和灸

2. **肾俞穴双点灸**　肾俞是肾气血在背部的输注部位，具有补肾强腰、调和阴阳的功效。患者可自觉热感深透至腹腔或扩散至腰骶部或向下肢传导，灸至热敏灸感消失（图3-10-2）。

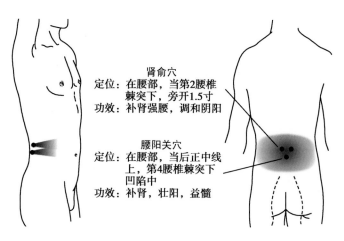

肾俞穴
定位：在腰部，当第2腰椎棘突下，旁开1.5寸
功效：补肾强腰，调和阴阳

腰阳关穴
定位：在腰部，当后正中线上，第4腰椎棘突下凹陷中
功效：补肾，壮阳，益髓

图3-10-2　肾俞穴双点灸、腰阳关穴单点灸

3．腰阳关穴单点灸　腰阳关位于督脉，具有补肾、壮阳、益髓的功效。患者可自觉热感深透至腹腔或扩散至腰骶部或向下肢传导至脚心发热，灸至热敏灸感消失（图 3-10-2）。

4．血海穴双点灸　血海乃脾经调血要穴，具有养血、活血、祛瘀的功效。部分患者的感传可直接到达下腹部；如感传仍不能上至腹部者，再取一支点燃的艾条悬灸感传所达部位的近心端点，进行温和灸，依次接力使感传到达下腹部，最后将两支艾条分别固定于血海和下腹部进行温和灸，灸至热敏灸感消失（图 3-10-3）。

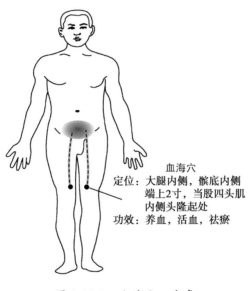

血海穴
定位：大腿内侧，髌底内侧端上2寸，当股四头肌内侧头隆起处
功效：养血，活血，祛瘀

图 3-10-3　血海穴双点灸

（三）量因人异，敏消量足

每次选取上述 1~2 组穴位，每天 1 次，每次每穴的施灸时间以热敏灸感消失为度。10 次为 1 个疗程，疗程间休息 2~5 天，共 2~3 个疗程。

（四）灸后防护，巩固疗效

1．大多数阳痿属心理性阳痿，热敏灸激发经气，疏通经络，疗效满意。

2．解除精神负担，调畅情绪，极其重要。忌滥服药物，忌盲乱投医，应到医院查明病因，正规治疗，更不可讳疾忌医。

【验案举例】

杨先生，42 岁，1 年前出现勃起功能障碍，并伴腰部酸痛，诊断为阳痿。经探查，在双肾俞探及穴位热敏，即行双点灸，立感热流渗透入腰部，并向四周扩散，5 分钟后热流汇合成片并感腰骶部酸胀，20 分钟后热流沿腰部传至小腹，小腹及前阴部酸胀舒适，灸感约持续 30 分钟后沿传导路线渐向双肾俞回缩，皮肤灼热，乃停止，遂完成 1 次灸疗。次日复诊，于腰阳关穴探及热敏，施温和灸，约 10 分钟后感热感深透至腹腔，持续 20 分钟左右热流渐回缩至腰阳关，皮肤灼热，乃停灸，完成 1 次热敏灸治疗。按上述方法探敏治疗 3 个疗程，共 30 次，性生活恢复正常，腰部酸痛未作，1 年后随访未见复发。

第十一节　慢性前列腺炎

慢性前列腺炎是男性前列腺组织的非特异性感染引起的炎症性疾病，是青壮年男性常见病，以发病缓慢、症状复杂、病程迁延、顽固难愈、容易复发为特征。慢性细菌性前列腺炎属于中医学"白浊""白淫""劳淋"范畴，慢性非细菌性前列腺炎可归属于"淋浊""精浊"等范畴。中医学认为本病与思欲不遂、房劳过度、相火妄动、酒色劳倦、湿热下注、败精瘀阻等因素有关。

【临床表现】

症状分为两类。一为下尿路刺激症状，二为炎症反应或反射性疼痛症状。表现为不同程度的尿频、尿急、尿痛，尿不尽感，尿道灼热，于晨起、尿末或大便时尿道有少量白色分泌物流出，会阴部、外生殖器区、下腹部、耻骨上区、腰骶及肛门周围坠胀、疼痛。

【灸法治则】

本病以清热利湿、理气活血为基本治疗原则。根据肾主生殖以及任脉、督脉、肝经的循行特点，选择相关穴位探感定位、辨敏施灸。

【治疗方案】

（一）探感选穴，准确定位

1. 高发穴区　热敏穴位高发区一般多位于关元、中极、肾俞、命门、次髎等穴区，对这些部位进行穴位热敏探查常能发现热敏穴位。

2. 探查手法　在本病热敏穴位高发区，按下述步骤分别依序进行回旋、雀啄、往返、温和灸四步操作。

回旋灸 —温热局部气血 2分钟→ 雀啄灸 —加强敏化 1分钟→ 往返灸 —激发经气 1分钟→ 温和灸 —发动传感 2分钟→ 出现热敏灸感 → 确定热敏穴位

3. 热敏灸感　灸关元、中极穴，灸感多为透热、传热；灸肾俞、命门、次髎穴，灸感多为透热、扩热、传热。

（二）循序激发，辨敏施灸

按照以下顺序，择优选穴施灸：

关元、中极穴双点灸→肾俞穴双点灸→命门、次髎穴温和灸。

上述热敏穴区不是每位患者全都出现，没有出现穴位热敏的就不做相应操作。

1. 关元、中极穴双点灸　关元、中极均位于任脉，合用具有培补元气、通利水道的作用。患者可自觉热感深透至腹腔并沿带脉传至腰骶部，灸至热敏灸感消失（图3-11-1）。

2. 肾俞穴双点灸　肾俞是肾气血在背部的输注部位，具有强腰脊、补阴阳的功效。患者可自觉热感透至深部并扩散至腰背部且向下腹部传导，灸至热敏灸感消失（图3-11-2）。

3. 命门、次髎穴温和灸　命门、次髎穴合用具有补益元气、通络止痛、利小便的功效。患者可自觉热感透至深部并扩散至腰背部且向下腹部传导，灸至热敏灸感消失（图3-11-3）。

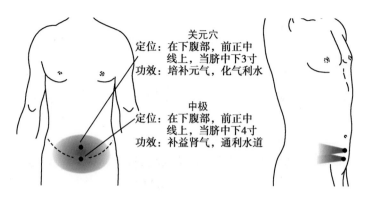

关元穴
定位：在下腹部，前正中
线上，当脐中下3寸
功效：培补元气，化气利水

中极
定位：在下腹部，前正中
线上，当脐中下4寸
功效：补益肾气，通利水道

图 3-11-1　关元、中极穴双点灸

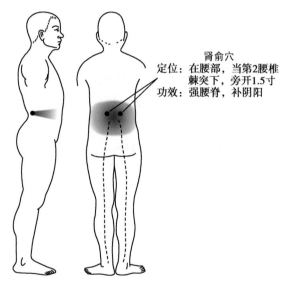

肾俞穴
定位：在腰部，当第2腰椎
棘突下，旁开1.5寸
功效：强腰脊，补阴阳

图 3-11-2　肾俞穴双点灸

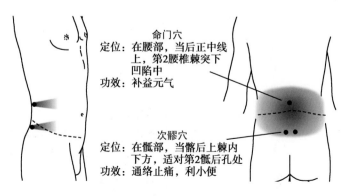

命门穴
定位：在腰部，当后正中线
上，第2腰椎棘突下
凹陷中
功效：补益元气

次髎穴
定位：在骶部，当髂后上棘内
下方，适对第2骶后孔处
功效：通络止痛，利小便

图 3-11-3　命门、次髎穴温和灸

（三）量因人异，敏消量足

每次选取上述 1~2 组穴位，每天 1 次，每次每穴的施灸时间以热敏灸感消失为度。10 次为 1 个疗程，疗程间休息 2~5 天，共 2~3 个疗程。

（四）灸后防护，巩固疗效

1. 慢性前列腺炎由于其病变部位较为特殊，药物治疗效果不显著，热敏灸能调节免疫、抗炎、改善局部血液循环，故有较好疗效。

2. 注意防寒保暖，禁酒，性生活适度，劳逸结合。

【验案举例】

胡先生，46 岁，1 年前无明显诱因出现夜尿频繁，阴囊部坠胀不适，并伴有轻微腰部酸软，尿道口偶有白色黏液溢出。诊断为慢性前列腺炎，曾多方求治，疗效不佳。经查，于中极、双侧肾俞穴探及穴位热敏。在双侧肾俞穴施双点灸，自觉热流徐徐入里，3 分钟后感热流呈片状扩散至腰背部，并向右腰外侧扩散，继扩散至右上腹部，感整个右上腹部温热舒适，该热流继续呈片状下传至中极穴处，5 分钟后感整个小腹滚热，自觉小腹热感明显高于腰背部，该灸感持续约 50 分钟后热流沿传导路线回缩至双肾俞穴，并感皮肤灼热，乃停灸，完成 1 次热敏灸治疗。按上述方法治疗 10 次后上症明显好转，继续热敏灸治疗 20 次，上述症状消失，1 年后随访，未见复发。

第十二节　偏头痛

偏头痛是由于神经、血管功能失调所引起的疾病，以一侧头部疼痛反复发作为主，常伴有恶心、呕吐、对光及声音过敏等特点。本病与遗传有关，部分患者可在头部、脑外伤后出现，某些脑神经递质可诱发，以年轻的成年女性居多，疼痛程度多为中、重度。本病属于中医学"头痛""头风"范畴，认为多与恼怒、紧张、风火痰浊有关。情志不遂，肝失疏泄，郁而化火；或恼怒急躁，肝阳上亢，风火循肝胆经脉上冲头部；或体内素有痰湿，随肝阳上冲而循经走窜，留滞于头部少阳经脉，使经络痹阻不通，故暴痛骤起。

【临床表现】

多在青春期起病，以女性多见，可有家族史；每次发作持续 4~72 小时不等，疼痛为单侧、搏动性，活动后头痛加重，可伴恶心、呕吐、畏光、畏声等；部分患者有抑郁、欣快、不安或嗜睡等精神症状以及厌食、口渴等消化道症状。

【灸法治则】

本病以疏调少阳，通络止痛为基本治疗原则。根据经脉循行特点，选择相关穴位探感定位、辨敏施灸。

【治疗方案】

（一）探感选穴，准确定位

1. 高发穴区　热敏穴位高发区一般多位于风池、率谷、日月、阳陵泉、足窍阴等穴区，对这些部位进行穴位热敏探查常能发现热敏穴位。

2. 探查手法　在本病热敏穴位高发区，按下述步骤分别依序进行回旋、雀啄、往返、温和灸四步操作。

回旋灸 $\xrightarrow[\text{2分钟}]{\text{温热局部气血}}$ 雀啄灸 $\xrightarrow[\text{1分钟}]{\text{加强敏化}}$ 往返灸 $\xrightarrow[\text{1分钟}]{\text{激发经气}}$ 温和灸 $\xrightarrow[\text{2分钟}]{\text{发动传感}}$ 出现热敏灸感 $\rightarrow$ 确定热敏穴位

3. 热敏灸感　灸风池穴，灸感多为透热、扩热；灸率谷穴，灸感多为透热、扩热、非热觉；灸日月穴，灸感多为透热、扩热；灸阳陵泉穴，灸感多为传热、透热；灸足窍阴穴，灸感多为传热。

（二）循序激发，辨敏施灸

按照以下顺序，择优选穴施灸：

风池穴双点灸→率谷穴双点灸→日月穴双点灸→阳陵泉穴双点灸→足

窍阴穴双点灸。

上述热敏穴区不是每位患者全都出现，没有出现穴位热敏的就不做相应操作。

1. **风池穴双点灸** 风池位于足少阳胆经，具有疏风解表、清利头目、通络止痛的功效。患者可自觉热感深透或扩散至头面侧部，灸至热敏灸感消失（图3-12-1）。

2. **率谷穴双点灸** 率谷位于足少阳胆经，具有祛风热、利头目的功效。患者可自觉热感深透颅内或扩散至头面侧部或自觉局部有紧、压、酸、胀、痛感，灸至热敏灸感消失（图3-12-2）。

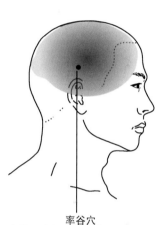

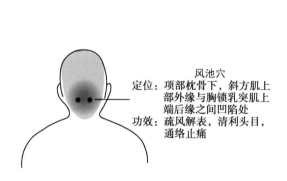

风池穴
定位：项部枕骨下，斜方肌上部外缘与胸锁乳突肌上端后缘之间凹陷处
功效：疏风解表，清利头目，通络止痛

率谷穴
定位：头部，耳尖直上入发际1.5寸处
功效：祛风热，利头目

图3-12-1 风池穴双点灸　　　　图3-12-2 率谷穴双点灸

3. **日月穴双点灸** 日月是胆的募穴，具有疏肝利胆、理气止痛的功效。患者可自觉热感深透或扩散至两胸侧，灸至热敏灸感消失（图3-12-3）。

4. **阳陵泉穴双点灸** 阳陵泉是足少阳胆经的合穴，具有疏利肝胆、理气止痛的功效。部分患者的感传可直接到达头面部；如感传仍不能上至头面部者，再取一支点燃的艾条悬于感传所达部位的近心端点，进行温和灸，依次接力使感传到达头面部，最后将两支艾条分别固定于阳陵泉和头面部进行温和灸，灸至热敏灸感消失（图3-12-4）。

5. **足窍阴穴双点灸** 足窍阴穴是足少阳胆经的井穴，具有平肝降逆、理气止痛的功效。部分患者的感传可直接到达头面部；如感传仍不能上至头面部者，再取一支点燃的艾条悬于感传所达部位的近心端点，进行温和灸，依次接力使感传到达头面部，最后将两支艾条分别固定于足窍阴和头面侧部进行温和灸，灸至热敏灸感消失（图 3-12-5）。

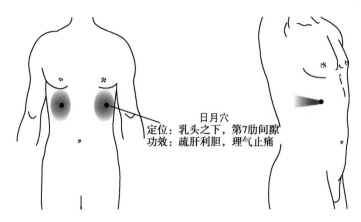

图 3-12-3　日月穴双点灸

日月穴
定位：乳头之下，第7肋间隙
功效：疏肝利胆，理气止痛

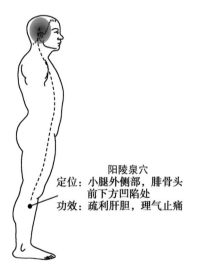

阳陵泉穴
定位：小腿外侧部，腓骨头
前下方凹陷处
功效：疏利肝胆，理气止痛

图 3-12-4　阳陵泉穴双点灸

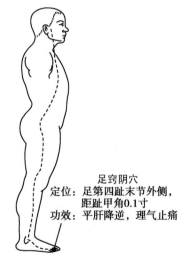

足窍阴穴
定位：足第四趾末节外侧，
距趾甲角0.1寸
功效：平肝降逆，理气止痛

图 3-12-5　足窍阴穴双点灸

（三）量因人异，敏消量足

每次选取上述 1~2 组穴位，每天 1 次，每次每穴的施灸时间以热敏灸感消失为度。10 次为 1 个疗程，疗程间休息 2~5 天，共 2~3 个疗程。

（四）灸后防护，巩固疗效

1. 热敏灸激发经气，疏通经络，对本病疗效确切，但调畅情绪很重要。

2. 注意劳逸结合，适当体育活动，避风寒，限食辛辣及烟酒，保持大便通畅。

【验案举例】

唐女士，48岁，6余年前无明显诱因出现左侧额颞部搏动性头痛，伴恶心、呕吐等。头痛反复发作，每年发作4~6次，每次发作持续5~7天。3天前左侧额颞部搏动性头痛发作，经治疗疗效不显，头颅CT检查未见异常，诊断为偏头痛。于左风池穴、左率谷穴探及穴位热敏，嘱侧卧，于左风池穴、左率谷穴同时施双点灸，数分钟后风池穴处感热流深透并向前扩散至左颞部，左率谷穴处感热扩散至整个左侧颞部，持续约40分钟热流渐回缩至左率谷穴并感皮肤灼热，乃停灸，立感左侧头颅温暖舒适，头痛立消，完成1次热敏灸治疗。次日复诊诉头痛减轻，已无恶心、呕吐等症状，按上述方法探敏治疗15次，头痛症状消除，半年后随访，未见复发。

第十三节　面神经麻痹

面神经麻痹又称面瘫，是指由于耳后茎乳孔内面神经发生非特异性炎症，造成面神经功能障碍，以口角㖞斜为主要症状的疾病。关于本病的发生机制目前尚不清楚，一般认为是一种非化脓性面神经炎，病因有两种可能：即面神经本身或其外周病变。面神经本身的因素认为系受风寒引起局部营养神经的血管发生痉挛，导致神经缺血、水肿及受压迫；也有认为是风湿性或病毒感染所致，如由疱疹病毒侵犯面神经所引起的面瘫称为亨特综合征。外周因素则有因茎乳孔内骨膜炎致使面神经受压或血循环障碍，造成面神经麻痹。本病属中医学"口眼㖞斜""卒口僻"等范畴，劳作过度，机体正气不足，脉络空虚，卫外不固，风寒或风热乘虚入中面部经络，致气血痹阻，经筋功能失调，筋肉失于约束，出现口眼㖞斜。

【临床表现】

起病突然，常于睡眠醒来时，发现一侧面部板滞、麻木、瘫痪，不能做蹙额、皱眉、露齿、鼓腮等动作；漱口漏水，进食时食物易滞留于病侧齿颊之间；病侧额纹、鼻唇沟消失，眼睑闭合不全，迎风流泪；少数于发病前几天可伴有麻痹，侧耳后、耳内疼痛或面部不适等前驱症状；还可出现病侧舌前 2/3 味觉减退或消失、听觉过敏等。

【灸法治则】

本病以祛风解表、温经通络为基本治疗原则，后期佐以扶正养筋，选择相关穴位探感定位、辨敏施灸。

【治疗方案】

（一）探感选穴，准确定位

1．高发穴区　热敏穴位高发区一般多位于翳风、阳白、下关、颊车、大椎、神阙、足三里等穴区，对这些部位进行穴位热敏探查常能发现热敏穴位。

2．探查手法　在本病热敏穴位高发区，按下述步骤分别依序进行回旋、雀啄、往返、温和灸四步操作。

回旋灸 $\xrightarrow[\text{2分钟}]{\text{温热局部气血}}$ 雀啄灸 $\xrightarrow[\text{1分钟}]{\text{加强敏化}}$ 往返灸 $\xrightarrow[\text{1分钟}]{\text{激发经气}}$ 温和灸 $\xrightarrow[\text{2分钟}]{\text{发动传感}}$ 出现热敏灸感 $\rightarrow$ 确定热敏穴位

3．热敏灸感　灸翳风、下关、颊车、阳白穴，灸感多为扩热、透热、非热觉；灸大椎穴，灸感多为透热、传热、扩热；灸神阙穴，灸感多为透热、扩热；灸足三里穴，灸感多为传热。

（二）循序激发，辨敏施灸

按照以下顺序，择优选穴施灸：

Ⅰ. 急性期面瘫的治疗操作

翳风穴患侧单点灸→下关穴患侧单点灸→颊车穴患侧单点灸→阳白穴患侧单点灸→大椎穴单点灸。

上述热敏穴区不是每位患者全都出现，没有出现穴位热敏的就不做相应操作。

1. **翳风穴患侧单点灸** 翳风位于手少阳三焦经，具有祛风解表、正口僻的功效。患者可自觉热感深透或非热觉感或扩散至患侧面部，灸至热敏灸感消失（图 3-13-1）。

2. **下关穴患侧单点灸** 下关位于足阳明胃经，具有祛风通络、利牙关的功效。患者可自觉热感透至深部并扩散至患侧面部，灸至热敏灸感消失（图 3-13-1）。

3. **颊车穴患侧单点灸** 颊车位于足阳明胃经，具有祛风通络、利牙关的功效。患者可自觉热感透至深部并扩散至患侧面部，灸至热敏灸感消失（图 3-13-1）。

4. **阳白穴患侧单点灸** 阳白位于足少阳胆经，具有祛风、通络的功效。患者可自觉热感深透或扩散至整个额部或自觉局部有紧、压、酸、胀感，灸至热敏灸感消失（图 3-13-2）。

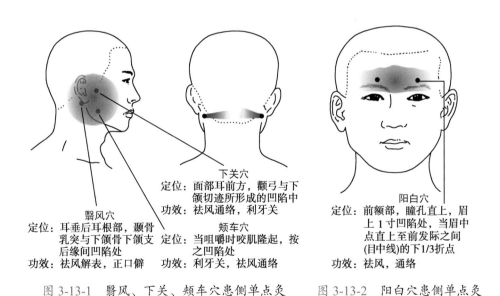

下关穴
定位：面部耳前方，颧弓与下颌切迹所形成的凹陷中
功效：祛风通络，利牙关

翳风穴
定位：耳垂后耳根部，颞骨乳突与下颌骨下颌支后缘间凹陷处
功效：祛风解表，正口僻

颊车穴
定位：当咀嚼时咬肌隆起，按之凹陷处
功效：利牙关，祛风通络

阳白穴
定位：前额部，瞳孔直上，眉上 1 寸凹陷处，当眉中点直上至前发际之间（目中线）的下 1/3 折点
功效：祛风，通络

图 3-13-1 翳风、下关、颊车穴患侧单点灸　图 3-13-2 阳白穴患侧单点灸

5. **大椎穴单点灸** 大椎穴为督脉穴位，具有祛风散寒、解表通络等功效。患者可觉热感透至深部并扩散至整个头项背部，灸至热敏灸感消失（图 3-13-3）。

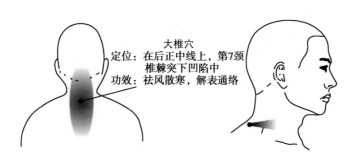

大椎穴
定位：在后正中线上，第7颈椎棘突下凹陷中
功效：祛风散寒，解表通络

图 3-13-3 大椎穴单点灸

Ⅱ. 恢复期面瘫的治疗操作

阳白穴患侧单点灸→下关穴患侧单点灸→颊车穴患侧单点灸→神阙穴单点灸→足三里穴双点灸。

上述热敏穴区不是每位患者全都出现，没有出现穴位热敏的就不做相应手法操作。

1. **阳白穴患侧单点灸** 阳白位于足少阳胆经，具有祛风、通络的功效。患者可自觉热感深透或扩散至整个额部或自觉局部有紧、压、酸、胀感，灸至热敏灸感消失（图 3-13-2）。

2. **下关穴患侧单点灸** 下关位于足阳明胃经，具有祛风通络、止痛的功效。患者可自觉热感透至深部并扩散至患侧面部，灸至热敏灸感消失（图 3-13-1）。

3. **颊车穴患侧单点灸** 颊车位于足阳明胃经，具有祛风通络、利牙关的功效。患者可自觉热感透至深部并扩散至患侧面部，灸至热敏灸感消失（图 3-13-1）。

4. **神阙穴单点灸** 神阙位于任脉，乃补益元气的要穴。患者可自觉热感深透至腹腔或沿两侧扩散至腰部，灸至热敏灸感消失（图 3-13-4）。

5. **足三里穴双点灸** 足三里是足阳明胃经的合穴，具有益气血、补脾胃的功效。部分患者的感传可直接到达腹部；如感传仍不能上至腹部者，再取一支点燃的艾条放置于感传所达部位的近心端点，进行温和灸，依次接力使感传到达腹部，最后将两支艾条分别固定于足三里和腹部进行温和灸，灸至热敏灸感消失（图 3-13-5）。

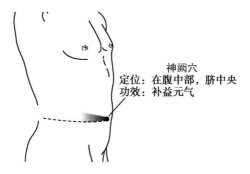

神阙穴
定位：在腹中部，脐中央
功效：补益元气

图 3-13-4　神阙穴单点灸

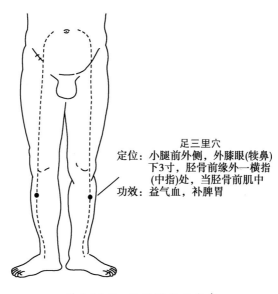

足三里穴
定位：小腿前外侧，外膝眼(犊鼻)
下3寸，胫骨前缘外一横指
(中指)处，当胫骨前肌中
功效：益气血，补脾胃

图 3-13-5　足三里穴双点灸

（三）量因人异，敏消量足

每次选取上述 2~3 组穴位，每天 1 次，每次每穴的施灸时间以热敏灸感消失为度。10 次为 1 个疗程，疗程间休息 2~5 天，共 2~3 个疗程。

（四）灸后防护，巩固疗效

1. 热敏灸对面瘫（急性期）能有效改善局部血液循环，促进面神经炎症水肿的消退和吸收，疗效可靠，治疗越早越好。对恢复期与后遗症期面瘫亦有一定疗效。

2. 治疗期间应避风寒，忌冷饮。

【验案举例】

程女士，46岁。1个月前出现口角左㖞，伴右耳后乳突部疼痛，现症：口角左㖞，鼓腮漏气，右额纹变浅，右眼闭合不全，已无乳突部疼痛。于右颊车穴探及穴位热敏，施单点灸时，感热明显扩散至整个右侧面部，灸感持续约30分钟后感施灸穴处皮肤灼热，遂停灸，完成1次热敏灸治疗。次日复诊，在右阳白穴探及穴位热敏，遂于右阳白穴施灸，约1分钟后感热流徐徐深透，渐扩散至右侧颞部，继施"接力"灸，热流渐扩散至右面颊部，右面颊部温热舒适，灸感持续约40分钟后热流渐回缩至右阳白穴并感皮肤灼热，乃停灸，完成热敏灸治疗。按上法治疗10次后，口角微向左㖞斜，右侧额纹加深，右眼基本闭合。继续按上法探敏治疗，每2日1次，同时嘱其在家中自灸神阙穴、足三里穴各20分钟，1个月后面瘫痊愈。

第十四节　三叉神经痛

三叉神经痛是一种原因未明的三叉神经分支分布区域内反复发作的阵发性剧烈疼痛。本病属中医学的"面痛""面颊痛""面风痛"等范畴，认为本病系外邪侵袭面部筋脉或血气痹阻而致。风寒之邪袭于阳明筋脉，寒性收引，凝滞筋脉，血气痹阻，发为面痛；风热邪毒浸淫面部筋脉，气血不畅，而致面痛；血气痹阻，久病入络，或因外伤，致气滞血瘀而发面痛。

【临床表现】

三叉神经支配区反复发作短暂性电击、刀割、烧灼、撕裂、针刺样疼痛，每次发作数秒至1~2分钟，突发、突止，间歇期可完全正常；疼痛多为一侧，亦可为双侧，有触发点，严重者伴同侧面肌抽搐；呈周期性发作，发作期可持续数天、数周至数月，而缓解期长短不一，可为数天至数年不等。

【灸法治则】

本病以通络止痛为基本治疗原则。根据疼痛局部的经脉循行特点选择相关穴位探感定位、辨敏施灸。

【治疗方案】

（一）探感选穴，准确定位

1. 高发穴区　热敏穴位高发区多位于下关、四白、夹承浆、风池、鱼腰等穴区，对这些部位进行穴位热敏探查常能发现热敏穴位。

2. 探查手法　在本病热敏穴位高发区，按下述步骤分别依序进行回旋、雀啄、往返、温和灸四步操作。

回旋灸 $\xrightarrow[\text{2分钟}]{\text{温热局部气血}}$ 雀啄灸 $\xrightarrow[\text{1分钟}]{\text{加强敏化}}$ 往返灸 $\xrightarrow[\text{1分钟}]{\text{激发经气}}$ 温和灸 $\xrightarrow[\text{2分钟}]{\text{发动传感}}$ 出现热敏灸感 $\longrightarrow$ 确定热敏穴位

3. 热敏灸感　灸下关、四白、夹承浆、鱼腰穴，灸感多为透热、扩热、非热觉；灸风池穴，灸感多为透热、扩热。

（二）循序激发，辨敏施灸

按照以下顺序，择优选穴施灸：

下关穴患侧单点灸→四白穴患侧单点灸→夹承浆穴患侧单点灸→风池穴双点灸→鱼腰穴患侧单点灸。

上述热敏穴区不是每位患者全都出现，没有出现穴位热敏的就不做相应操作。

1. 下关穴患侧单点灸　下关位于足阳明胃经，具有祛风通络、止痛的功效。患者可自觉热感深透并向四周扩散，灸至热敏灸感消失（图 3-14-1）。

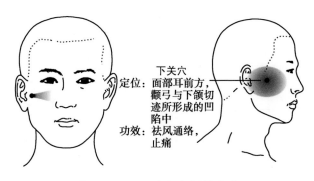

图 3-14-1   下关穴患侧单点灸

2．四白穴患侧单点灸   四白穴位于足阳明胃经，具有祛风、止痛的功效。患者可自觉热感深透并向四周扩散，灸至热敏灸感消失（图 3-14-2）。

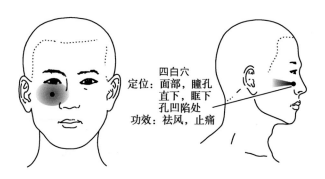

图 3-14-2   四白穴患侧单点灸

3．夹承浆穴患侧单点灸   夹承浆具有祛风止痛的功效。患者可自觉热感深透并向四周扩散，灸至热敏灸感消失（图 3-14-3）。

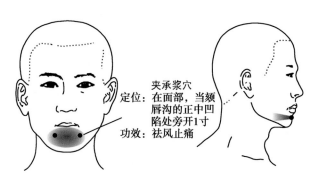

图 3-14-3   夹承浆穴患侧单点灸

4. **风池穴双点灸**　风池位于足少阳胆经，具有祛风散寒、清利头目的功效。患者可自觉热感深透并向四周扩散，灸至热敏灸感消失（图 3-14-4）。

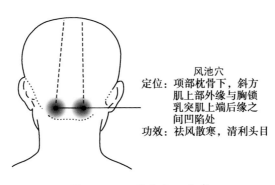

风池穴
定位：项部枕骨下，斜方
肌上部外缘与胸锁
乳突肌上端后缘之
间凹陷处
功效：祛风散寒，清利头目

图 3-14-4　风池穴双点灸

5. **鱼腰穴患侧单点灸**　鱼腰乃经外奇穴，具有通络止痛的功效。患者可自觉热感深透并向四周扩散，灸至热敏灸感消失（图 3-14-5）。

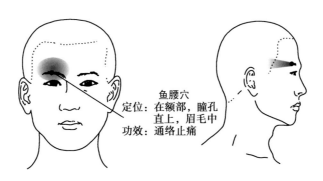

鱼腰穴
定位：在额部，瞳孔
直上，眉毛中
功效：通络止痛

图 3-14-5　鱼腰穴患侧单点灸

（三）量因人异，敏消量足

每次选取上述 1~2 组穴位，每天 1 次，每次每穴的施灸时间以热敏灸感消失为度。10 次为 1 个疗程，疗程间休息 2~5 天，共 2~3 个疗程。

（四）灸后防护，巩固疗效

1. 热敏灸治疗本病有通络镇痛作用，但难以根治。
2. 保持乐观情绪，避免急躁、焦虑。

余女士，48岁，2年前因情志抑郁致右侧面颊部出现阵发性针刺样剧痛，每天发作2～3次，每次持续近1分钟，诊断为三叉神经痛，口服卡马西平能缓解。近1个月来，发作次数明显增多，疼痛时间延长。经查，在双风池穴、右下关穴探及穴位热敏。先于双风池穴施双点灸，约半分钟后，感热流徐徐深透，3分钟后感热流汇合成片并向颅内渗透，该灸感持续约30分钟后，热流渐回缩至双风池穴。继在右下关穴施热敏灸，感热流深透并向四周扩散至整个右侧面颊，灸感持续约20分钟，热流回缩至施灸表面，并感皮肤灼热，遂停灸，完成1次热敏灸治疗。次日复诊诉灸后右面部疼痛缓解，发作次数减少，每次持续时间仅数秒钟至半分钟。嘱畅情志，少吃辛辣食物。经过20次热敏灸治疗后，右面部疼痛消失，半年后随访未见复发。

第十五节　面肌痉挛

面肌痉挛为一侧面部肌肉间断性不自主阵挛性抽动或无痛性强直。本病发生的病因尚不清楚，可能与炎症、面神经根处因蛛网膜炎而形成粘连、面神经受动静脉压迫及精神因素等有关，部分患者继发于面神经炎。面肌痉挛中医称"面风"，认为是由于素体阴亏或体弱气虚引起阴虚、血少、筋脉失养生风，或各种原因致瘀血阻滞于络脉而致面部经筋功能失调，产生不自主抽动。

【临床表现】

抽搐常先从下眼睑开始，逐渐扩展到半侧面肌，以口角肌肉的抽搐最为明显；精神紧张或疲倦可使症状加重，睡眠时停止发作；抽搐为阵发性，不能自行控制，每次抽搐时间数秒钟至数分钟或更长。

【灸法治则】

本病以活血息风、疏通经筋为基本治疗原则。根据经脉循行特点选择相关穴位探感定位、辨敏施灸。

【治疗方案】

（一）探感选穴，准确定位

1. 高发穴区　热敏穴位高发区一般多位于百会、率谷、风池、下关、手三里、阳陵泉等穴区，对这些部位进行穴位热敏探查常能发现热敏穴位。

2. 探查手法　在本病热敏穴位高发区，按下述步骤分别依序进行回旋、雀啄、往返、温和灸四步操作。

回旋灸 → 温热局部气血 / 2分钟 → 雀啄灸 → 加强敏化 / 1分钟 → 往返灸 → 激发经气 / 1分钟 → 温和灸 → 发动传感 / 2分钟 → 出现热敏灸感 → 确定热敏穴位

3. 热敏灸感　灸百会穴，灸感多为透热、传热；灸率谷穴，灸感多为透热、扩热、非热觉；灸风池穴，灸感多为透热、扩热；灸下关穴，灸感多为透热、扩热；灸手三里穴，灸感多为传热；灸阳陵泉穴，灸感多为传热、透热。

（二）循序激发，辨敏施灸

按照以下顺序，择优选穴施灸：

百会穴单点灸→率谷穴患侧单点灸→风池穴双点灸→下关穴患侧单点灸→手三里穴双点灸→阳陵泉穴双点灸。

上述热敏穴区不是每位患者全都出现，没有出现穴位热敏的就不做相应操作。

1. 百会穴单点灸　百会穴乃督脉与足太阳经的交会穴，具有宁神、开窍的功效。患者可自觉热感深透至颅内或沿督脉向前向后传导，灸至热敏灸感消失（图3-15-1）。

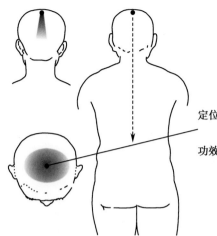

图 3-15-1　百会穴单点灸

2. 率谷穴患侧单点灸　率谷位于足少阳胆经，具有祛风热、利头目的功效。患者可自觉热感深透颅内或扩散至头面侧部或自觉局部有紧、压、酸、胀、痛感，灸至热敏灸感消失（图 3-15-2）。

3. 风池穴双点灸　风池位于足少阳胆经，具有祛风止痉的功效。患者可自觉热感深透并向四周扩散，灸至热敏灸感消失（图 3-15-3）。

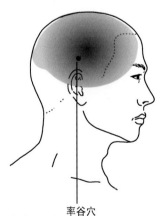

率谷穴
定位：头部，耳尖直上入发际
　　　1.5寸处
功效：祛风热，利头目

图 3-15-2　率谷穴患侧单点灸

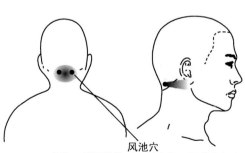

风池穴
定位：项部枕骨下，斜方肌上部外缘与胸
　　　锁乳突肌上端后缘之间凹陷处
功效：祛风止痉

图 3-15-3　风池穴双点灸

4. **下关穴患侧单点灸** 下关穴位于足阳明胃经，具有祛风、通络止痉的功效。患者可自觉热感深透并向四周扩散，灸至热敏灸感消失（图 3-15-4）。

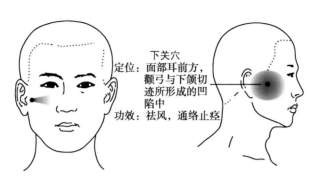

定位：面部耳前方，颧弓与下颌切迹所形成的凹陷中

功效：祛风，通络止痉

图 3-15-4 下关穴患侧单点灸

5. **手三里穴双点灸** 手三里位于手阳明大肠经，具有通络、止痉的功效。部分患者的感传可直接到达面部；如感传仍不能上至面部，再取一支点燃的艾条放置于感传所达部位的近心端点，进行温和灸，依次接力使感传到达面部，最后将两支艾条分别固定于手三里和面部进行温和灸，灸至热敏灸感消失（图 3-15-5）。

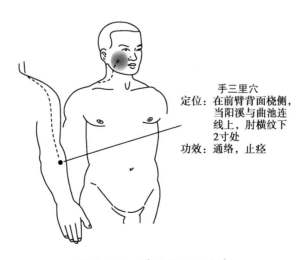

手三里穴

定位：在前臂背面桡侧，当阳溪与曲池连线上，肘横纹下2寸处

功效：通络，止痉

图 3-15-5 手三里穴双点灸

6. 阳陵泉穴双点灸　阳陵泉是足少阳胆经的合穴，具有清泄肝胆、舒筋活络的功效。部分患者的感传可直接到达面部，如感传仍不能上至面部，再取一支点燃的艾条放置于感传所达部位的近心端点，进行温和灸，依次接力使感传到达面部，最后将两支艾条分别固定于阳陵泉和面部进行温和灸，灸至热敏灸感消失（图 3-15-6）。

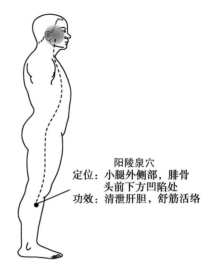

阳陵泉穴
定位：小腿外侧部，腓骨头前下方凹陷处
功效：清泄肝胆，舒筋活络

图 3-15-6　阳陵泉穴双点灸

（三）量因人异，敏消量足

每次选取上述 1～2 组穴位，每天 1 次，每次每穴的施灸时间以热敏灸感消失为度。10 次为 1 个疗程，疗程间休息 2～5 天，共 2～3 个疗程。

（四）灸后防护，巩固疗效

1. 热敏灸对风寒阻络型有一定疗效。但本症较顽固，易于反复发作。

2. 本症受情绪影响较大，平时应注意情志调养，避免七情过甚。不吃辛辣、煎炒油炸和刺激性食品。

【验案举例】

符先生，52 岁。3 年前无明显诱因出现左侧口角阵发性抽动，始 1 个月仅抽动 3～5 次，持续时间仅数分钟。近 1 个月来症状逐渐加重，现整个左面颊部均出现抽动，每日抽动数 10 次，持续时间延长，每次几分钟。热敏探查发现左侧手三里、左侧阳陵泉穴出现传热现象。予左手三里、左阳陵泉穴单点灸，以活血息风，疏通经筋。于左侧手三里穴行单点灸，即感热流沿左上肢向上传导，经施"接力"灸，热流上传于左面颊，左面颊有蚁行感，灸感持续约 40 分钟后左面颊蚁行感消失，热流渐回缩至左侧手三里穴，并感皮肤灼热，乃停灸。换灸左侧阳陵泉穴，5 分钟后感热流呈片状沿左大腿外侧上传于腹部，经施"接力"灸，热流即呈线状上传于左面颊部，该灸感持续约 25 分钟后渐沿传导路线回缩至左侧阳陵泉穴，并感皮肤灼热，遂停灸，完成 1 次热敏灸治疗。次日复诊，诉面肌仅在睡前抽动数分钟。继按上法治疗，嘱调情志。治疗 20 次后，面肌抽动消失，患者痊愈。嘱睡前自灸阳陵泉穴半小时，每日 1 次，连续 20 天，以巩固疗效。3 个月后随访，未见复发。

第十六节　枕神经痛

枕神经痛又称上颈神经痛，是指位于后头部枕大神经或枕小神经与耳大神经分布区的阵发性疼痛。常由受凉、上呼吸道感染或坐卧时头颈部姿势不良、颈椎病及椎管内肿瘤等原因刺激或压迫枕神经导致。枕神经痛属中医学"太阳头痛"范畴，与足太阳、督脉关系密切，因外感风寒，寒邪阻滞经络，寒性收引，筋脉拘急而痛；或枕部外伤，瘀血阻络，或肝郁气滞，血行不畅，瘀血阻滞经脉而痛；或素体虚弱，久病或劳累过度伤及气血，气血不足，筋脉失养而痛。

【临床表现】

疼痛位于头后、头后下部，放散到项部、头顶部，呈阵发性发作；疼痛性质似针刺或刀割样放射痛，有时为跳痛；向对侧转头时而被诱发，打喷嚏、咳嗽时加重；头枕、项部两侧可触及压痛点。

【灸法治则】

本病以疏通经络、活血止痛为基本治疗原则。根据局部穴位，配合远端选穴特点选择相关穴位探感定位、辨敏施灸。

【治疗方案】

（一）探感选穴，准确定位

1. 高发穴区　热敏穴区高发区一般多位于枕项部压痛点、风池、玉枕、大椎、阳陵泉等穴区，对这些部位进行穴位热敏探查常能发现热敏穴位。

2. 探查手法 在本病热敏穴位高发区，按下述步骤分别依序进行回旋、雀啄、往返、温和灸四步操作。

回旋灸 $\xrightarrow[\text{2分钟}]{\text{温热局部气血}}$ 雀啄灸 $\xrightarrow[\text{1分钟}]{\text{加强敏化}}$ 往返灸 $\xrightarrow[\text{1分钟}]{\text{激发经气}}$ 温和灸 $\xrightarrow[\text{2分钟}]{\text{发动传感}}$ 出现热敏灸感 $\rightarrow$ 确定热敏穴位

3. 热敏灸感 灸压痛点，灸感多为透热、扩热、非热觉；灸风池穴，灸感多为透热、扩热；灸玉枕穴，灸感多为透热、扩热、非热觉；灸大椎穴，灸感多为透热、传热、扩热；灸阳陵泉穴，灸感多为传热、透热。

（二）循序激发，辨敏施灸

按照以下顺序，择优选穴施灸：

枕项部压痛点单点灸→风池穴双点灸→玉枕穴患侧单点灸→大椎穴单点灸→阳陵泉穴双点灸。

上述热敏穴区不是每位患者全都出现，没有出现穴位热敏的就不做相应操作。

1. 枕项部压痛点单点灸 患者可自觉热感透向深部并向四周扩散或自觉局部有紧、压、酸、胀、痛感，灸至热敏灸感消失（图 3-16-1）。

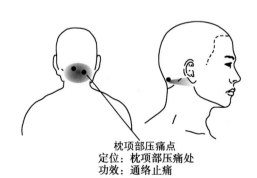

枕项部压痛点
定位：枕项部压痛处
功效：通络止痛

图 3-16-1 枕项部压痛点单点灸

2. 风池穴双点灸 风池位于足少阳胆经，具有通络止痛的功效。患者可自觉热感深透并向四周扩散，灸至热敏灸感消失（图 3-16-2）。

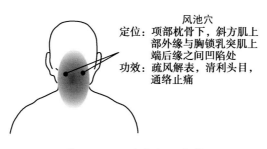

图 3-16-2　风池穴双点灸

3．玉枕穴患侧单点灸　玉枕位于足太阳膀胱经，具有清利头目、通络止痛的功效。患者可自觉热感透向深部并向四周扩散或自觉局部有紧、压、酸、胀、痛感，灸至热敏灸感消失（图 3-16-3）。

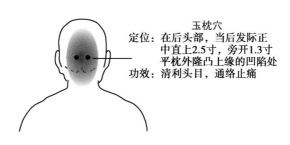

图 3-16-3　玉枕穴患侧单点灸

4．大椎穴单点灸　大椎穴为督脉穴位，具有祛风散寒、解表通络等功效。患者可觉热感透至深部并扩散至整个头项背部，灸至热敏灸感消失（图 3-16-4）。

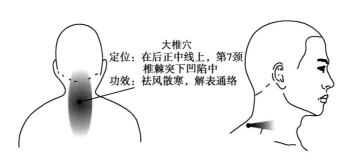

图 3-16-4　大椎穴单点灸

5. 阳陵泉穴双点灸　阳陵泉是足少阳胆经的合穴，具有清泄肝胆、通络止痛的功效。部分患者的感传可直接到达头部；如感传仍不能上至头部者，再取一支点燃的艾条放置于感传所达部位的近心端点，进行温和灸，依次接力使感传到达头部，最后将两支艾条分别固定于阳陵泉和头部进行温和灸，以热敏灸感消失为度（图 3-16-5）。

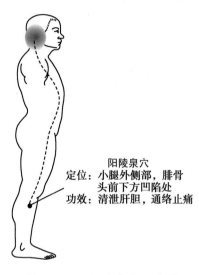

阳陵泉穴
定位：小腿外侧部，腓骨
头前下方凹陷处
功效：清泄肝胆，通络止痛

图 3-16-5　阳陵泉穴双点灸

（三）量因人异，敏消量足

每次选取上述 2 组穴位，每天 1 次，每次每穴的施灸时间以热敏灸感消失为度。5 次为 1 个疗程，疗程间休息 2 天，共 2～3 个疗程。

（四）灸后防护，巩固疗效

1. 热敏灸能迅速消除局部炎症水肿，对枕神经痛疗效显著。
2. 注意保暖，避免风寒侵袭。

【验案举例】

单先生，32 岁。6 个月前工作紧张而出现后枕部紧痛，咳嗽、喷嚏时加剧，左枕部有一明显压痛点，医院诊断为枕神经痛。每于天气变化、情绪紧张或感冒而诱发疼痛。昨日枕部疼痛又发，颈椎 CT 检查示无明显异常。在左风池穴、左玉枕穴探查出现透热现象。双点灸左风池穴、左玉枕穴，以疏通经络、活血止痛。在左风池穴、左玉枕穴施双点灸，5分钟后两股热流扩散并汇合成片，10分钟后热流向大脑深部渗透，自觉头颅皮温渐升高，由温热感渐觉滚热，该灸感持续约20分钟后渐回缩至上述两穴，并感皮肤灼热，乃停灸，完成1次治疗。次日告知疼痛减轻，继按上述方法探敏治疗5次，疼痛消失。

第十七节 带状疱疹后遗神经痛

带状疱疹后遗神经痛是一种由于带状疱疹病毒导致后根神经节的炎症、变性引起的，以皮肤疱疹愈合4~6周后皮肤仍然存在持续性疼痛为主要表现的周围神经疾病。与发病年龄有关，小于40岁患者很少发生，60岁以上患者发生率为50%，70岁以上患者发生率为75%，10%~25%的后遗神经痛患者疼痛可持续超过1年。中医学认为本病多由于热毒郁火未净、血虚肝旺、气阴不足三种原因造成局部气血凝滞，痹阻经络，以致经络挛急而造成"不通则痛"和局部肌肤失养导致"不荣则痛"。

【临床表现】

病前大多数有发热、全身倦怠等前驱症状；皮肤感受觉呈现明显的激惹征，尤其是痛觉异常敏感；皮肤损害表现为初起皮肤潮红，继而出现簇集性粟粒大小丘疹、丘疱疹，迅速变为水疱，皮损沿神经呈单侧分布，排列呈带状；神经过敏痛为本病主要的特征，疼痛的性质大多数为剧烈的自发性刀割样痛、闪电样痛或烧灼样痛，坐卧不安，夜不能寐。

【灸法治则】

本病以理气、通络、止痛为基本治疗原则。根据经气所过、主治所及等理论，选择相关穴位探感定位、辨敏施灸。

【治疗方案】

（一）探感选穴，准确定位

1. **高发穴区**　肋间神经区域带状疱疹后遗神经痛患者热敏穴位高发区一般多位于同神经节段背俞穴、心俞、至阳、膈俞等穴区，对这些部位进行穴位热敏探查常能发现热敏穴位。

2. **探查手法**　在本病热敏穴位高发区，按下述步骤分别依序进行回旋、雀啄、往返、温和灸四步操作。

回旋灸 $\xrightarrow[\text{2分钟}]{\text{温热局部气血}}$ 雀啄灸 $\xrightarrow[\text{1分钟}]{\text{加强敏化}}$ 往返灸 $\xrightarrow[\text{1分钟}]{\text{激发经气}}$ 温和灸 $\xrightarrow[\text{2分钟}]{\text{发动传感}}$ 出现热敏灸感 $\rightarrow$ 确定热敏穴位

3. **热敏灸感**　灸病痛局部或同节段背俞穴，灸感多为透热、传热、非热觉；灸心俞穴，灸感多为透热、扩热、传热、非热觉；灸至阳、膈俞穴，灸感多为透热、扩热、传热。

（二）循序激发，辨敏施灸

按照以下顺序，择优选穴施灸：

病痛局部或同节段背俞穴单点灸→心俞穴双点灸→至阳穴单点灸→膈俞穴双点灸。

上述热敏穴区不是每位患者全都出现，没有出现穴位热敏的就不做相应操作。

1. **病痛局部或同节段背俞穴单点灸**　患者可自觉热感透向深部，向四周扩散并传至远部或自觉麻木、疼痛，灸至热敏灸感消失（图 3-17-1）。

2. **心俞穴双点灸**　心俞是心气输注于背部的部位，患者可自觉热感透向深部，向四周扩散并传至远部或自觉麻木、疼痛，灸至热敏灸感消失（图 3-17-2）。

3. **至阳穴单点灸**　至阳位于督脉，具有温督、理气、止痛的作用。患者可自觉热感传至病痛附近区域，灸至热敏灸感消失（图 3-17-3）。

4. **膈俞穴双点灸**　膈俞乃血会，具有活血化瘀、通络止痛的作用。部分患者的感传可直接到达病痛处，如感传仍不能上至病痛处，再取一支

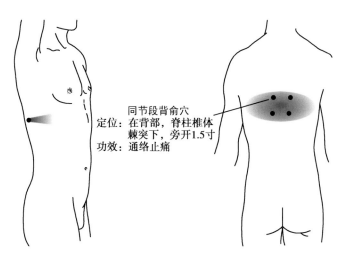

图 3-17-1 病痛局部或同节段背俞穴单点灸

同节段背俞穴
定位：在背部，脊柱椎体棘突下，旁开1.5寸
功效：通络止痛

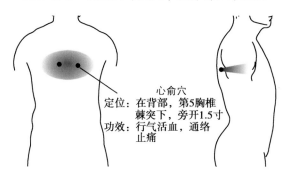

图 3-17-2 心俞穴双点灸

心俞穴
定位：在背部，第5胸椎棘突下，旁开1.5寸
功效：行气活血，通络止痛

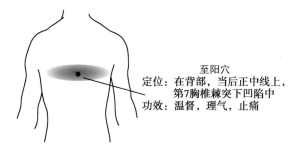

图 3-17-3 至阳穴单点灸

至阳穴
定位：在背部，当后正中线上，第7胸椎棘突下凹陷中
功效：温督，理气，止痛

点燃的艾条放置于感传所达部位的端点，进行温和灸，依次接力使感传到达病痛处，最后将两支艾条分别固定于膈俞和病痛局部进行温和灸，灸至热敏灸感消失（图 3-17-4）。

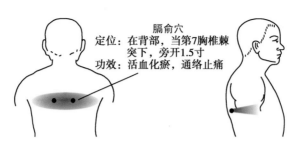

膈俞穴
定位：在背部，当第7胸椎棘
突下，旁开1.5寸
功效：活血化瘀，通络止痛

图 3-17-4　膈俞穴双点灸

（三）量因人异，敏消量足

每次选取上述 1～2 组穴位，每天 1 次，每次每穴的施灸时间以热敏灸感消失为度。10 次为 1 个疗程，疗程间休息 2～5 天，共 2～3 个疗程。

（四）灸后防护，巩固疗效

1. 热敏灸治疗本症有通络镇痛作用，但早期正规治疗是关键，可减轻神经损害，减少后遗神经痛的发生。

2. 发病后饮食应清淡，调畅情志，不要过分紧张。

【验案举例】

崔先生，65 岁。患者诉 8 个月前无明显诱因出现前胸左侧皮肤疼痛不适，3 天后疼痛加重，烧灼样疼痛，痛如火燎，伴发热，皮肤感觉异常。几天后逐渐出现一条带状小疱，从上而下，约 7cm 长，疼痛难忍，至附近医院皮肤科就诊，各项检查后诊断为"带状疱疹"。经治疗（具体用药不详）疱疹逐渐发脓并结痂，体温正常，但仍经常有烧灼样皮肤疼痛，有时疼痛伴有发紧感，睡眠时疼痛常能缓解，但白天疼痛难以忍受，经中西医治疗效果不佳。现来我科求诊，查：前胸约左侧第 6 肋间处有一长约 6cm 的带状结痂后皮损，色暗红，接触性疼痛，舌质淡苔黄，脉滑数。诊断为带状疱疹后遗神经痛。经查，于左心俞、左膈俞穴探及穴位热敏，于左心俞穴施温和灸，立感热流扩散至整个肩背部，酸胀温热，5 分钟后，温热感沿侧胸向左前胸扩散，灸感持续约 20 分钟后渐回缩至左心俞，继灸 5 分钟后，左心俞穴皮肤灼热，乃停灸。改灸左膈俞穴，立感热流深透入里，1 分钟后热流呈线状向左侧胸部扩散，数分钟后感热流继续向左前胸扩散，5 分钟后整个左前胸温热感，灸感持续约 20 分钟后渐回缩至左膈俞穴，并感皮肤灼热，遂停灸，完成 1 次治疗。次日复诊，患者诉前胸部疼痛稍减，按上述方法治疗 20 次，痊愈。

第十八节　脑梗死

脑梗死，又称缺血性卒中，是指各种原因所致脑部血液供应障碍，导致局部脑组织缺血、缺氧性坏死，而出现相应神经功能缺损的一类临床综合征。中医学认为本病属于本虚标实之证，在本为阴阳失调，气机逆乱；在标为风火相煽，痰浊壅塞，瘀血内阻。常见的病因有忧思恼怒，饮酒无度，或恣食肥甘，纵欲劳累，或起居不慎等。

【临床表现】

常突然起病，不省人事，半身不遂，口眼㖞斜，言语不利，偏身麻木；部分患者发病前有肢体麻木感，说话不清，一过性眼前发黑，头晕或眩晕、恶心等短暂脑缺血的症状；半身不遂可以是单个肢体或一侧肢体，可以是上肢比下肢重或下肢比上肢重，并可出现吞咽困难，说话不清，恶心、呕吐，头痛，眩晕，耳鸣等。

【灸法治则】

本病以扶正祛邪、益气活血为基本治疗原则，根据脑为元神之府，督脉总领一身阳气等理论，选择相关穴位探感定位、辨敏施灸。

【治疗方案】

（一）探感选穴，准确定位

1. 高发穴区　热敏穴位高发区多位于百会、风池、神阙、手三里、阳陵泉等穴区。对这些部位进行穴位热敏探查常能发现热敏穴位。

2. 探查手法　在本病热敏穴位高发区，按下述步骤分别依序进行回旋、雀啄、往返、温和灸四步操作。

回旋灸 $\xrightarrow[\text{2分钟}]{\text{温热局部气血}}$ 雀啄灸 $\xrightarrow[\text{1分钟}]{\text{加强敏化}}$ 往返灸 $\xrightarrow[\text{1分钟}]{\text{激发经气}}$ 温和灸 $\xrightarrow[\text{2分钟}]{\text{发动传感}}$ 出现热敏灸感 $\rightarrow$ 确定热敏穴位

3．**热敏灸感** 灸百会穴，灸感多为透热、传热；灸风池穴，灸感多为透热、传热、扩热；灸神阙穴，灸感多为透热；灸手三里穴，灸感多为传热；灸阳陵泉穴，灸感多为传热、透热。

（二）循序激发，辨敏施灸

按照以下顺序，择优选穴施灸：

百会穴单点灸→风池穴双点灸→神阙穴单点灸→手三里穴双点灸→阳陵泉穴双点灸。

上述热敏穴区不是每位患者全都出现，没有出现穴位热敏的就不做相应操作。

1．**百会穴单点灸** 百会穴乃督脉与足太阳膀胱经的交会穴，具有宁神、开窍的功效。患者可自觉热感深透至颅内或沿督脉向前向后传导，灸至热敏灸感消失（图 3-18-1）。

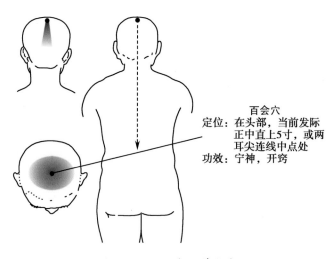

百会穴
定位：在头部，当前发际正中直上5寸，或两耳尖连线中点处
功效：宁神，开窍

图 3-18-1　百会穴单点灸

2. **风池穴双点灸** 风池乃祛风要穴，具有息风通络、开窍的功效。患者可自觉热感深透或向四周扩散或沿督脉向前向后传导，灸至热敏灸感消失（图 3-18-2）。

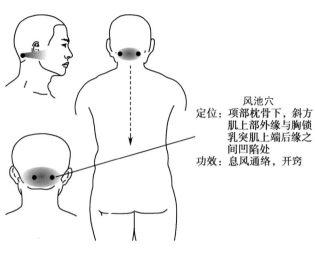

风池穴
定位：项部枕骨下，斜方
 肌上部外缘与胸锁
 乳突肌上端后缘之
 间凹陷处
功效：息风通络，开窍

图 3-18-2 风池穴双点灸

3. **神阙穴单点灸** 神阙位于任脉，乃补益元气的要穴。患者可自觉热感深透至腹腔，灸至热敏灸感消失（图 3-18-3）。

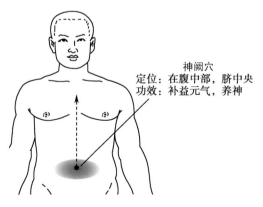

神阙穴
定位：在腹中部，脐中央
功效：补益元气，养神

图 3-18-3 神阙穴单点灸

4. **手三里穴双点灸** 手三里为阳明多气多血之经穴，具有活血通络的作用。部分患者的感传可直接到达头部；如感传仍不能上至头部者，再取一支点燃的艾条放置于感传所达部位的端点，进行温和灸，依次接力使感传到达头部，最后将两支艾条分别固定于手三里和头部进行温和灸，灸至热敏灸感消失（图 3-18-4）。

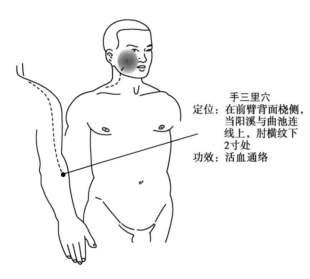

手三里穴
定位：在前臂背面桡侧，当阳溪与曲池连线上，肘横纹下2寸处

功效：活血通络

图 3-18-4　手三里穴双点灸

5. **阳陵泉穴双点灸** 阳陵泉是足少阳胆经的合穴，具有清泄肝胆、舒筋活络的功效。部分患者的感传可直接到达头部；如感传仍不能上至头部者，再取一支点燃的艾条放置于感传所达部位的端点，进行温和灸，依次接力使感传到达头部，最后将两支艾条分别固定于阳陵泉和头部进行温和灸，灸至热敏灸感消失（图 3-18-5）。

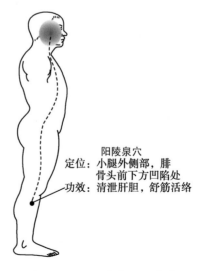

阳陵泉穴
定位：小腿外侧部，腓骨头前下方凹陷处
功效：清泄肝胆，舒筋活络

（三）量因人异，敏消量足

每次选取上述 3～4 个穴位，每天 1

图 3-18-5　阳陵泉穴双点灸

次，每次每穴的施灸时间以热敏灸感消失为度。10 次为 1 个疗程，疗程间休息 2~5 天，共 2~3 个疗程。

（四）灸后防护，巩固疗效

1. 热敏灸对脑梗死疗效肯定，治疗越早越好。坚定康复信心，避免情绪波动，心态平和，有利康复。

2. 有"三高"症（高血糖、高血脂、高血压）的患者应定期检查，做到无病先防，有病早治，有效预防复发。

【验案举例】

焦女士，59 岁。3 天前无明显诱因出现左侧肢体活动不利，当日到医院就诊，诊断为脑梗死。现神清，左侧肢体活动不利，无胸闷、憋气等症。CT 示右脑基底部梗死。探查发现百会穴透热和传热现象，左手三里穴、左阳陵泉穴有传热现象。于百会穴施单点灸，感热流直入大脑内部，继则传向右侧颞部，而后折向前额及左颞部，立感整个头颅温暖舒适。灸感持续 25 分钟后热流回缩至百会穴皮肤表面，施灸点头皮出现灼热感后停灸此穴。换灸左手三里穴处，热感沿手臂外侧成带状上传于头顶处，20 分钟后灸感减弱消失。继灸左阳陵泉穴，10 分钟后阳陵泉穴处热感徐徐上传至腹，而且左上臂出现温热感，灸感维持 30 分钟左右减弱消失，施灸点皮肤出现灼热感后停灸，结束 1 次热敏灸治疗。继续热敏灸治疗 20 次，每天 1 次，症状逐渐消失，20 天后肢体活动恢复正常。

第十九节　失眠

失眠是以入睡和 / 或睡眠维持困难所致的睡眠质量或数量达不到正常生理需求而影响白天社会功能的一种主观体验，是最常见的睡眠障碍性疾患。西医学认为本病与睡眠 – 觉醒调节机制紊乱及心理、社会因素有关，病因尚不明确。中医称失眠为"不寐""不得眠"，多因情志所伤，饮食不节，久病、年迈成虚，禀赋不足，心虚胆怯所致。其主要病机为脏腑阴阳失调，气血失和，以致心神失养或心神不安，阳不入阴，阴不含阳，神不守舍；或跷脉功能失调，阳跷脉亢盛，阴跷脉失于对其制约，阴不制阳，而致失眠。

【临床表现】

临床上可见夜间入睡困难、易醒、早醒、醒后不能再睡、睡眠时间明显减少，常伴有头痛、头晕、心慌、健忘、多梦等症状，导致白昼工作、学习、记忆及其他功能低下。

【灸法治则】

本病以养心安神为基本治疗原则。根据心主神、脑为元神之府、督脉入脑等理论，选择相关穴位探感定位、辨敏施灸。

【治疗方案】

（一）探感选穴，准确定位

1. 高发穴区　热敏穴位高发区一般多位于百会、心俞、至阳、神阙、涌泉等穴区。对这些部位进行穴位热敏探查常能发现热敏穴位。

2. 探查手法　在本病热敏穴位高发区，按下述步骤分别依序进行回旋、雀啄、往返、温和灸四步操作。

回旋灸 —温热局部气血 2分钟→ 雀啄灸 —加强敏化 1分钟→ 往返灸 —激发经气 1分钟→ 温和灸 —发动传感 2分钟→ 出现热敏灸感 → 确定热敏穴位

3. 热敏灸感　灸百会穴，灸感多为透热、传热；灸心俞穴，灸感多为透热、扩热、表面不（微）热深部热；灸至阳穴，灸感多为透热、传热；灸神阙穴，灸感多为透热、表面不（微）热深部热；灸涌泉穴，灸感多为透热、扩热。

（二）循序激发，辨敏施灸

按照以下顺序，择优选穴施灸：

百会穴单点灸→心俞穴双点灸→至阳穴单点灸→神阙穴单点灸→涌泉

穴双点灸。

上述热敏穴区不是每位患者全都出现，没有出现穴位热敏的就不做相应操作。

1. 百会穴单点灸 百会穴乃督脉与足太阳膀胱经的交会穴，具有养神、定志的功效。患者可自觉热感深透至脑内，或向前额或向后项沿督脉传导，灸至热敏灸感消失（图 3-19-1）。

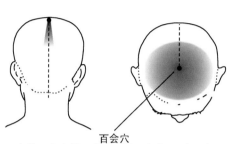

百会穴
定位：在头部，当前发际正中直上5寸，或两耳尖连线中点处
功效：养神，定志

图 3-19-1 百会穴单点灸

2. 心俞穴双点灸 心俞是心气输注于背部的穴位，具有补心、宁心、安神的功效。患者可自觉热感深透至胸腔，或向上肢传导，或出现表面不（微）热深部热现象，灸至热敏灸感消失（图 3-19-2）。

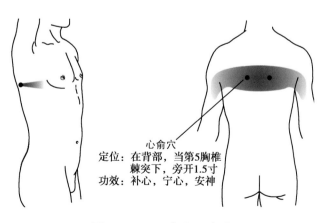

心俞穴
定位：在背部，当第5胸椎棘突下，旁开1.5寸
功效：补心，宁心，安神

图 3-19-2 心俞穴双点灸

3. 至阳穴单点灸 至阳位于督脉，具有益阳通督、宁心安神的功效。患者可自觉热感透至胸腔或沿督脉向上向下传导或扩散至整个背部，灸至热敏灸感消失（图 3-19-3）。

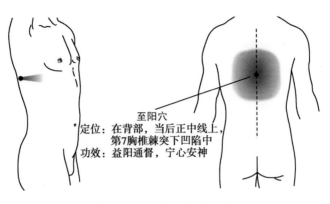

至阳穴
定位：在背部，当后正中线上，
第7胸椎棘突下凹陷中
功效：益阳通督，宁心安神

图 3-19-3　至阳穴单点灸

4. 神阙穴单点灸 神阙位于任脉，乃补益元气的要穴。患者可自觉热感深透至腹腔，或出现表面不（微）热深部热现象，灸至热敏灸感消失（图 3-19-4）。

5. 涌泉穴双点灸 涌泉是足少阴肾经的井穴，具有泄热、养阴、安神的功效。患者多出现透热或扩热等现象，灸至热敏灸感消失（图 3-19-5）。

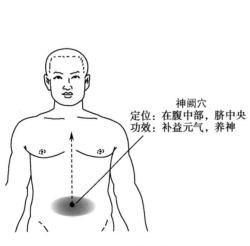

神阙穴
定位：在腹中部，脐中央
功效：补益元气，养神

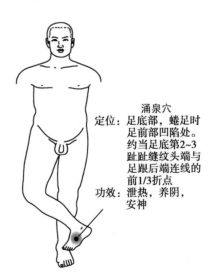

涌泉穴
定位：足底部，蜷足时
足前部凹陷处。
约当足底第2~3
趾趾缝纹头端与
足跟后端连线的
前1/3折点
功效：泄热，养阴，
安神

图 3-19-4　神阙穴单点灸　　　图 3-19-5　涌泉穴双点灸

（三）量因人异，敏消量足

每次选取上述 2 组穴位，每天 1 次，每次每穴的施灸时间以热敏灸感消失为度。10 次为 1 个疗程，疗程间休息 2～5 天，共 2～3 个疗程。

（四）灸后防护，巩固疗效

1. 热敏灸能安神定志，对治疗失眠疗效较好，且无药物的不良反应，但对长期依赖安眠药的患者则效果较差。

2. 养成良好的睡眠习惯，生活有规律，可睡前温水泡脚，晚餐不宜过饱，睡前不饮茶和咖啡等饮料。

【验案举例】

陶女士，55 岁，入睡困难已 2 年。常整夜不能入睡，入睡后多梦，白天精神差，经治疗效果不佳。在双心俞穴探及穴位热敏，即于双心俞穴施双点灸，立感两股热流扩散并汇合成片，5 分钟后右心俞穴扩热不显，并感皮肤灼热，乃停灸。而左心俞穴沿后背成片状向腋下传导，10 分钟后向上肢内侧传导至肘尖，灸感持续约 30 分钟后热流沿其传导路线回缩至左心俞穴，仍有透热现象，15 分钟后感左心俞穴皮肤灼热后停灸，完成 1 次热敏灸治疗。第二日复诊，大约睡 4 小时，晨起精神状态佳。继按上述方案探敏治疗 15 次后，每晚能入睡 5～6 小时，白天精神尚可。

第二十节　过敏性鼻炎

过敏性鼻炎是指鼻黏膜接触变应原后，由免疫球蛋白介导的炎症反应及其引发的一系列鼻部症状。本病在任何年龄都可发生，但多见于 15～40 岁的青壮年，小儿患者也不少。本病好发于春秋季。目前，本病发病率呈现上升趋势，据国外统计，其发病率在 10%～20%，在我国则发病率更高，可达到 37.74%。本病属中医学"鼻鼽"范畴，多由感受风邪，或禀赋不足，阳气虚弱，肺、脾、肾三脏虚损，卫表不固，机体受到风邪外袭，导致肺气失宣、鼻窍不利而为病。

【临床表现】

有半年以上典型的过敏病史；喷嚏每天数次阵发性发作，多在晨起时或夜晚接触变应原后立刻发作；流大量清水样鼻涕，有时可不自觉从鼻孔滴下；鼻塞轻重程度不一，间歇性或持续性，单侧、双侧或两侧交替，表现不一；大多数感觉鼻内发痒，花粉症可伴有眼睛、外耳道、软腭等处发痒；有不同程度的嗅觉减退。

【灸法治则】

本病以温经通窍，益气固表为基本治疗原则。根据肺主呼吸、开窍于鼻的理论，选择相关穴位探感定位、辨敏施灸。

【治疗方案】

（一）探感选穴，准确定位

1．高发穴区　热敏穴位高发区一般多位于上印堂、通天、风池、肺俞、神阙等穴区，对这些部位进行穴位热敏探查常能发现热敏穴位。

2．探查手法　在本病热敏穴位高发区，按下述步骤分别依序进行回旋、雀啄、往返、温和灸四步操作。

$$回旋灸 \xrightarrow[\text{2分钟}]{\text{温热局部气血}} 雀啄灸 \xrightarrow[\text{1分钟}]{\text{加强敏化}} 往返灸 \xrightarrow[\text{1分钟}]{\text{激发经气}} 温和灸 \xrightarrow[\text{2分钟}]{\text{发动传感}} 出现热敏灸感 \rightarrow 确定热敏穴位$$

3．热敏灸感　灸上印堂穴，灸感多为扩热、非热觉；灸通天穴，灸感多为透热、非热觉；灸风池穴，灸感多为透热、扩热、传热；灸肺俞穴，灸感多为透热、扩热、传热；灸神阙穴，灸感多为透热、扩热。

（二）循序激发，辨敏施灸

按照以下顺序，择优选穴施灸：

上印堂穴单点灸→通天穴双点灸→风池穴双点灸→肺俞穴双点灸→神

阙穴单点灸。

　　上述热敏穴区不是每位患者全都出现，没有出现穴位热敏的就不做相应操作。

　　1．上印堂穴单点灸　上印堂穴为经外奇穴，位于额面部，具有祛风解表、通鼻窍的作用。患者可自觉热感扩散至整个额部或额部紧压感，灸至热敏灸感消失（图 3-20-1）。

　　2．通天穴双点灸　通天穴位于足太阳膀胱经，具有疏风解表、宣通鼻窍的作用。患者可自觉热感深透或扩散或紧压感，灸至热敏灸感消失（图 3-20-2）。

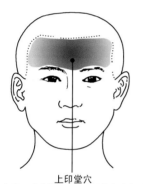

上印堂穴
定位： 在额部，当两眉头之中间为
印堂穴，在印堂穴上1寸
功效： 祛风解表，通鼻窍

图 3-20-1　上印堂穴单点灸

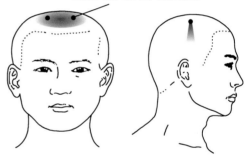

通天穴
定位： 前发际正中直上4寸，旁开1.5寸
功效： 疏风解表，宣通鼻窍

图 3-20-2　通天穴双点灸

　　3．风池穴双点灸　风池穴具有疏风解表、清利头目、宣通鼻窍的作用。患者可自觉热感深透或向四周扩散或沿督脉上下传导，灸至热敏灸感消失（图 3-20-3）。

　　4．肺俞穴双点灸　肺俞是肺气输注于背部的部位，可治本脏之疾，具有疏风散寒、宣利肺气的作用。患者可自觉热感透至胸腔或扩散至整个背部或热感向上肢传导，灸至热敏灸感消失（图 3-20-4）。

　　5．神阙穴单点灸　神阙位于任脉，乃补益元气的要穴。患者可自觉热感深透至腹腔，灸至热敏灸感消失（图 3-20-5）。

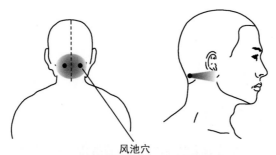

风池穴

定位：项部枕骨下，斜方肌上部外缘与胸
　　　锁乳突肌上端后缘之间凹陷处
功效：疏风解表，清利头目，宣通鼻窍

图 3-20-3　风池穴双点灸

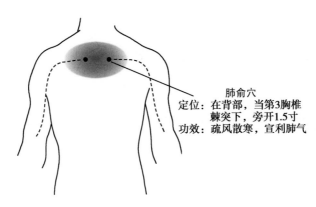

肺俞穴

定位：在背部，当第3胸椎
　　　棘突下，旁开1.5寸
功效：疏风散寒，宣利肺气

图 3-20-4　肺俞穴双点灸

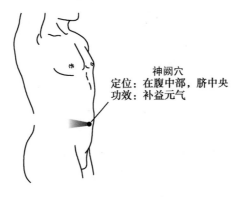

神阙穴

定位：在腹中部，脐中央
功效：补益元气

图 3-20-5　神阙穴单点灸

（三）量因人异，敏消量足

每次选取上述 2~3 组穴位，每天 1 次，每次每穴的施灸时间以热敏灸感消失为度。10 次为 1 个疗程，疗程间休息 2~5 天，共 2~3 个疗程。

（四）灸后防护，巩固疗效

1. 热敏灸温阳通气，增强免疫力，能有效治疗过敏性鼻炎。
2. 尽量远离变应原，注意气候变化，防寒保暖，加强锻炼，增强抵抗力。

【验案举例】

康先生，50 岁，晨起流清涕、鼻塞、打喷嚏 6 年。近 1 年来症状加重，医院诊断为过敏性鼻炎。右肺俞穴、上印堂穴探及穴位热敏。对右肺俞穴施单点灸，温热感逐渐扩散，几分钟后感整个背部温热舒适，约 5 分钟后热流继续向内渗透，徐徐注入胸腔内，该灸感持续约 40 分钟后，热感范围变小，并感表面皮肤有灼热痛感，遂停灸。换灸上印堂穴，自觉热感扩散至整个前额，并觉前额紧压感，非常舒适，灸感持续约 20 分钟后渐回缩并感施灸点皮肤灼热，完成 1 次热敏灸治疗。继续按上述方案探敏治疗 10 次，症状消失。6 个月后随访，未见复发。

第二十一节　荨麻疹

荨麻疹俗称"风疹块"，是以异常瘙痒，皮肤出现成块、成片状风团为主要表现的疾病。其病因目前尚不完全清楚，主要因素是机体敏感性增强，皮肤、黏膜小血管扩张及通透性增加而出现的一种局限性水肿反应，产生红斑、风团，伴瘙痒。中医认为本病病位在肌肤腠理，多与风邪侵袭，或与胃肠积热有关。腠理不固，风邪侵袭，遏于肌肤，营卫不和，或素有胃肠积热，复感风邪，均可使病邪内不得疏泄，外不得透达，郁于腠理而发为本病。

【临床表现】

突然出现大小不等的红色或白色风团，数小时后又迅速消失，并不断成批发出。每日发出一批或几批，持续 1 周至 1 个月左右停止发出；慢性者反复发作，长达数周、数月甚至数年；黏膜也可受累：发生在胃肠道可有腹痛及腹泻，如生在喉头黏膜可有闷气、呼吸困难，甚至引起窒息；常有进食某种蛋白质类食物史或药物过敏史。如鱼、虾等海鲜；或对冷空气过敏；或体内有肠寄生虫、慢性病灶；或和日光，热，摩擦及压力等物理因素有关。

【灸法治则】

本病以祛风止痒治标，调和营血治本为基本治疗原则。根据肺主皮毛、肺与大肠相表里、督脉主一身之阳、脾主运化水湿等理论，选择相关穴位探感定位、辨敏施灸。

【治疗方案】

（一）探感选穴，准确定位

1. 高发穴区　热敏穴位高发区一般多位于肺俞、至阳、神阙、曲池、血海、三阴交等穴区，对这些部位进行穴位热敏探查常能发现热敏穴位。

2. 探查手法　在本病热敏穴位高发区，按下述步骤分别依序进行回旋、雀啄、往返、温和灸四步操作。

回旋灸 $\xrightarrow[\text{2分钟}]{\text{温热局部气血}}$ 雀啄灸 $\xrightarrow[\text{1分钟}]{\text{加强敏化}}$ 往返灸 $\xrightarrow[\text{1分钟}]{\text{激发经气}}$ 温和灸 $\xrightarrow[\text{2分钟}]{\text{发动传感}}$ 出现热敏灸感 $\longrightarrow$ 确定热敏穴位

3. 热敏灸感　灸肺俞、至阳穴，灸感多为透热、扩热、传热；灸神阙穴，灸感多为透热、扩热；灸曲池穴，灸感多为透热、传热；灸血海穴，灸感多为透热、传热；灸三阴交穴，灸感多为透热、传热。

（二）循序激发，辨敏施灸

按照以下顺序，择优选穴施灸：

肺俞穴双点灸→至阳穴单点灸→神阙穴单点灸→曲池穴双点灸→血海穴双点灸→三阴交穴双点灸。

上述热敏穴区不是每位患者全都出现，没有出现穴位热敏的就不做相应操作。

1. 肺俞穴双点灸　肺俞是肺气输注于背部的部位，可治本脏之疾，具有疏风散寒、宣利肺气的作用。患者可自觉热感透至胸腔或扩散至整个背部或热感向上肢传导，灸至热敏灸感消失（图3-21-1）。

2. 至阳穴单点灸　至阳位于督脉，具有温督通阳、固实卫表的作用。患者可自觉热感透至胸腔或沿背部正中向上传导或向上肢传至肘关节，灸至热敏灸感消失（图3-21-1）。

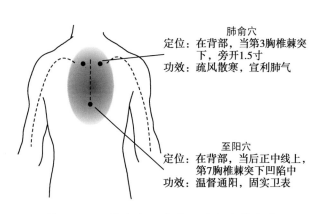

肺俞穴
定位：在背部，当第3胸椎棘突
　　　下，旁开1.5寸
功效：疏风散寒，宣利肺气

至阳穴
定位：在背部，当后正中线上，
　　　第7胸椎棘突下凹陷中
功效：温督通阳，固实卫表

图 3-21-1　肺俞穴双点灸、至阳穴单点灸

3. 神阙穴单点灸　神阙位于任脉，乃补益元气的要穴。患者可自觉热感深透至腹腔，灸至热敏灸感消失（图3-21-2）。

4. 曲池穴双点灸　曲池位于手阳明大肠经，具有解表、祛风、退热的作用。患者可自觉热感深透或向上或向下沿手阳明大肠经传导，灸至热敏灸感消失（图3-21-3）。

5. 血海穴双点灸　血海乃治疗皮肤病的要穴，"治风先治血，血行风自灭"，具有调血祛瘀的功效。患者可自觉热感深透或向上或向下沿足太阴脾经传导，灸至热敏灸感消失（图3-21-4）。

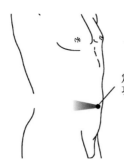

神阙穴
定位：在腹中部，脐中央
功效：补益元气

图 3-21-2　神阙穴单点灸

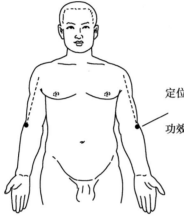

曲池穴
定位：在肘横纹外侧端，屈
　　　肘，当尺泽与肱骨外
　　　上髁连线中点
功效：解表，祛风，退热

图 3-21-3　曲池穴双点灸

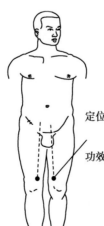

血海穴
定位：大腿内侧，髌底内侧
　　　端上2寸，当股四头肌
　　　内侧头隆起处
功效：调血祛瘀

图 3-21-4　血海穴双点灸

6. 三阴交穴双点灸 三阴交是足三阴经交会之穴，具有调血、补脾、养阴的功效。患者可自觉热感深透或向上或向下沿足太阴脾经传导，灸至热敏灸感消失（图3-21-5）。

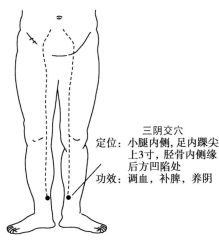

三阴交穴
定位：小腿内侧，足内踝尖
上3寸，胫骨内侧缘
后方凹陷处
功效：调血，补脾，养阴

图 3-21-5 三阴交穴双点灸

（三）量因人异，敏消量足

每次选取上述 2～3 组穴位，每天 1 次，每次每穴的施灸时间以热敏灸感消失为度。10 次为 1 个疗程，疗程间休息 2～5 天，共 2～3 个疗程。

（四）灸后防护，巩固疗效

1. 热敏灸祛风解表，活血通阳，调节免疫，改善内环境，对本症有一定疗效。但应积极寻找并去除病因。

2. 保持生活规律，加强体育锻炼，增强体质，适应寒热变化。

【验案举例】

黄女士，21 岁。荨麻疹病史 3 年。双上肢成团状红色皮疹伴瘙痒 1 天，口干、心烦。查体见双上肢成团状红色皮疹。热敏探查发现神阙穴、双肺俞穴透热和传热现象。予神阙穴、双肺俞穴温和灸，以祛风止痒，调和营血。神阙施单点灸时，患者立感热流向下腹部扩散，感下腹部温暖舒适，灸感持续约 30 分钟热流渐回缩至神阙穴，并感局部皮肤灼热，乃停灸神阙穴。换灸双肺俞穴，于数分钟后感热流如"水注"向皮肤深部灌注，感胸腔深部温热，并沿后背正中向上呈片状扩散，约 5 分钟后整个肩背部感到温热，灸感持续约 40 分钟后热流渐回缩至双侧肺俞穴，并感皮肤灼热后停灸，完成 1 次热敏灸治疗。继续按上述治疗方案探敏治疗 12 次，同时嘱每晚睡前自灸神阙穴 30 分钟，上述症状消失，3 个月后随访无复发。

🐚 第二十二节　颈椎病

颈椎病是指因颈椎退行性变引起颈椎管或椎间孔变形、狭窄，刺激、压迫颈部脊髓、神经根、交感神经造成其结构或功能损害所引起的一系列症状。最新观点认为，颈椎病的发生是退变或损伤导致颈椎动静力学平衡失调，出现异位压迫或化学刺激或免疫反应而引起。颈椎病的分类目前并不十分统一，常见分类为颈型、神经根型、椎动脉型、交感神经型、脊髓型、其他型等 6 型。中医学称本病为"项痹"，认为感受外邪、跌仆损伤、动作失度，可使项部经络气血运行不畅，故颈部疼痛、僵硬、酸胀；肝肾不足，气血亏损，督脉空虚，筋骨失养，气血不能养益脑窍，而出现头痛、头晕、耳鸣、耳聋；经络受阻，气血运行不畅，导致上肢疼痛麻木等症状。颈椎病主要与督脉和手、足太阳经密切相关。

【临床表现】

颈型：颈部症状如枕项部疼痛，肌肉僵硬，活动受限，局部压痛；X 线片提示生理曲度变化及不稳；除外颈部其他疾患。

神经根型：其主要症状病变在颈椎第 5 节以上者可见颈肩痛或颈枕痛及枕部麻木等；在颈椎第 5 节以下者可见颈僵，活动受限，有一侧或两侧颈、肩、臂放射痛，并伴有手指麻木，上肢发沉、无力，持物坠落等症状。

椎动脉型：常见症状为当头颈活动到某一位置时，突然发生眩晕及下肢麻木无力而摔倒，意识往往清楚；椎动脉造影对诊断有帮助。

交感神经型：主要表现为主观症状，如枕部疼痛、头沉、头晕或偏头痛、心慌、胸闷、肢凉或手足发热、四肢酸胀等。

脊髓型：其临床表现可见上肢或下肢、一侧或两侧的麻木、酸软无力，颈颤臂抖，甚者可表现为不同程度的全痉挛性瘫痪，如活动不便、步态笨拙、走路不稳，以致卧床不起，甚至呼吸困难，四肢僵硬等。

其他型：其他型如食管型颈椎病，颈椎椎体前鸟嘴样增生压迫食管引起吞咽困难等；此经食管钡剂造影可证实。

【灸法治则】

热敏灸对颈型、神经根型、椎动脉型三型较适宜。本病以活血通经，舒筋活络为基本治疗原则。根据"经气所过，主治所及"原则，以督脉、足太阳经、手太阳经、手阳明经穴和夹脊穴为主，选择相关穴位探感定位、辨敏施灸。

【治疗方案】

（一）探感选穴，准确定位

1. 高发穴区　热敏穴位高发区一般多位于颈夹脊、肩井、风池、大椎、神庭、肺俞穴等穴区，对这些部位进行穴位热敏探查常能发现热敏穴位。

2. 探查手法　在本病热敏穴位高发区，按下述步骤分别依序进行回旋、雀啄、往返、温和灸四步操作。

回旋灸 $\xrightarrow[\text{2分钟}]{\text{温热局部气血}}$ 雀啄灸 $\xrightarrow[\text{1分钟}]{\text{加强敏化}}$ 往返灸 $\xrightarrow[\text{1分钟}]{\text{激发经气}}$ 温和灸 $\xrightarrow[\text{2分钟}]{\text{发动传感}}$ 出现热敏灸感 $\rightarrow$ 确定热敏穴位

3. 热敏灸感　灸颈夹脊穴，灸感多为透热、扩热、非热觉；灸肩井穴，灸感多为透热、扩热、非热觉；灸风池、大椎穴，灸感多为透热、扩热；灸肺俞穴，灸感多为透热、扩热；灸神庭穴，灸感多为扩热、传热。

（二）循序激发，辨敏施灸

按照以下顺序，择优选穴施灸：

颈型：颈夹脊穴压痛点单点灸→肩井穴压痛点单点灸→风池、大椎穴温和灸；

神经根型：颈夹脊穴压痛点单点灸→肩井穴压痛点单点灸→大椎、肺俞穴温和灸；

椎动脉型：神庭、大椎穴双点灸。

上述热敏穴区不是每位患者全都出现，没有出现穴位热敏的就不做相应操作。

Ⅰ. 颈型

1. 颈夹脊穴压痛点单点灸　患者可自觉热感透向项背部并向四周扩散或自觉项背部有紧、压、酸、胀、痛感，灸至热敏灸感消失（图3-22-1）。

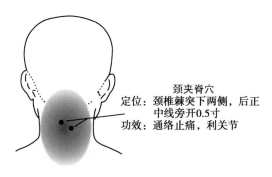

颈夹脊穴
定位：颈椎棘突下两侧，后正中线旁开0.5寸
功效：通络止痛，利关节

图 3-22-1　颈夹脊穴压痛点单点灸

2. 肩井穴压痛点单点灸　患者可自觉热感向项背部及上肢扩散或自觉肩部有紧、压、酸、胀、痛感，灸至热敏灸感消失（图3-22-2）。

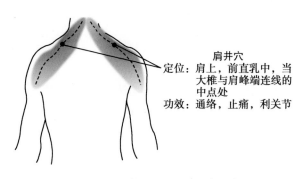

肩井穴
定位：肩上，前直乳中，当大椎与肩峰端连线的中点处
功效：通络，止痛，利关节

图 3-22-2　肩井穴压痛点单点灸

3．风池、大椎穴温和灸　风池、大椎穴均为头颈部要穴，合用能疏风解表、通络止痛。患者可自觉热感沿督脉传至项背部，灸至热敏灸感消失（图 3-22-3）。

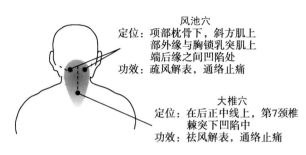

风池穴
定位：项部枕骨下，斜方肌上部外缘与胸锁乳突肌上端后缘之间凹陷处
功效：疏风解表，通络止痛

大椎穴
定位：在后正中线上，第7颈椎棘突下凹陷中
功效：祛风解表，通络止痛

图 3-22-3　风池、大椎穴温和灸

Ⅱ．神经根型

1．颈夹脊穴压痛点单点灸　自觉热感透向项背部并向四周扩散或自觉项背部有紧、压、酸、胀、痛感，灸至热敏灸感消失（图 3-22-4）。

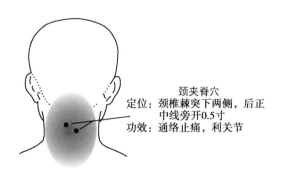

颈夹脊穴
定位：颈椎棘突下两侧，后正中线旁开0.5寸
功效：通络止痛，利关节

图 3-22-4　颈夹脊穴压痛点单点灸

2．肩井穴压痛点单点灸　自觉热感透向项背部及向上肢扩散或自觉肩部有紧、压、酸、胀、痛感，灸至热敏灸感消失（图 3-22-5）。

3．大椎、肺俞穴温和灸　大椎、肺俞穴合用重在疏风、解表、散寒、止痛。患者可自觉热感向项背部及上肢扩散传导至腕部；如感传不能至腕部，可再取一支点燃的艾条放置于感传所达部位的端点，进行温和灸，依次接力使感传到达腕部，灸至热敏灸感消失（图 3-22-6）。

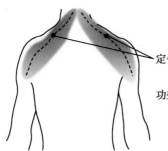

肩井穴
定位：肩上，前直乳中，当
大椎与肩峰端连线的
中点处
功效：通络，止痛，利关节

图 3-22-5　肩井穴压痛点单点灸

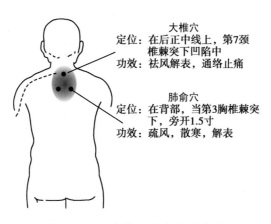

大椎穴
定位：在后正中线上，第7颈
椎棘突下凹陷中
功效：祛风解表，通络止痛

肺俞穴
定位：在背部，当第3胸椎棘突
下，旁开1.5寸
功效：疏风，散寒，解表

图 3-22-6　大椎、肺俞穴温和灸

Ⅲ. 椎动脉型

神庭、大椎穴双点灸　神庭、大椎均位于督脉，合用能祛风、通络、止痛。患者自觉热感透向穴位深部或发生扩热、传热，灸至热敏灸感消失（图 3-22-7）。

（三）量因人异，敏消量足

每次选取上述 2～3 组穴位，每天 1～2 次，每次每穴的施灸时间以热敏灸感消失为度。10 次为 1 个疗程，疗程间休息 2～5 天，共 2～3 个疗程。

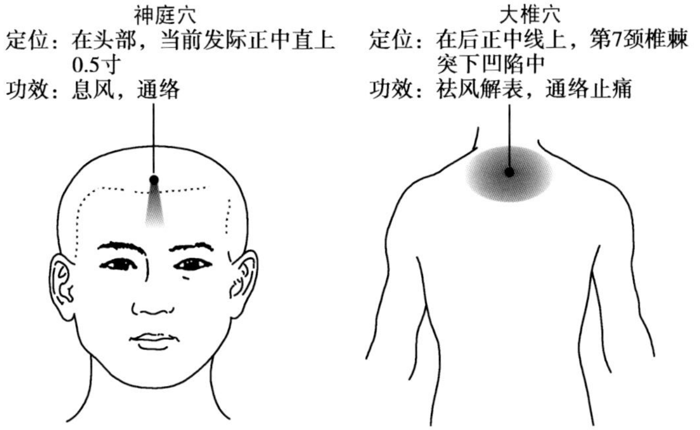

神庭穴
定位：在头部，当前发际正中直上
0.5寸
功效：息风，通络

大椎穴
定位：在后正中线上，第7颈椎棘
突下凹陷中
功效：祛风解表，通络止痛

图 3-22-7 神庭、大椎穴双点灸

（四）灸后防护，巩固疗效

1. 热敏灸能祛寒化湿、温通经脉，对于颈椎病的治疗、预防均有良好效果。

2. 低枕平卧休息，劳逸结合，减少颈部劳损，防风寒，适当进行颈项功能锻炼。

【验案举例】

姚女士，28岁。颈项部酸痛2年，加重伴头晕1周。患者就诊前1周因伏案工作时间较长而引起颈项部酸痛，时伴头晕症状，X线片示颈椎退行性变。在双侧风池穴探及穴位热敏，施行双点灸，5分钟后感热流徐徐入里，并扩散成片，整个后枕部温热舒适。40分钟后热流渐回缩至双侧风池穴，并感皮肤灼热，遂停灸，完成1次热敏灸治疗，患者灸后即感头晕症状减轻。第2日又在大椎处探及穴位热敏，故在双侧风池穴、大椎穴施灸，患者感热向里渗透，并感三处热流汇合沿督脉向上传导直至神庭穴处，30分钟后热流回缩至风池穴，并感皮肤灼热，遂停灸，完成1次热敏灸治疗。后按上法探敏治疗，每日1次，连续治疗10天，症状消失，3个月后随访无复发。

第二十三节 肩周炎

肩周炎是肩周围肌肉、肌腱、滑囊及关节囊的慢性损伤性炎症。肩周炎并非单一病因的疾病，其发生与组织退行性变、慢性劳损、外伤及风寒湿邪侵袭有关。本病中医称"漏肩风"，多因体虚、劳损、风寒侵袭肩部，使经气不利所致。肩部感受风寒，阻痹气血；或劳作过度、外伤，损及筋脉，气滞血瘀；或年老气血不足，筋骨失养，皆可使肩部脉络气血不利，不通则痛。肩部主要归手三阳所主，内外因素导致肩部经络阻滞不通或失养是本病的主要病机。

【临床表现】

主要表现为肩部疼痛，活动受限。早期其痛可向颈部和上臂放散，或呈弥散性疼痛，静止痛为其特征，表现为日轻夜重，晚间常可痛醒，晨起肩关节稍活动后疼痛可减轻。由于疼痛，肩关节活动明显受限。后期病变组织产生粘连，功能障碍加重，而疼痛程度减轻。

【灸法治则】

本病以祛风散寒、疏通经络、活血止痛为基本治疗原则。根据局部配合远端穴位理论，以手太阳、手阳明、手少阳经穴为主，选择相关穴位探感定位、辨敏施灸。

【治疗方案】

（一）探感选穴，准确定位

1. 高发穴区　热敏穴位高发区一般多位于肩部压痛点、膏肓、肩井、肩髃等穴区。对这些部位进行穴位热敏探查常能发现热敏穴位。

2. 探查手法　在本病热敏穴位高发区，按下述步骤分别依序进行回旋、雀啄、往返、温和灸四步操作。

回旋灸 → 温热局部气血 2分钟 → 雀啄灸 → 加强敏化 1分钟 → 往返灸 → 激发经气 1分钟 → 温和灸 → 发动传感 2分钟 → 出现热敏灸感 → 确定热敏穴位

3．**热敏灸感** 灸肩部压痛点、肩髃穴，灸感多为透热、扩热、非热觉；灸膏肓穴，灸感多为传热、透热；灸肩井穴，灸感多为透热、扩热、传热、非热觉。

（二）循序激发，辨敏施灸

按照以下顺序，择优选穴施灸：

肩部压痛点、肩髃穴双点灸→膏肓穴患侧单点灸→肩井穴患侧单点灸。

上述热敏穴区不是每位患者全都出现，没有出现穴位热敏的就不做相应操作。

1．**肩部压痛点、肩髃穴双点灸** 患者可自觉热感透向深部并向四周扩散或自觉酸、胀、痛感，灸至热敏灸感消失（图 3-23-1）。

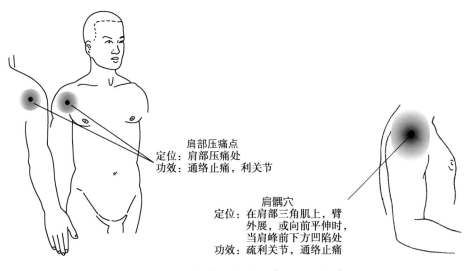

图 3-23-1 肩部压痛点、肩髃穴双点灸

2．**膏肓穴患侧单点灸** 膏肓位于足太阳膀胱经，具有通经理气、疏利关节的作用。患者可自觉热感沿腋下及上臂后内侧传至肘关节，灸至热敏灸感消失（图 3-23-2）。

3．**肩井穴患侧单点灸** 患者可自觉热感透向深部并向四周扩散或有紧、压、酸、胀、痛感或热感沿上肢传导；部分患者的感传可直接到腕部；如感传仍不能传至腕部，再取一支点燃的艾条分别放置于肩髃、臂臑、曲池、手三里、外关穴进行温和灸，依次接力使感传到达手背部，最后将两支艾条分别固定于肩井穴和手三里穴进行温和灸，灸至热敏灸感消失（图 3-23-3，图 3-23-4）。

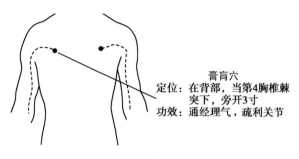

膏肓穴
定位：在背部，当第4胸椎棘突下，旁开3寸
功效：通经理气，疏利关节

图 3-23-2　膏肓穴患侧单点灸

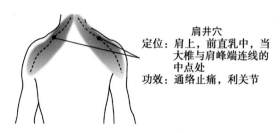

肩井穴
定位：肩上，前直乳中，当大椎与肩峰端连线的中点处
功效：通络止痛，利关节

图 3-23-3　肩井穴患侧单点灸

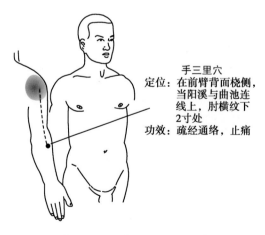

手三里穴
定位：在前臂背面桡侧，当阳溪与曲池连线上，肘横纹下2寸处
功效：疏经通络，止痛

图 3-23-4　手三里穴温和灸

（三）量因人异，敏消量足

每次选取上述 1～2 组穴位，每天 1 次，每次每穴的施灸时间以热敏灸感消失为度。10 次为 1 个疗程，疗程间休息 2～5 天，共 2～3 个疗程。

（四）灸后防护，巩固疗效

1. 热敏灸疏通经络以消炎镇痛，亦可行无痛瘢痕灸，治疗肩周炎往往能收到奇特疗效。

2. 肩周炎经治疗疼痛缓解后，应积极进行肩关节的功能锻炼，促进康复。

【验案举例】

李女士，66 岁，左肩关节酸胀疼痛、活动受限 1 个月，诊断为肩周炎。在患者左肩外侧压痛点、肩髃穴区可探及穴位热敏，遂施行双点灸，5 分钟后患者感压痛点局部透热，且酸胀明显，肩髃穴区出现透热现象，患者感热徐徐向里渗透，持续时间达 30 分钟，后感透热及酸胀现象消失，遂停灸。灸后患者即感肩部温暖舒适，疼痛稍解。第 2 天复诊，左肩关节活动度增加，疼痛较前减轻。按上法探敏治疗 15 次后，左肩关节已无疼痛，活动基本正常，3 个月后随访无复发。

第二十四节　腰椎间盘突出症

腰椎间盘突出症主要是由于腰椎间盘退行性改变，椎间盘纤维环破裂，髓核突出，刺激或压迫相邻组织如脊神经根、脊髓等，从而产生腰部疼痛，一侧或双下肢麻木、疼痛等临床症状。本病多由损伤、劳损及受寒等所致。以 L4～L5、L5～S1 间隙发病率最高，占腰椎间盘突出症的 90%～96%，一般多个腰椎间盘同时发病者较少，占 5%～22%。本病属于中医学的"腰痛"范畴，中医学认为外伤或劳损可致瘀血阻滞筋脉，不通则痛；或寒湿、湿热之邪侵犯腰部经络，导致经脉不通；肝肾亏虚，肾主骨，筋骨失养，遂致本病。根据经络学说，足太阳膀胱经夹脊抵于腰，督脉贯脊循行于腰部，足少阴肾经"贯脊属肾"，又有腰为肾之府之称，故腰痛多与足太阳经、督脉和足少阴经脉、经筋病变有关。

【临床表现】

常有腰部外伤、慢性劳损或感受寒湿史；腰部及臀部感觉疼痛不适；一侧下肢或两侧下肢麻木、放射性疼痛，咳嗽喷嚏时疼痛加重。

【灸法治则】

本病以祛风散寒、活血通经、疏调经筋为基本治疗原则。根据循经远端配穴理论，主要在督脉、足太阳、足少阳经穴等选择相关穴位探感定位、辨敏施灸。

【治疗方案】

（一）探感选穴，准确定位

1. 高发穴区　热敏穴位高发区一般多位于至阳、命门、腰俞、腰部压痛点、关元俞等穴区，对这些部位进行穴位热敏探查常能发现热敏穴位。

2. 探查手法　在本病热敏穴位高发区，按下述步骤分别依序进行回旋、雀啄、往返、温和灸四步操作。

回旋灸 —温热局部气血→ 雀啄灸 —加强敏化→ 往返灸 —激发经气→ 温和灸 —发动传感→ 出现热敏灸感 → 确定热敏穴位
　　　　　2分钟　　　　　　　　1分钟　　　　　　　1分钟　　　　　　　2分钟

3. 热敏灸感　灸至阳、命门、腰俞穴，灸感多为透热、传热；灸腰部压痛点，灸感多为透热、扩热、非热觉；灸关元俞，灸感多为扩热、传热、透热、非热觉。

（二）循序激发，辨敏施灸

按照以下顺序，择优选穴施灸：

至阳、命门、腰俞穴循经往返灸和接力灸→腰部压痛点单点灸→关元俞患侧单点灸。

　　上述热敏穴区不是每位患者全都出现，没有出现穴位热敏的就不做相应操作。

　　1. 至阳、命门、腰俞穴循经往返灸和接力灸　振奋督脉阳气。至阳、命门、腰俞穴均位于督脉，合用共奏补肾气、强腰脊、通络止痛的功效。患者可觉热感沿背腰骶部督脉传导，灸至热敏灸感消失（图3-24-1）。

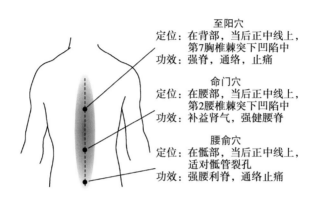

至阳穴
定位：在背部，当后正中线上，
第7胸椎棘突下凹陷中
功效：强脊，通络，止痛

命门穴
定位：在腰部，当后正中线上，
第2腰椎棘突下凹陷中
功效：补益肾气，强健腰脊

腰俞穴
定位：在骶部，当后正中线上，
适对骶管裂孔
功效：强腰利脊，通络止痛

图3-24-1　至阳、命门、腰俞穴循经往返灸和接力灸

　　2. 腰部压痛点单点灸　患者可自觉热感透向深部甚至腹腔或向四周扩散或自觉局部有紧、压、酸、胀、痛感或向下肢传导，灸至热敏灸感消失（图3-24-2）。

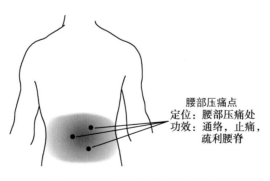

腰部压痛点
定位：腰部压痛处
功效：通络，止痛，
疏利腰脊

图3-24-2　腰部压痛点单点灸

　　3. 关元俞患侧单点灸　关元俞和承扶、委中、阳陵泉、昆仑穴位于足太阳膀胱经和足少阳胆经，合用主要起到通经活络、利腰脊止痛的功

效。患者可自觉热感透向深部并向四周扩散或有紧、压、酸、胀、痛感或热感沿下肢传导；部分患者的感传可直接到达足跟部；如感传仍不能传至足跟部，再取一支点燃的艾条分别放置于承扶、委中、阳陵泉、昆仑穴进行温和灸，依次接力使感传到达足跟部，最后将两支艾条分别固定于昆仑和关元俞进行温和灸，灸至热敏灸感消失（图3-24-3）。

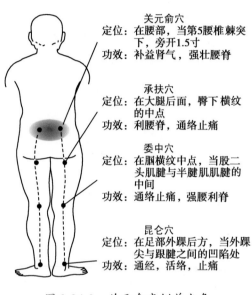

关元俞穴
定位：在腰部，当第5腰椎棘突下，旁开1.5寸
功效：补益肾气，强壮腰脊

承扶穴
定位：在大腿后面，臀下横纹的中点
功效：利腰脊，通络止痛

委中穴
定位：在腘横纹中点，当股二头肌腱与半腱肌肌腱的中间
功效：通络止痛，强腰利脊

昆仑穴
定位：在足部外踝后方，当外踝尖与跟腱之间的凹陷处
功效：通经，活络，止痛

图 3-24-3 关元俞患侧单点灸

（三）量因人异，敏消量足

每次选取上述1~2组穴位，每天1次，每次每穴的施灸时间以热敏灸感消失为度。10次为1个疗程，疗程间休息2~5天，共1~2个疗程。

（四）灸后防护，巩固疗效

1. 热敏灸疏通经气，消炎镇痛，改善循环，对急性期与恢复期的腰椎间盘突出症非手术治疗，具有独特的疗效优势。

2. 急性期应睡硬板床，卧床休息，以减少突出物对神经根的刺激。症状明显好转后，可逐步进行背肌锻炼，并在护腰带保护下下地做轻微活动。

【验案举例】

王先生，45 岁，有腰椎间盘突出症病史。10 天前因受寒腰部疼痛又发，右腰部疼痛伴右下肢放射痛，虽经牵引、按摩及药物治疗，疗效不佳。在右关元俞处探及穴位热敏。于右关元俞施单点灸，数分钟后右足背局部感到温热，灸感持续约 15 分钟后，感热流下传至右阳陵泉穴附近，非常舒适。灸感持续长达 2 小时后热流渐回缩至右关元俞并感皮肤灼热，乃停灸，完成 1 次热敏灸治疗。灸后腰部疼痛明显减轻，右下肢外侧无放射痛。继续按上述治疗方案探敏治疗 12 次后，患者诉腰部已无任何不适，下肢活动自如。半年后随访，未见复发。

第二十五节　膝关节骨性关节炎

膝关节骨性关节炎是指关节软骨出现原发性或继发性退行性改变，并伴软骨下骨质增生，从而使关节逐渐被破坏及产生畸形，影响膝关节功能的一种退行性疾病。中医将本病称为"骨痹"，认为肾为先天之本而主骨，骨的病变属于肾；因此，骨关节炎的发病主要由于年老体衰，肝肾亏虚，气血凝滞，复感风寒湿热之邪而经络气血阻滞，迁延日久，邪实正虚日益加重而形成骨痹。

【临床表现】

膝关节疼痛或僵硬感，行走和上下楼梯时疼痛明显；膝关节活动受限、肿胀，行走时膝关节摇摆不稳；晨僵，清晨一开始活动时，感膝盖发硬、沉重、迟钝且疼痛；膝关节活动时有骨响声。

【灸法治则】

本病以养肾柔筋通络为基本治疗原则。针灸治疗的基本目的是缓解疼痛、改善功能、延缓疾病的进程及保护关节功能。根据《内经》"在骨守骨，在筋守筋"的理论，以局部选穴为主，配合循经选择相关穴位探感定位、辨敏施灸。

【治疗方案】

（一）探感选穴，准确定位

1. 高发穴区　热敏穴位高发区一般多位于局部压痛点、内膝眼、外膝眼、鹤顶、梁丘、阴陵泉、血海、阳陵泉等穴区。对这些部位进行穴位热敏探查常能发现热敏穴位。

2. 探查手法　在本病热敏穴位高发区，按下述步骤分别依序进行回旋、雀啄、往返、温和灸四步操作。

回旋灸 $\xrightarrow[2分钟]{温热局部气血}$ 雀啄灸 $\xrightarrow[1分钟]{加强敏化}$ 往返灸 $\xrightarrow[1分钟]{激发经气}$ 温和灸 $\xrightarrow[2分钟]{发动传感}$ 出现热敏灸感 $\rightarrow$ 确定热敏穴位

3. 热敏灸感　灸膝部压痛点，灸感多为透热、扩热、非热觉；灸内、外膝眼穴，灸感多为透热、扩热；灸鹤顶穴，灸感多为透热、扩热；灸梁丘、阴陵泉穴，灸感多为传热、透热；灸血海、阳陵泉穴，灸感多为传热、透热。

（二）循序激发，辨敏施灸

按照以下顺序，择优选穴施灸：

膝部压痛点单点灸→内、外膝眼穴患侧双点灸→鹤顶穴单点灸→梁丘、阴陵泉穴双点灸→血海、阳陵泉穴双点灸。

上述热敏穴区不是每位患者全都出现，没有出现穴位热敏的就不做相应操作。

1. 膝部压痛点单点灸　患者可自觉热感透至膝关节内或扩散至整个膝关节或局部有酸、胀、痛感，灸至热敏灸感消失（图 3-25-1）。

2. 内、外膝眼穴患侧双点灸　内、外膝眼均位于髌骨底，具有通络止痛、利关节的作用。患者可自觉热感透至膝关节内并扩散至整个膝关节，灸至热敏灸感消失（图 3-25-2）。

3. 鹤顶穴单点灸　鹤顶是经外奇穴，具有行气活血、通络止痛的功

效。患者可自觉热感透至膝关节内并扩散至整个膝关节，灸至热敏灸感消失（图 3-25-3）

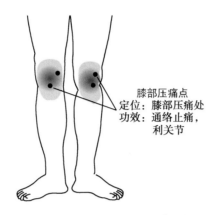

膝部压痛点
定位：膝部压痛处
功效：通络止痛，
利关节

图 3-25-1 膝部压痛点单点灸

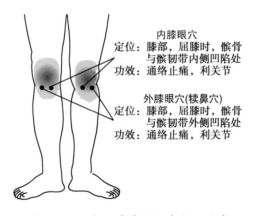

内膝眼穴
定位：膝部，屈膝时，髌骨
与髌韧带内侧凹陷处
功效：通络止痛，利关节

外膝眼穴(犊鼻穴)
定位：膝部，屈膝时，髌骨
与髌韧带外侧凹陷处
功效：通络止痛，利关节

图 3-25-2 内、外膝眼穴患侧双点灸

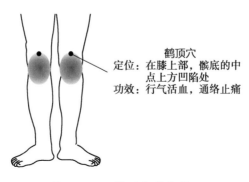

鹤顶穴
定位：在膝上部，髌底的中
点上方凹陷处
功效：行气活血，通络止痛

图 3-25-3 鹤顶穴单点灸

4．梁丘、阴陵泉穴双点灸　梁丘是胃经郄穴，阴陵泉是脾经合穴，两者合用具有祛风湿、利关节的作用。患者可自觉热感透至膝关节内并扩散至整个膝关节，灸至热敏灸感消失（图 3-25-4）。

5．血海、阳陵泉穴双点灸　血海能够调血祛瘀、通络止痛，阳陵泉具有舒筋、通络、利关节的作用。患者可自觉热感透至膝关节内并扩散至整个膝关节，灸至热敏灸感消失（图 3-25-5）。

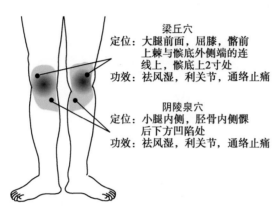

梁丘穴
定位：大腿前面，屈膝，髂前
　　　上棘与髌底外侧端的连
　　　线上，髌底上2寸处
功效：祛风湿，利关节，通络止痛

阴陵泉穴
定位：小腿内侧，胫骨内侧髁
　　　后下方凹陷处
功效：祛风湿，利关节，通络止痛

图 3-25-4　梁丘、阴陵泉穴双点灸

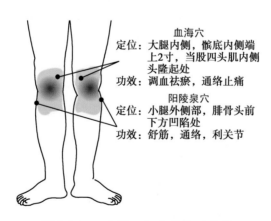

血海穴
定位：大腿内侧，髌底内侧端
　　　上2寸，当股四头肌内侧
　　　头隆起处
功效：调血祛瘀，通络止痛

阳陵泉穴
定位：小腿外侧部，腓骨头前
　　　下方凹陷处
功效：舒筋，通络，利关节

图 3-25-5　血海、阳陵泉穴双点灸

（三）量因人异，敏消量足

每次选取上述 1～2 组穴位，每天 1 次，每次每穴的施灸时间以热敏灸感消失为度。10 次为 1 个疗程，疗程间休息 2～5 天，共 2～3 个疗程。

（四）灸后防护，巩固疗效

1. 热敏灸疏通经气，消炎镇痛，改善循环，对膝关节骨性关节炎（伴肿胀）疗效可靠，可作为保守治疗的首选疗法。

2. 注意膝关节的防寒保暖，增强体质，减轻体重，避免久行、久立。

【验案举例】

何先生，56 岁，右膝关节酸痛、肿胀 3 年。现行走不便，下蹲困难，诊断为膝关节骨性关节炎。在右内膝眼穴处探及穴位热敏，当即对右内膝眼穴施单点灸，于数秒钟后感热流如"水注"向皮肤深部灌注，约 5 分钟后，感热流内传至整个膝关节深部，并感膝关节深部酸痛。40 分钟后，膝关节深部酸痛感消失，但仍有热感，50 分钟后热感消失，并感皮肤灼热疼痛，右内膝眼穴停灸，结束 1 次热敏灸治疗。灸后感右膝关节疼痛明显减轻，休息时不感疼痛。按上述治疗方案治疗 10 次，平地步行时不感疼痛，膝关节肿胀明显减轻，仅于上下楼梯时稍感右膝关节酸痛，下蹲已无困难。继续按以上方案探敏治疗 20 次，右膝关节行走时已无不适。

第二十六节　肌筋膜疼痛综合征

肌筋膜疼痛综合征又称肌筋膜炎，由于肌肉和筋膜的无菌性炎症刺激体表小神经而出现疼痛。主要发生在颈部和腰背部肌筋膜，也可发生在四肢等活动频繁的肌肉群。本病多发生于潮湿寒冷环境下野外工作者，慢性劳损为另一个重要的发病因素，见于腰背部长期超负荷劳动的人群。本病属中医学"痹证"范畴，多由久卧湿地，贪凉或劳累后复感寒邪，风寒湿邪侵入机体，寒凝血滞，使肌筋气血运行不畅，经络痹阻不通；或劳作过度，筋脉受损，气血阻滞脉络；或素体虚弱，气血不足，筋脉失荣所致。

【临床表现】

其疼痛有以下 3 种：

（1）激痛点：其痛点较为固定，按压时，一触即发，产生剧痛，并向肢体远处传导。

（2）区域性疼痛：疼痛的部位常分布在一定的范围之内。

（3）区域疼痛的部位肌肉按压时有种绷紧带状感，沿绷紧带状区走行的某一点的剧烈点状触痛。

【灸法治则】

本病以疏通筋脉，活血止痛为基本原则。根据《内经》"在筋守筋"的理论，以局部阿是穴及经穴为主，如选择颈部、肩背部的阿是穴，手太阳、手少阳、手阳明经的背部腧穴。背部夹脊穴、足太阳膀胱经穴、督脉穴也是常选用的穴位。

【治疗方案】

（一）探感选穴，准确定位

1. 高发穴区　热敏穴位高发区多位于局部痛点穴、天柱、膏肓、至阳、腰阳关、大肠俞、手三里、阳陵泉等穴区，对这些部位进行穴位热敏探查常能发现热敏穴位。

2. 探查手法　在本病热敏穴位高发区，按下述步骤分别依序进行回旋、雀啄、往返、温和灸四步操作。

回旋灸 $\xrightarrow[\text{2分钟}]{\text{温热局部气血}}$ 雀啄灸 $\xrightarrow[\text{1分钟}]{\text{加强敏化}}$ 往返灸 $\xrightarrow[\text{1分钟}]{\text{激发经气}}$ 温和灸 $\xrightarrow[\text{2分钟}]{\text{发动传感}}$ 出现热敏灸感 $\rightarrow$ 确定热敏穴位

3. 热敏灸感　灸项背部压痛点，灸感多为透热、扩热、非热觉；灸天柱穴，灸感多为透热；灸膏肓、至阳穴，灸感多为透热、扩热、传热；灸腰骶部压痛点，灸感多为透热、扩热、非热觉；灸腰阳关、大肠俞穴，灸感多为透热、传热、扩热；灸上肢压痛点，灸感多为透热、扩热、非热觉；灸手三里穴，灸感多为传热、透热；灸下肢压痛点，灸感多为透热、传热、非热觉；灸阳陵泉穴，灸感多为传热、透热。

（二）循序激发，辨敏施灸

按照以下顺序，择优选穴施灸：

项背部：项背部压痛点温和灸→天柱穴双点灸→膏肓穴患侧单点灸→至阳穴单点灸。

腰骶部：腰骶部压痛点温和灸→腰阳关穴单点灸→大肠俞穴患侧单点灸。

上肢：上肢压痛点单点灸→手三里穴患侧单点灸。

下肢：下肢压痛点单点灸→阳陵泉穴患侧单点灸。

上述热敏穴区不是每位患者全都出现，没有出现穴位热敏的就不做相应操作。

Ⅰ. 项背部

1. **项背部压痛点温和灸** 患者可自觉热感透向深部并向四周扩散或自觉局部有紧、压、酸、胀、痛感，灸至热敏灸感消失（图 3-26-1）。

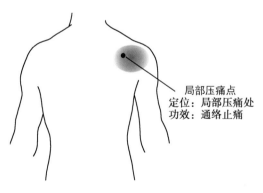

局部压痛点
定位：局部压痛处
功效：通络止痛

图 3-26-1 项背部压痛点温和灸

2. **天柱穴双点灸** 天柱穴属足太阳膀胱经，有通络止痛的功效。患者可觉热感向颅内渗透，灸至热敏灸感消失（图 3-26-2）。

3. **膏肓穴患侧单点灸** 膏肓位于足太阳膀胱经，具有通络止痛的作用。患者可自觉热感透向深部并向四周扩散或传至上肢；部分患者的感传可到达腕关节；如感传仍不能下至腕关节，再取一支点燃的艾条放置于感传所达部位的远心端点，进行温和灸，依次接力使感传到达腕关节，最后将两支艾条分别固定于膏肓和腕关节进行温和灸，灸至热敏灸感消失（图 3-26-3）。

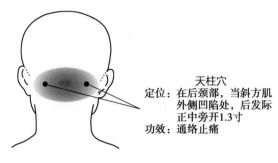

天柱穴
定位：在后颈部，当斜方肌
外侧凹陷处，后发际
正中旁开1.3寸
功效：通络止痛

图 3-26-2 天柱穴双点灸

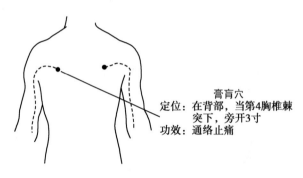

膏肓穴
定位：在背部，当第4胸椎棘
突下，旁开3寸
功效：通络止痛

图 3-26-3 膏肓穴患侧单点灸

4. 至阳穴单点灸 至阳位于督脉，具有温督、通阳、止痛的功效。患者可自觉热感深透或沿督脉向上向下传导或传至病痛部位，灸至热敏灸感消失（图 3-26-4）。

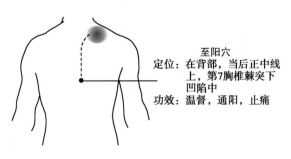

至阳穴
定位：在背部，当后正中线
上，第7胸椎棘突下
凹陷中
功效：温督，通阳，止痛

图 3-26-4 至阳穴单点灸

Ⅱ. 腰骶部

1. **腰骶部压痛点温和灸**　患者可自觉热感透向深部并向四周扩散或自觉局部有紧、压、酸、胀、痛感，灸至热敏灸感消失（图 3-26-5）。

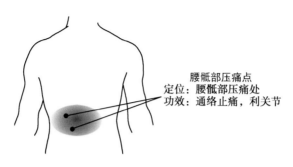

腰骶部压痛点
定位：腰骶部压痛处
功效：通络止痛，利关节

图 3-26-5　腰骶部压痛点温和灸

2. **腰阳关穴单点灸**　腰阳关位于督脉，具有温督散寒、通络止痛的作用。患者可自觉热感深透或沿督脉向上向下传导或传至病痛部位，灸至热敏灸感消失（图 3-26-6）。

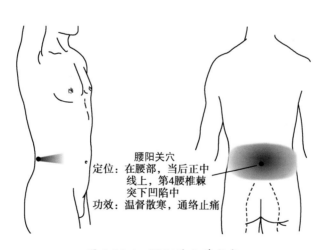

腰阳关穴
定位：在腰部，当后正中线上，第4腰椎棘突下凹陷中
功效：温督散寒，通络止痛

图 3-26-6　腰阳关穴单点灸

3. **大肠俞穴患侧单点灸**　大肠俞位于足太阳膀胱经，具有理气、通络、止痛的功效。患者可自觉热感透向深部并向四周扩散或传至下肢；部分患者的感传可到达踝关节；如感传仍不能下至踝关节，再取一支点燃的

艾条放置于感传所达部位的远心端点，进行温和灸，依次接力使感传到达踝关节，最后将两支艾条分别固定于大肠俞和踝关节进行温和灸，灸至热敏灸感消失（图3-26-7）。

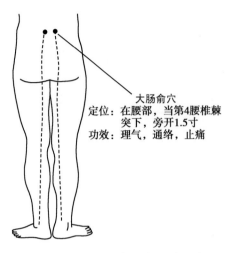

大肠俞穴
定位：在腰部，当第4腰椎棘
突下，旁开1.5寸
功效：理气，通络，止痛

图 3-26-7　大肠俞穴患侧单点灸

Ⅲ．上肢

1. **上肢压痛点单点灸**　患者可自觉热感透向深部并向四周扩散或自觉局部有紧、压、酸、胀、痛感，灸至热敏灸感消失（图3-26-8）。

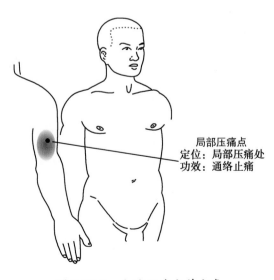

局部压痛点
定位：局部压痛处
功效：通络止痛

图 3-26-8　上肢压痛点单点灸

2．手三里穴患侧单点灸　手三里位于手阳明大肠经，具有疏经通络、消肿止痛的功效。患者可自觉热感深透或向上或向下沿手阳明大肠经传导，灸至热敏灸感消失（图3-26-9）。

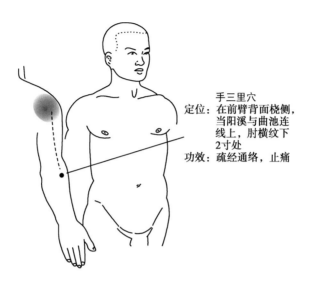

手三里穴

定位：在前臂背面桡侧，当阳溪与曲池连线上，肘横纹下2寸处

功效：疏经通络，止痛

图 3-26-9　手三里穴患侧单点灸

Ⅳ．下肢

1．下肢压痛点单点灸　患者可自觉热感透向深部并向四周扩散或自觉局部有紧、压、酸、胀、痛感，灸至热敏灸感消失（图3-26-10）。

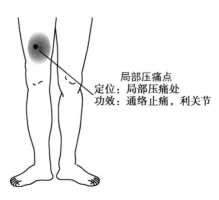

局部压痛点

定位：局部压痛处

功效：通络止痛，利关节

图 3-26-10　下肢压痛点单点灸

2．阳陵泉穴患侧单点灸　阳陵泉为胆经的合穴、属筋会，具有舒筋通络、止痛的作用。患者可自觉热感深透或向上或向下沿足少阳胆经传导，灸至热敏灸感消失（图3-26-11）。

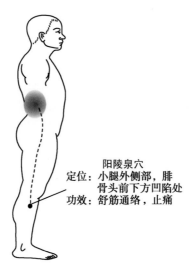

阳陵泉穴
定位：小腿外侧部，腓骨头前下方凹陷处
功效：舒筋通络，止痛

图3-26-11　阳陵泉穴患侧单点灸

（三）量因人异，敏消量足

每次于疼痛邻近区域选取上述2~3组穴位，每天1次，每次每穴的施灸时间以热敏灸感消失为度。10次为1个疗程，疗程间休息2~5天，共2个疗程。

（四）灸后防护，巩固疗效

1．热敏灸治疗本病疗效好，应早诊断早治疗。如已出现肌肉硬结，疗程会延长，必要时加穴位注射。

2．避风寒，慎起居，夏天不要贪凉席地而卧。

【验案举例】

赵某，女，38岁。患者1年前夜卧受寒后晨起感左侧颈项部酸胀疼痛不适，不能俯仰转颈，稍用力即感头枕部疼痛难忍，经针刺治疗后症状消失，后常因受寒而反复发作，热敷可稍缓解。5天前因吹空调受凉后颈项部疼痛剧烈，治疗后未见缓解。查体：舌质淡、苔白腻，脉浮紧，左侧颈项部肌肉僵硬，左侧天柱穴区明显压痛，颈椎 X 线正侧位片未见明显异常。经探查，天柱穴区可探及穴位热敏，即于天柱穴施行单点灸，约 1 分钟后感觉热流慢慢扩散开，并向枕内渗透，5 分钟后感觉整个后颈项部温热舒适，持续约 35 分钟后热感回缩至皮肤，皮肤灼热，遂停灸，完成 1 次热敏灸治疗。治疗后颈项部松软舒适，次日复诊，自诉颈项部酸胀疼痛感明显减轻，按上述方法继续探敏治疗 10 次，酸胀疼痛感消失，3 个月后随访，未闻复发。

第二十七节　肱骨外上髁炎

肱骨外上髁炎是肘部肌腱附着处慢性损伤性炎症，出现肘关节外上方及前臂的放射性疼痛不适感。一般起病缓慢，常反复发作，无明显外伤史，主要与长期旋转前臂、屈伸肘关节及肘部受震荡等因素有关。本病中医称"肘劳"或"伤筋"，病因主要为慢性劳损，前臂在反复地做拧、拉、旋转等动作时，可使肘部的筋脉慢性损伤，迁延日久，气血阻滞，脉络不通，不通则痛。肘外部主要归手三阳经所主，故手三阳经筋受损是本病的主要病机。

【临床表现】

本病好发于网球运动员、提琴手、水电工、家庭妇女等；肘外方痛：肘关节外侧疼痛，尤以前臂旋转、腕关节活动时明显，可沿前臂肌肉向下放射疼痛不适感，拧毛巾、扫地等动作时加重，握物无力，手不能平举重物。

【灸法治则】

本病以舒筋通络，止痛为基本治疗原则。在选穴上主要以局部选穴为主，可配合循经远端配穴，选择相关穴位探感定位，辨敏施灸。

【治疗方案】

（一）探感选穴，准确定位

1. **高发穴区** 热敏穴位高发区多位于局部压痛点、厥阴俞、手三里、阳陵泉（健侧）等穴区。对这些部位进行穴位热敏探查常能发现热敏穴位。

2. **探查手法** 在本病热敏穴位高发区，按下述步骤分别依序进行回旋、雀啄、往返、温和灸四步操作。

回旋灸 $\xrightarrow[\text{2分钟}]{\text{温热局部气血}}$ 雀啄灸 $\xrightarrow[\text{1分钟}]{\text{加强敏化}}$ 往返灸 $\xrightarrow[\text{1分钟}]{\text{激发经气}}$ 温和灸 $\xrightarrow[\text{2分钟}]{\text{发动传感}}$ 出现热敏灸感 $\rightarrow$ 确定热敏穴位

3. **热敏灸感** 灸局部压痛点，灸感多为透热、传热、非热觉；灸厥阴俞穴，灸感多为透热、扩热；灸手三里穴，灸感多为传热、透热；灸阳陵泉穴，灸感多为传热、透热。

（二）循序激发，辨敏施灸

按照以下顺序，择优选穴施灸：

局部压痛点单点灸→厥阴俞穴双点灸→手三里穴单点灸→阳陵泉穴健侧单点灸。

上述热敏穴区不是每位患者全都出现，没有出现穴位热敏的就不做相应操作。

1. **局部压痛点单点灸** 患者可自觉热感透向深部并向四周扩散或自觉深部有紧、压、酸、胀、痛感，灸至热敏灸感消失（图3-27-1）。

2. **厥阴俞穴双点灸** 厥阴俞位于足太阳膀胱经，具有祛风寒、通络止痛的功效。患者可自觉热感沿腋下及上臂后外侧传至肘关节处，灸至热敏灸感消失（图3-27-2）。

3. **手三里穴单点灸** 手三里位于手阳明大肠经，具有疏经通络、消肿止痛的功效。患者可自觉热感深透，或向上或向下沿手阳明大肠经传导，灸至热敏灸感消失（图3-27-3）。

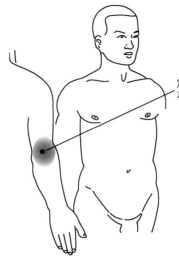

局部压痛点
定位：局部压痛处
功效：通络止痛，利关节

图 3-27-1 局部压痛点单点灸

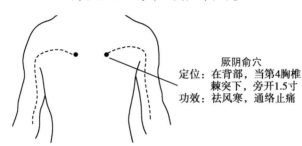

厥阴俞穴
定位：在背部，当第4胸椎
棘突下，旁开1.5寸
功效：祛风寒，通络止痛

图 3-27-2 厥阴俞穴双点灸

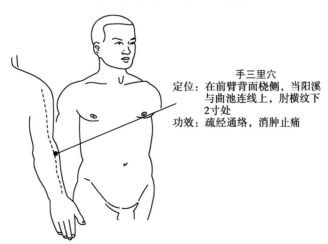

手三里穴
定位：在前臂背面桡侧，当阳溪
与曲池连线上，肘横纹下
2寸处
功效：疏经通络，消肿止痛

图 3-27-3 手三里穴单点灸

4．阳陵泉穴健侧单点灸　阳陵泉为胆经的合穴、属筋会，具有舒筋通络、止痛的作用。患者可自觉热感透向深部，或向上或向下沿足少阳胆经传导，或自觉局部有紧、压、酸、胀、痛感，灸至热敏灸感消失（图3-27-4）。

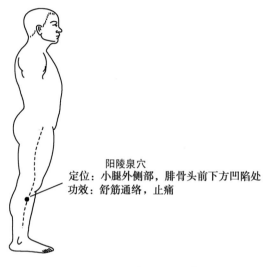

阳陵泉穴
定位：小腿外侧部，腓骨头前下方凹陷处
功效：舒筋通络，止痛

图 3-27-4　阳陵泉穴健侧单点灸

（三）量因人异，敏消量足

每次选取上述 1 ~ 2 组穴位，每天 1 次，每次每穴的施灸时间以热敏灸感消失为度。10 次为 1 个疗程，疗程间休息 2 ~ 5 天，共 2 个疗程。

（四）灸后防护，巩固疗效

1．热敏灸对无菌性炎症有较好的消炎镇痛作用。治愈后仍要防止肘部吹风、着凉，避免过劳，以免复发。

2．从事反复伸屈肘关节工作的中老年人，应注意劳逸结合，适度进行有针对性的锻炼。

【验案举例】

李女士，59 岁，右肘关节疼痛 2 个月，患者因常干家务引起右肘关节疼痛无力，提热水瓶、拧毛巾、扫地时疼痛加剧，局部压痛明显。在患者局部压痛处、手三里区可探及穴位热敏，遂施行双点灸，5 分钟后患者感压痛点的艾热向里渗透并向四周扩散，自觉压痛点深部有胀感，手三里有热徐徐向里渗透，患者感右肘关节温暖舒适，40 分钟后透热、扩热现象消失，患者感局部皮肤灼热，遂停灸。第 2 天复诊，右肘关节疼痛减轻，继续按上法探敏治疗 15 次，肘关节疼痛消失。3 个月后随访未复发。

第二十八节　强直性脊柱炎

强直性脊柱炎是一种主要侵犯脊柱，并累及骶髂关节和周围关节的慢性进行性炎性疾病。本病属中医"大偻""骨痹"范畴，多由肝肾亏虚，阳气不足，督脉失养，复感寒湿外邪，气血运行不畅，而致体内痰湿内生，瘀血阻络而致。

【临床表现】

强直性脊柱炎早期可无任何临床症状，有些患者在早期可表现出轻度的全身症状，如乏力、消瘦、长期或间断低热、厌食、轻度贫血等。以患者逐渐出现腰背部或骶髂部疼痛和 / 或发僵，夜间疼痛加重，翻身困难，晨起或久坐后起立时腰部发僵明显，但活动后减轻等为主要临床表现。

【灸法治则】

本病以祛寒化湿，活血通络，温脾益肾为基本治疗原则。在选穴上主要以局部选穴为主，可配合循经远端配穴，选择相关穴位探感定位，辨敏施灸。

【治疗方案】

（一）探感选穴，准确定位

1. 高发穴区　热敏穴位高发区多位于至阳、命门、腰俞、肾俞、足三里等穴区，对这些部位进行穴位热敏探查常能发现热敏穴位。

2. 探查手法 在本病热敏穴位高发区，按下述步骤分别依序进行回旋、雀啄、往返、温和灸四步操作。

回旋灸 →(温热局部气血 / 2分钟)→ 雀啄灸 →(加强敏化 / 1分钟)→ 往返灸 →(激发经气 / 1分钟)→ 温和灸 →(发动传感 / 2分钟)→ 出现热敏灸感 → 确定热敏穴位

3. 热敏灸感 灸至阳、命门、腰俞穴，灸感多为透热、传热；灸肾俞穴，灸感多为透热、扩热、传热；灸足三里穴，灸感多为传热、透热。

（二）循序激发，辨敏施灸

按照以下顺序，择优选穴施灸：

至阳、命门、腰俞穴循经往返灸和接力灸→肾俞穴双点灸→足三里穴双点灸。

上述热敏穴区不是每位患者全都出现，没有出现穴位热敏的就不做相应操作。

1. 至阳、命门、腰俞穴循经往返灸和接力灸 至阳、命门、腰俞穴皆为督脉要穴，督脉主一身阳气，三穴合用，温督通阳。患者可自觉热感沿头项背腰部督脉传导，灸至热敏灸感消失（图 3-28-1）。

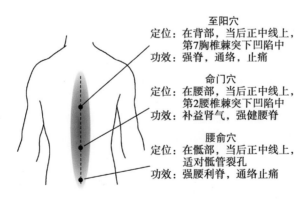

至阳穴
定位：在背部，当后正中线上，第7胸椎棘突下凹陷中
功效：强脊，通络，止痛

命门穴
定位：在腰部，当后正中线上，第2腰椎棘突下凹陷中
功效：补益肾气，强健腰脊

腰俞穴
定位：在骶部，当后正中线上，适对骶管裂孔
功效：强腰利脊，通络止痛

图 3-28-1 至阳、命门、腰俞穴循经往返灸和接力灸

2. 肾俞穴双点灸 肾俞是肾气血在背部的输注部位，具有补肾强腰、调和阴阳的功效。患者可自觉热感深透至腹腔或扩散至腰骶部或向下肢传导，灸至热敏灸感消失（图 3-28-2）。

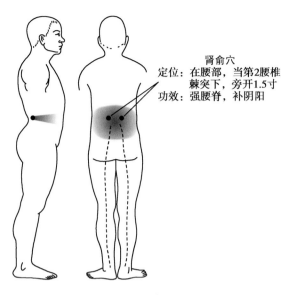

肾俞穴
定位：在腰部，当第2腰椎
棘突下，旁开1.5寸
功效：强腰脊，补阴阳

图 3-28-2　肾俞穴双点灸

3. 足三里穴双点灸　足三里是足阳明胃经的合穴，具有调理脾胃、补中益气的功效。部分患者的感传可直接到达腹部；如感传仍不能上至腹部者，再取一支点燃的艾条放置于感传所达部位的近心端点，进行温和灸，依次接力使感传到达腹部，最后将两支艾条分别固定于足三里和腹部进行温和灸，灸至热敏灸感消失（图 3-28-3）。

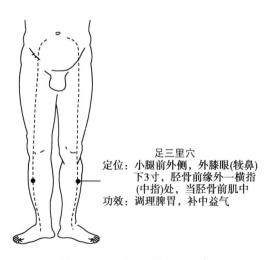

足三里穴
定位：小腿前外侧，外膝眼(犊鼻)
下3寸，胫骨前缘外一横指
(中指)处，当胫骨前肌中
功效：调理脾胃，补中益气

图 3-28-3　足三里穴双点灸

（三）量因人异，敏消量足

每次选取上述 1~2 组穴位，每天 1 次，每次每穴的施灸时间以热敏灸感消失为度。10 次为 1 个疗程，疗程间休息 2~5 天，共 2 个疗程。

（四）灸后防护，巩固疗效

1. 强直性脊柱炎是以疼痛、功能障碍、关节变形为主要表现的慢性炎症性病症，常规疗法效果平平。热敏灸具有温阳化湿、活血通络的作用，坚持 3 个月以上的治疗，疗效肯定。

2. 症状缓解后，巩固治疗很重要。可以辅助足三里麦粒灸强身健体，远期疗效更好。

【验案举例】

魏先生，36 岁。10 年前因背痛和晨起发僵，髋关节两侧交替疼痛，活动后减轻，在医院检查显示 HLA-B27 阳性，同时伴有低热、乏力、食欲减退、消瘦等症状，诊断为强直性脊柱炎。开始疼痛为间歇性，以后发展为持续性，曾注射过注射用重组人 Ⅱ 型肿瘤坏死因子受体 – 抗体融合蛋白（益赛普）及口服布洛芬、美洛昔康，后又口服中药 1 年多，症状无改善，无法正常生活和工作，于是接受热敏灸治疗。探查发现至阳穴附近出现透热现象，温和灸至阳穴 5 分钟后感觉热感向深部渗透至胸腔，持续 30 分钟。之后在双肾俞附近探查出传热，继续施灸传至腰骶部，持续 50 分钟。完成本次治疗，髋关节疼痛减轻。第 2 天复诊，在足三里穴区探查到传热现象，施接力灸，热感传至胯部。治疗 20 次后，腰胯部疼痛明显减轻，胯部功能活动明显好转，便坚持按疗程治疗（1 个疗程 10 天，停 2 天）。经 4 个多疗程治疗后，右腿已能伸直睡觉，并能站直腰走路，晨僵症状也消失，生活可以自理了。按上述方法继续热敏灸 25 次，症状基本消失。此后，一直坚持麦粒灸足三里保健，至今已 6 年，疼痛未再发，活动正常，精气神好。

第二十九节　干燥综合征

干燥综合征是一种侵犯外分泌腺体，尤以侵犯唾液腺和泪腺为主的慢性自身免疫性疾病。主要表现为口、眼干燥，也可有多器官、多系统损害。受累器官中有大量淋巴细胞浸润，血清中多种自身抗体阳性。本综合征也称为自身免疫性外分泌腺病、舍格伦综合征、口眼干燥关节炎综合征，常与其他风湿病或自身免疫性疾病重叠。本病中医属"燥痹"范畴，病因包括先天禀赋不足和后天致病因素，病机为阴液不足、气血亏虚、津液输布障碍、燥毒瘀互结，导致脏腑功能失调、阴阳失衡。

【临床表现】

临床上主要表现为干燥性角结膜炎和口腔干燥症，如口干、猖獗龋、涎腺炎、眼干涩等，还可累及内脏器官；全身症状可见乏力、低热等。

【灸法治则】

本病以益气生津为基本治疗原则。在选穴上主要以局部选穴为主，可配合循经远端配穴，选择相关穴位探感定位，辨敏施灸。

【治疗方案】

（一）探感选穴，准确定位

1. 高发穴区　热敏穴位高发区多位于中脘、神阙、关元等穴区，对这些部位进行穴位热敏探查常能发现热敏穴位。

2. 探查手法　在本病热敏穴位高发区，按下述步骤分别依序进行回旋、雀啄、往返、温和灸四步操作。

$$回旋灸 \xrightarrow[\text{2分钟}]{\text{温热局部气血}} 雀啄灸 \xrightarrow[\text{1分钟}]{\text{加强敏化}} 往返灸 \xrightarrow[\text{1分钟}]{\text{激发经气}} 温和灸 \xrightarrow[\text{2分钟}]{\text{发动传感}} 出现热敏灸感 \rightarrow 确定热敏穴位$$

3. 热敏灸感　灸中脘穴，灸感多为透热、扩热；灸神阙、关元穴，灸感多为透热。

（二）循序激发，辨敏施灸

按照以下顺序，择优选穴施灸：

中脘穴单点灸→关元穴单点灸→神阙穴单点灸。

上述热敏穴区不是每位患者全都出现，没有出现穴位热敏的就不做相应操作。

1. 中脘穴单点灸　中脘位于任脉，胃募穴，具有健脾益气的功效。患者可自觉热感透至腹腔内或扩散至整个上腹部，灸至热敏灸感消失（图 3-29-1）。

2. 关元穴单点灸　关元亦居任脉，是足三阴经的交会穴，具有益气生津的功效。患者可自觉热感透至腹腔内，灸至热敏灸感消失（图 3-29-1）。

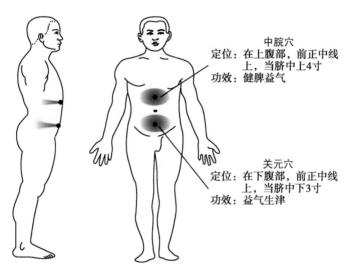

中脘穴
定位：在上腹部，前正中线
　　　上，当脐中上4寸
功效：健脾益气

关元穴
定位：在下腹部，前正中线
　　　上，当脐中下3寸
功效：益气生津

图 3-29-1　中脘穴、关元穴单点灸

3. 神阙穴单点灸　神阙为任脉禁针宜灸要穴，具有益气养阴的功效。患者可自觉热感透至腹腔，灸至热敏灸感消失（图 3-29-2）。

（三）量因人异，敏消量足

每次选取上述 1~2 组穴位，每天 1 次，每次每穴的施灸时间以热敏灸感消失为度。10 次为 1 个疗程，疗程间休息 2~5 天，共 2 个疗程。

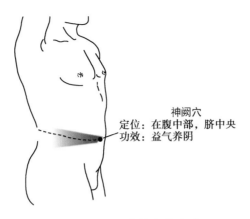

神阙穴
定位：在腹中部，脐中央
功效：益气养阴

图 3-29-2 神阙穴单点灸

（四）灸后防护，巩固疗效

1. 热敏灸能温补阳气，活血通络，阳生阴长，可达到益气生津之功效，对于阳虚型干燥综合征有显著疗效。

2. 可适当增加室内湿度，适当使用人工泪液滴眼，加强锻炼，保持心态平和。

【验案举例】

王先生，54 岁，双眼干涩、喜眨眼，需用人工泪液滴眼（7~8 次 /d）才能缓解 1 年。伴口干，稍进干食需喝水才能下咽，纳稍差，大便干，冬天手足不温，某省级医院诊断为干燥综合征。经查，可在中脘、关元穴处探及穴位热敏，第 1 天悬灸中脘穴时，约 20 分钟热感在上腹部开始扩散，同时渐渐透入胃脘，约 40 分钟灸感减弱，第 1 次治疗结束。第 2 天探查中脘与关元穴，关元穴更敏感，于是选取关元穴悬灸治疗，15 分钟后热感从两侧扩散至腰部，同时渐渐透入腹腔，且有明显舒畅感，约 50 分钟灸感消失。第 3 天患者自诉眼目干涩与口干稍有减轻，患者认为热敏灸治疗方案有效，于是坚持治疗。按照上述方案灸至 1 个月时，眼睛干涩、喜眨眼及口干症状好转。共治疗 3 个月，每周 3~4 次，患者偶有眨眼，口干、眼干明显改善，使用人工泪液滴眼 1~2 次 /d。3 个月后随访，效果稳定。

第三十节　癌性胸腹水

　　癌性胸腹水，也称为恶性胸腹腔积液，是中晚期癌症常见的并发症之一，也是部分患者的主要临床症状或体征，严重的胸腹水甚至可危及生命。本病属中医学"痰饮""臌胀"范畴。《素问·至真要大论》云："诸病水液，澄澈清冷，皆属于寒。"说明多由于脾肾阳虚、三焦水道不利，水液潴留，积为胸腹水。

【临床表现】

　　癌性胸腔积液常见于肺癌、乳腺癌，其次为恶性淋巴瘤、卵巢癌、恶性胸膜间皮瘤（多为血性积液）、食管癌、胃癌、贲门癌及病因不明的恶性肿瘤。主要表现为呼吸困难、胸痛、胸闷、气喘、咳嗽、体重下降、厌食等，少数患者起初无症状。癌性腹水常见于卵巢癌、肝癌、胃癌、胰腺癌、肠癌、子宫内膜癌等。主要表现为腹胀、纳差、乏力、消瘦、口干、口苦、黑便、双下肢水肿、大小便不利等。

【灸法治则】

　　本病以温阳利水为基本治疗原则。在选穴上主要以任脉选穴为主，可配合循经远端配穴，选择相关穴位探感定位，辨敏施灸。

【治疗方案】

（一）探感选穴，准确定位

　　1. 高发穴区　热敏穴位高发区多位于膻中、中脘、水分、关元、中极、脾俞等穴区。对这些部位进行穴位热敏探查常能发现热敏穴位。

　　2. 探查手法　在本病热敏穴位高发区，按下述步骤分别依序进行回旋、雀啄、往返、温和灸四步操作。

回旋灸 —温热局部气血 2分钟→ 雀啄灸 —加强敏化 1分钟→ 往返灸 —激发经气 1分钟→ 温和灸 —发动传感 2分钟→ 出现热敏灸感 → 确定热敏穴位

3. **热敏灸感**　灸膻中穴，灸感多为透热、扩热、传热；灸中脘穴，灸感多为透热、扩热；灸水分、关元、中极穴，灸感多为透热、扩热；灸脾俞穴，灸感多为透热、扩热。

（二）循序激发，辨敏施灸

按照以下顺序，择优选穴施灸：

膻中、中脘穴双点灸→水分穴单点灸→关元、中极双点灸→脾俞穴双点灸。

上述热敏穴区不是每位患者全都出现，没有出现穴位热敏的就不做相应操作。

1. **膻中、中脘穴双点灸**　膻中属任脉，心包募穴，八会穴之气会，具有宽胸理气、宣肺行水的功效，可出现热感扩散至胸部，或出现热流沿任脉上下循行，灸至热敏灸感消失。中脘位于任脉，胃募穴，具有宣肺利水的功效，可觉热感透至腹腔内或扩散至整个上腹部，灸至热敏灸感消失（图 3-30-1）。

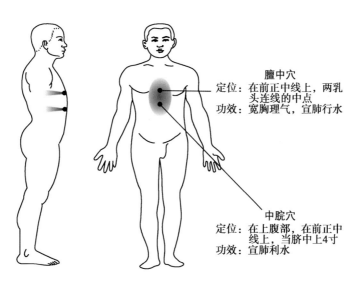

图 3-30-1　膻中、中脘穴双点灸

膻中穴
定位：在前正中线上，两乳头连线的中点
功效：宽胸理气，宣肺行水

中脘穴
定位：在上腹部，在前正中线上，当脐中上4寸
功效：宣肺利水

2. **水分穴单点灸**　水分属任脉，具有益气行水的功效，可出现热感渗透至腹腔内，灸至热敏灸感消失（图 3-30-2）。

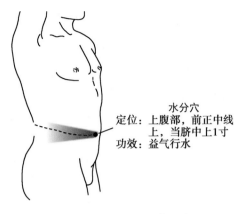

水分穴
定位：上腹部，前正中线
上，当脐中上1寸
功效：益气行水

图 3-30-2　水分穴单点灸

3．关元、中极穴双点灸　关元居任脉，是足三阴经的交会穴，具有培补元气、化气利水的功效。中极亦居任脉，具有补益肾气、通利水道的功效。患者可自觉热感透至腹腔内，灸至热敏灸感消失（图 3-30-3）。

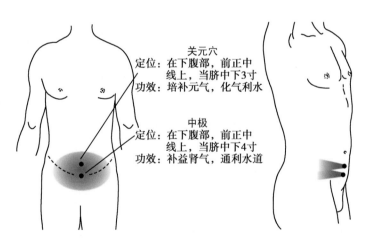

关元穴
定位：在下腹部，前正中
线上，当脐中下3寸
功效：培补元气，化气利水

中极
定位：在下腹部，前正中
线上，当脐中下4寸
功效：补益肾气，通利水道

图 3-30-3　关元、中极穴双点灸

4．脾俞穴双点灸　脾俞是脾气输注于背部的部位，可治本脏之疾，具有温脾益气、运化水湿的功效。患者常可觉热感透至深部或扩散至整个腰背部，灸至热敏灸感消失（图 3-30-4）。

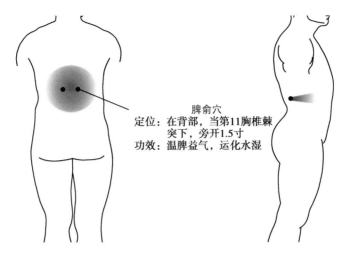

脾俞穴
定位：在背部，当第11胸椎棘突下，旁开1.5寸
功效：温脾益气，运化水湿

图 3-30-4　脾俞穴双点灸

（三）量因人异，敏消量足

每次选取上述 1～2 组穴位，每天 1 次，每次每穴的施灸时间以热敏灸感消失为度。10 次为 1 个疗程，疗程间休息 2～5 天，共 2 个疗程。

（四）灸后防护，巩固疗效

1. 癌性胸腹水多为脾肾阳虚，三焦水道不利，多选择具有温阳利水功效的热敏穴位，对改善癌性胸腹水大有裨益，从而提高晚期肿瘤患者生活质量，延长患者生命。

2. 癌性胸腹水患者多正气虚，扶正祛邪要坚持常灸。

【验案举例】

姚女士，77 岁，因确诊肺腺癌 3 个月余，胸闷喘憋半月入院治疗。入院症见：胸闷喘憋，活动后加重，伴全身乏力，不欲饮食，恶风怕冷，进食后恶心呕吐，纳眠差，大便干，小便基本正常。查体：老年女性，神志清，精神不振，胸廓稍饱满，双肺呼吸音低，双侧胸部触觉语颤减弱，叩诊浊音，心音低，心律齐，各个瓣膜区未闻及杂音。舌质暗，苔薄，脉细弦。胸部彩超示：左侧大量胸腔积液（最大液深 11cm）。患者行热敏灸治疗，在中脘、关元、水分、中极、膻中穴区有明显透热现象，以膻中、水分穴透热最为显著，故在膻中穴、水分穴双点灸，感热流如水注深透至胸腔及腹腔，并向背腰部传导，施灸过程中患者微微汗出，感非常舒适，灸感持续约 40 分钟后热流回缩至膻中、水分穴，并感皮肤灼热后停止施灸。改于关元、中极穴处施灸，8 分钟后患者自诉热流由腹部向胸部传导，35 分钟后热流回缩至腹部并感施灸点皮肤灼热，乃停灸，完成 1 次热敏灸治疗。次日复诊，患者诉胸闷喘憋减轻，进食后恶心呕吐感好转，解水样大便，泻后未有不适，反感全身轻松，按上述方法继续治疗 1 周后腹泻自行停止。治疗 1 个疗程（10 天）后复查彩超：左侧胸腔中量积液（最大液深 8.2cm）。其间未行其他任何治疗，继续按上述方法治疗 2 个疗程（20 天）后，患者无明显胸闷、喘憋，全身乏力好转，进食后偶有恶心呕吐，食欲、睡眠均较前好转，再次复查胸部彩超，提示左侧胸腔中量积液（最大液深 6.6cm）。继续上述方法治疗 3 个疗程后，患者胸闷喘憋基本消失，恶心呕吐感明显减轻，食欲好转，全身乏力较前明显好转，复查胸部彩超，提示左侧胸腔少量积液（最大液深 3.4cm）。半年后随访，患者一般情况良好，胸闷喘憋未再发作，生活基本能自理，食量可，夜寐可，二便基本正常。

第四章

保健篇

第一节　脑保健

【保健对象】

1. 从事脑力活动强度较大，易产生脑疲劳的人群。
2. 出现脑疲劳综合征的人群。

【自我判断】

1. 易醒多梦，早晨醒来不愿起床，走路乏力，下肢发沉；不愿多讲话，声音细而短，自觉有气无力。
2. 不想参加社交，不愿见陌生人。
3. 坐下后不愿起来，时常呆想发愣。
4. 说话、工作时常出错，记忆力下降，反应迟钝，视疲劳，哈欠不断。
5. 提不起精神，想用茶或者咖啡提神。
6. 口苦、无味、食欲差。
7. 心理紧张，心绪不宁，烦躁、易怒，思维紊乱，注意力分散等。

【热敏探查】

对本病的穴位热敏高发部位百会、风池、命门、关元等穴区进行穴位热敏探查，标记热敏穴位。

【施灸手法】

1. **百会穴单点灸**　保健者可自觉热感扩散，或透至脑内，或头皮重、压、紧，灸至热敏灸感消失（图4-1-1）。
2. **风池穴双点灸**　保健者可觉热感向头顶方向传导，或向深部渗透，灸至热敏灸感消失（图4-1-2）。
3. **命门穴单点灸**　保健者可觉热感直透腹腔或出现表面不热深部热现象，或沿督脉传导，灸至热敏灸感消失（图4-1-3）。
4. **关元穴单点灸**　保健者可觉热感直透腹腔或出现表面不热深部热现象，灸至热敏灸感消失（图4-1-4）。

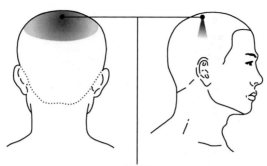

百会穴
定位：在头部，当前发际正中直上5寸，
或两耳尖连线中点处
功效：健脑，安神

图 4-1-1　百会穴单点灸

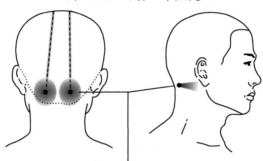

风池穴
定位：项部枕骨下，斜方肌上部外缘与胸
锁乳突肌上端后缘之间凹陷处
功效：祛风解表，清利头目，利五官七窍

图 4-1-2　风池穴双点灸

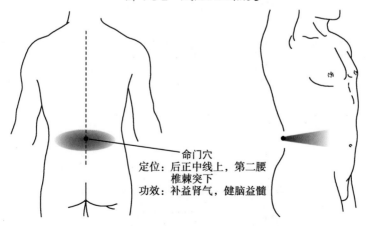

命门穴
定位：后正中线上，第二腰
椎棘突下
功效：补益肾气，健脑益髓

图 4-1-3　命门穴单点灸

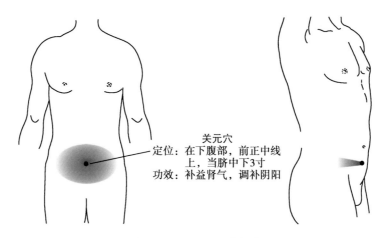

关元穴
定位：在下腹部，前正中线
上，当脐中下3寸
功效：补益肾气，调补阴阳

图 4-1-4 关元穴单点灸

【建议灸量】

每次选取上述 1~2 组穴位，每穴施灸时间以热敏灸感消失为度，每周 2~3 次，每月不少于 10 次。

【灸后防护】

1. 热敏灸能改善大脑血液循环，帮助消除脑疲劳。同时要保证睡眠时间，注意避免长时间的紧张工作，让大脑得到充分的休息。

2. 积极参加户外运动，多吃碱性食物，如海带、绿叶蔬菜、水果、豆类，少吃酸性食物，如肉类、糖类；补充一些富含维生素 B、维生素 E、蛋白质和必需的脂肪酸及矿物质的干果。

【验案举例】

张先生，40 岁，近 3 个月来，经常感觉提不起精神，有气无力，不愿讲话，有时说话、写文章常出错，记忆力也明显下降，不易入睡，且多梦，早晨醒来不愿起床，也不想参加社交活动，自觉口苦、无味。吃过中药，也做脑保健操，效果不佳，影响日常工作生活。热敏探查发现百会、双风池穴有明显扩热、传热、透热现象，于是对风池穴行双点灸，在百会穴施"接力"灸。双风池穴感明显扩热、传热，5 分钟后热流汇合一片，15 分钟后感热流呈线状上传于百会穴附近，即在百会穴施"接力"灸，热感深透颅内，数分钟后整个头颅均有温热感，灸感持续约25分钟后渐回缩并感百会穴皮肤灼热后停灸，完成1次艾灸保健。首诊艾灸后，即感头脑清爽，全身轻松。继续保健灸3次，睡眠改善。按上述方法进行热敏灸保健，每2天1次，1个月后症状消失。嘱其注意劳逸结合，避免用脑过度，经常做脑保健操，锻炼身体，积极参加户外活动，3个月后随访，效果稳定。

第二节　睡眠保健

【保健对象】

多梦、易醒、睡眠不实影响第2天工作生活的人群。

【自我判断】

1. 入睡困难，易醒，晨醒过早，睡眠不实。
2. 常感到头昏脑涨、精神萎靡、倦怠无力、纳谷不香、食欲缺乏、注意力不集中、记忆力减退。

【热敏探查】

对本病的穴位热敏高发部位百会、心俞、关元、涌泉等穴区进行穴位热敏探查，标记热敏穴位。

【施灸手法】

1. **百会穴单点灸**　保健者可自觉热感深透至脑内，或向前额或向后项沿督脉传导，灸至热敏灸感消失（图4-2-1）。
2. **心俞穴双点灸**　保健者可自觉热感深透至胸腔，或向上肢传导，或出现表面不（微）热深部热现象，灸至热敏灸感消失（图4-2-2）。
3. **关元穴单点灸**　保健者可自觉热感深透至腹腔，或出现表面不（微）热深部热现象，灸至热敏灸感消失（图4-2-3）。

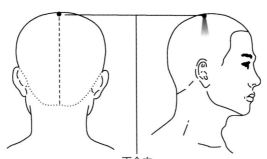

百会穴
定位：在头部，当前发际正中直上
5寸，或两耳尖连线中点处
功效：安神定志，清利头目

图 4-2-1 百会穴单点灸

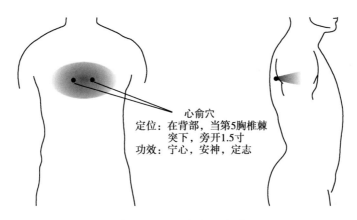

心俞穴
定位：在背部，当第5胸椎棘
突下，旁开1.5寸
功效：宁心，安神，定志

图 4-2-2 心俞穴双点灸

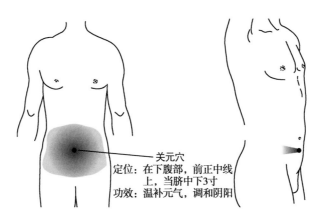

关元穴
定位：在下腹部，前正中线
上，当脐中下3寸
功效：温补元气，调和阴阳

图 4-2-3 关元穴单点灸

4. 涌泉穴双点灸　保健者多可自觉透热或扩热等现象，灸至热敏灸感消失（图 4-2-4）。

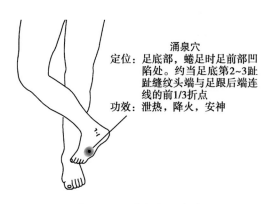

涌泉穴
定位：足底部，蜷足时足前部凹陷处。约当足底第2~3趾趾缝纹头端与足跟后端连线的前1/3折点
功效：泄热，降火，安神

图 4-2-4　涌泉穴双点灸

【建议灸量】

每次选取上述 1~2 组穴位，每穴施灸时间以热敏灸感消失为度，每周 2~3 次，每月不少于 10 次。

【灸后防护】

1. 热敏灸通过激发经气，调节脑细胞的兴奋与抑制过程，调整生物节律，对睡眠具有良好的调节作用。

2. 保持心态平和，劳逸适度；睡前可以适当散步，用温水泡脚；也可适量进补一些滋养心阴的食物，如冰糖莲子羹、小米红枣粥、藕粉或桂圆肉等。

【验案举例】

余女士，59 岁，近半年来入睡困难，易醒多梦，出现记忆力减退，精神不振。热敏探查发现关元穴区穴位热敏，即对关元穴施单点灸，2 分钟后感热流向下腹深部灌注，5 分钟后自觉整个腹腔滚烫温热，该灸感持续约 20 分钟后消失，并感皮肤灼热，遂停灸。次日感精神好，睡眠佳。在双心俞穴探及穴位热敏，即行双点灸，觉热感深透至胸腔，3 分钟后自觉整个胸腔温热舒适，10 分钟后热流呈片状向双上肢内侧传导，以左侧腋下及左上臂内侧明显，该灸感持续约 30 分钟后渐回缩至双心俞穴，2 分钟后感皮肤灼痛，乃停灸。按上述方法进行热敏灸保健 10 次后，能自然入睡，白天精神佳。嘱自灸关元穴，每晚 1 次，每月热敏灸保健 4 次，连续 2 个月，以巩固效果。

第三节 颈椎保健

【保健对象】

1. 长期伏案工作或面对电脑工作时间较长，颈椎易劳损的人群。
2. 经常有颈部不适感的人群。

【自我判断】

颈、项、肩部酸紧痛，活动受限，肩背部沉重，局部肌肉僵硬，上肢乏力。

【热敏探查】

对本病的穴位热敏高发部位风府、大椎、至阳、颈夹脊压痛点、肩井穴压痛点等穴区进行穴位热敏探查，标记热敏穴位。

【施灸手法】

1. 风府、大椎、至阳穴循经往返灸和接力灸　振奋督脉阳气。保健者可自觉热感沿头项背腰部督脉传导，灸至热敏灸感消失（图 4-3-1）。
2. 颈夹脊压痛点单点灸　保健者可自觉热感透向深部并向四周扩散或自觉项背部有紧、压、酸、胀、痛感，灸至热敏灸感消失（图 4-3-2）。
3. 肩井穴压痛点单点灸　保健者可自觉热感透向深部或自觉肩部有紧、压、酸、胀、痛感，或向上肢传导，灸至热敏灸感消失（图 4-3-3）。

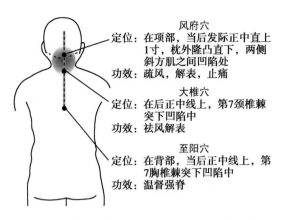

风府穴
定位：在项部，当后发际正中直上
1寸，枕外隆凸直下，两侧
斜方肌之间凹陷处
功效：疏风，解表，止痛

大椎穴
定位：在后正中线上，第7颈椎棘
突下凹陷中
功效：祛风解表

至阳穴
定位：在背部，当后正中线上，第
7胸椎棘突下凹陷中
功效：温督强脊

图 4-3-1　风府、大椎、至阳穴循经往返灸和接力灸

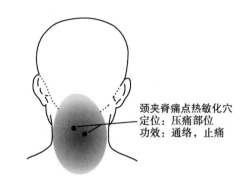

颈夹脊痛点热敏化穴
定位：压痛部位
功效：通络，止痛

图 4-3-2　颈夹脊压痛点单点灸

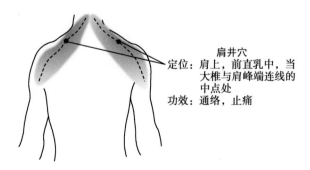

肩井穴
定位：肩上，前直乳中，当
大椎与肩峰端连线的
中点处
功效：通络，止痛

图 4-3-3　肩井穴压痛点单点灸

【建议灸量】

每次选取上述 1 ~ 2 组穴位，每穴施灸时间以热敏灸感消失为度，每周 2 ~ 3 次，每月不少于 10 次。

【灸后防护】

1. 颈椎保健的热敏穴位主要分布在颈、肩、背 3 个部位。在相应高发部位探查热敏穴位，并在此部位上进行热敏灸，激发经气的感传，疏通颈部经脉，调气和血，从而消除局部肌肉疲劳，预防和缓解颈椎的劳损，达到颈椎保健的目的。

2. 生活习惯的改变是颈椎保健的基础，避免长时间伏案工作，加强体育锻炼，配合颈椎保健操。睡眠时低枕平卧，避风寒。

【验案举例】

胡女士，45 岁，因长期伏案工作，最初感后颈项部酸胀、发紧，休息后可缓解，后颈项部酸胀逐渐加重，工作 10 分钟即感脖子发僵、发硬、疼痛，肩背部沉重感，自觉肌肉变硬，右上肢无力，伴头晕，遂来行热敏灸保健。在大椎、至阳、右肩井穴探查到穴位热敏，即在大椎、至阳穴区行循经往返灸，数分钟后感热流徐徐入里，10 分钟后热流沿督脉向上扩散至整个后颈项部，感整个颈项滚热，自觉舒适异常，轻松感，灸感持续约 30 分钟后，热流渐回缩至大椎穴并感灸处皮肤灼热，乃停灸大椎穴。此时至阳穴仍有透热现象，续灸该穴约 10 分钟后热流渐回缩，并感灸处皮肤灼热后停灸。继在右肩井穴上施热敏灸，数分钟后感热流呈片状传于右颈外侧，感右颈项部温热，灸感持续约 30 分钟后热流沿传导路线回缩至右肩井穴，并感右肩井穴皮肤灼热后停灸，完成 1 次热敏灸保健。次日即感症状明显减轻，继续热敏灸保健 15 次后，症状消失。嘱其注意劳逸结合，坚持做颈项保健操，3 个月后未见复发。

第四节　腰椎保健

【保健对象】

从事电脑工作、开长途车的人员，运动员，以及经常出现腰酸、腰痛等腰部不适症状的中老年人群。

【自我判断】

1. 腰或腰骶部酸楚、疼痛，反复发作，疼痛可随气候变化或劳累而变化，时轻时重，缠绵不愈。

2. 腰部可有压痛。

【热敏探查】

对本病的穴位热敏高发部位腰俞、命门、至阳、腰部压痛点、大肠俞、关元俞等穴区进行穴位热敏探查，标记热敏穴位。

【施灸手法】

1. 腰俞、命门、至阳穴循经往返灸和接力灸　振奋督脉阳气。保健者可自觉热感沿背腰部督脉传导，灸至热敏灸感消失（图 4-4-1）。

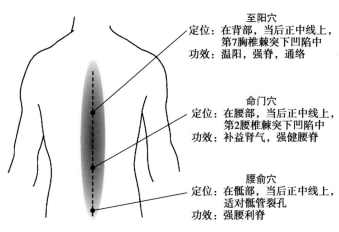

至阳穴
定位：在背部，当后正中线上，
第7胸椎棘突下凹陷中
功效：温阳，强脊，通络

命门穴
定位：在腰部，当后正中线上，
第2腰椎棘突下凹陷中
功效：补益肾气，强健腰脊

腰俞穴
定位：在骶部，当后正中线上，
适对骶管裂孔
功效：强腰利脊

图 4-4-1　腰俞、命门、至阳穴循经往返灸和接力灸

2．**腰部压痛点单点灸** 保健者可自觉热感透向深部甚至腹腔，或向四周扩散，或自觉局部有紧、压、酸、胀、痛感，或向下肢传导，灸至热敏灸感消失（图4-4-2）。

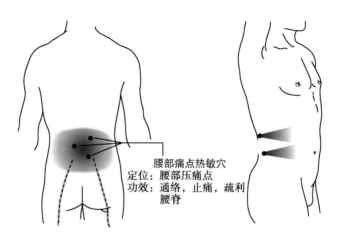

图 4-4-2 腰部压痛点单点灸

3．**大肠俞穴双点灸** 保健者可自觉热感透向深部甚至腹腔，或向四周扩散，或自觉局部有紧、压、酸、胀、痛感，或向下肢传导，灸至热敏灸感消失（图4-4-3）。

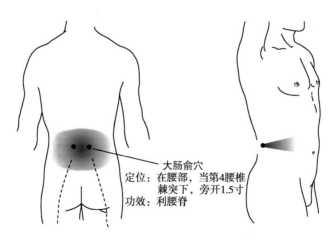

图 4-4-3 大肠俞穴双点灸

4．关元俞穴双点灸　保健者可自觉热感透向深部甚至腹腔，或沿两侧扩散至腰部，灸至热敏灸感消失（图4-4-4）。

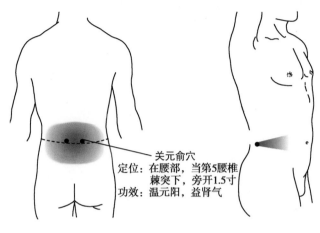

关元俞穴
定位：在腰部，当第5腰椎棘突下，旁开1.5寸
功效：温元阳，益肾气

图4-4-4　关元俞穴双点灸

【建议灸量】

每次选取上述1~2组穴位，每穴施灸时间以热敏灸感消失为度，每周2~3次，每月不少于10次。

【灸后防护】

1．热敏灸可以激发经气感传，疏通经络，调气活血，舒筋通脉，消炎解痉止痛，缓解腰肌紧张度，消除局部肌肉疲劳，预防和缓解腰椎的劳损。

2．必须纠正不良生活习惯，如久坐、久立、久行，避风寒。发作时最好睡硬板床，可配合腰椎保健操，有利于腰背肌力的恢复。

【验案举例】

高女士，42岁，6个月前自觉腰背酸胀不适。近1个月来感觉弯腰困难，且左下肢牵拉性酸胀，影响睡眠。在双大肠俞穴探及穴位热敏，即于双大肠俞穴施双点灸，数分钟后感腰背部片状温热，以左侧为甚，5分钟后，感热流向内扩散至整个腰背部，全身温热舒适，自觉昏昏欲睡，20分钟后感热流向下传至左大腿，约10分钟后自述左膝关节上至施灸点均有温热感，异常舒适。上述灸感持续长达 1 小时后热流渐回缩至腰背部大肠俞穴处，并感皮肤灼热、无透热现象后停灸，完成 1 次热敏灸保健。灸后腰部疼痛及左下肢牵拉酸胀感明显减轻。嘱卧硬板床休息，继续按上述方案热敏灸保健 15 次后，腰部已无任何不适，下肢活动自如。嘱其平时工作时经常变换体位，经常锻炼身体，6 个月后随访未复发。

第五节　膝关节保健

【保健对象】

1. 经常有膝关节酸痛不适、屈伸不利感或肥胖的中老年人群。
2. 虽无明显症状，但双膝关节 X 线片示双膝关节退行性改变。

【自我判断】

1. 多发生在 50 岁以后，女性多于男性。
2. 经常有膝关节酸痛不适，常在关节负重时，如上下楼或下蹲起立时表现明显。
3. 初期，休息后关节酸痛不适可缓解，但随时间推移，即使休息时表现也较明显，晨起或久坐起立时甚至出现膝部僵硬。

【热敏探查】

对本病的热敏穴位高发部位如膝关节局部压痛点、内膝眼、外膝眼、梁丘、阴陵泉、血海、阳陵泉等穴区进行穴位热敏探查，标记热敏穴位。

【施灸手法】

1. 局部压痛点单点灸　保健者可自觉热感透至膝关节内或扩散至整个膝关节或局部有酸、胀、痛感，灸至热敏灸感消失（图 4-5-1）。
2. 梁丘、血海穴双点灸　保健者可自觉热感透至膝关节内并扩散至整个膝关节，灸至热敏灸感消失（图 4-5-2）。

3．内、外膝眼穴双点灸　保健者可自觉热感透至膝关节内并扩散至整个膝关节，灸至热敏灸感消失（图4-5-3）。

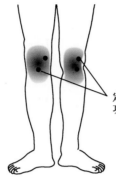

图 4-5-1　局部压痛点单点灸

内膝部痛点热敏化穴
定位：局部出现热敏的压痛点
功效：通络止痛，利关节

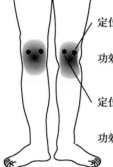

图 4-5-2　梁丘、血海穴双点灸

梁丘穴
定位：大腿前面，屈膝，髂前上棘与髌底外侧端的连线上，髌底上2寸处
功效：祛风湿，利关节，通络止痛

血海穴
定位：大腿内侧，髌底内侧端上2寸，当股四头肌内侧头隆起处
功效：活血祛瘀，通络止痛

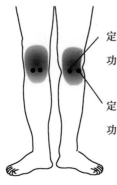

图 4-5-3　内、外膝眼穴双点灸

内膝眼穴
定位：膝部，屈膝时，髌骨与髌韧带内侧凹陷处
功效：通络止痛，疏利关节

外膝眼穴(犊鼻穴)
定位：膝部，屈膝时，髌骨与髌韧带外侧凹陷处
功效：通络止痛，疏利关节

4. 阴陵泉、阳陵泉穴双点灸　保健者可自觉热感透至膝关节内并扩散至整个膝关节，灸至热敏灸感消失（图 4-5-4）。

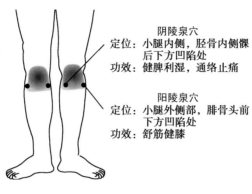

阴陵泉穴
定位：小腿内侧，胫骨内侧髁
后下方凹陷处
功效：健脾利湿，通络止痛

阳陵泉穴
定位：小腿外侧部，腓骨头前
下方凹陷处
功效：舒筋健膝

图 4-5-4　阴陵泉、阳陵泉穴双点灸

【建议灸量】

每次选取上述 1～2 组穴位，每穴施灸时间以热敏灸感消失为度，每周 2～3 次，每月不少于 10 次。

【灸后防护】

1. 正气虚弱、风寒湿邪侵袭关节经络而致关节酸痛、肿胀、屈曲不利，活动不便。热敏灸激发经气感传，行气活血，经气所过，主治所及，可改善膝关节周围软组织劳损。

2. 注意膝关节的防寒保暖，可适当参加各种运动锻炼，如散步、太极拳、游泳等。避免久行、久立。肥胖者应减肥，最大限度减轻膝关节负担。

【验案举例】

章先生，61 岁，自觉左膝关节酸痛不适 1 年多，早晨起床时疼痛较重，轻度活动后酸痛消失。近日左膝关节酸痛明显加重，下蹲困难，经热敷后酸痛可减轻，休息按摩后可缓解，但反复发作影响生活，故来行热敏灸保健。在左内膝眼穴探及穴位热敏，予左内膝眼穴单点灸，于数秒钟后感热流向皮肤深部灌注，约 5 分钟后，感热流下传至左阴陵泉穴附近，立刻在左阴陵泉穴施接力灸，感热流深入皮肤深部，自觉整个膝关节处温热，20 分钟后，感左阴陵泉穴处皮肤灼痛，无透热现象，遂停灸左阴陵泉穴。30 分钟后，热流回缩至左膝眼穴处，继灸 10 分钟后自感皮肤灼热疼痛，无透热现象，停止热敏灸，完成 1 次保健。灸后感左膝关节酸痛明显减轻。按上述方案热敏灸 7 次，平地行走时不感酸痛，但上下楼梯时仍有左膝关节不适感，下蹲稍感困难。继续按原方案热敏灸 10 次后，左膝关节行走时无明显不适。随访半年未复发。

第六节　前列腺保健

【保健对象】

长时间开车、经常酗酒、性生活过度，出现小便不畅，偶有滴白，下腹部或会阴部胀痛不适或夜尿次数增多，排尿费力的中老年人群。

【自我判断】

1. 少腹、会阴、睾丸部时有坠胀不适感。
2. 可出现尿频，夜尿次数增多，排尿费力，多见于老年人群。
3. 可伴有性功能减低、精神状态不佳，严重者常出现头晕、头痛、失眠、多梦、精神抑郁等表现。

【热敏探查】

对本病的穴位热敏高发部位中极、关元、阴陵泉、命门等穴区进行穴位热敏探查，标记热敏穴位。

【施灸手法】

1. 中极穴或关元穴单点灸　保健者可自觉热感透向深部甚至腹腔，或向四周扩散，或表面不（微）热深部热等，灸至热敏灸感消失（图 4-6-1）。
2. 阴陵泉穴双点灸　保健者可自觉热感沿大腿向上传导；部分保健者的感传可直接到达下腹部；如感传仍不能上至下腹部者，再取一支点燃的艾条放置于感传所达部位的近心端点，进行接力灸，依次接力使感传到达下腹部，最后将两支艾条分别固定于阴陵泉和下腹部进行温和灸，灸至热敏灸感消失（图4-6-2）。

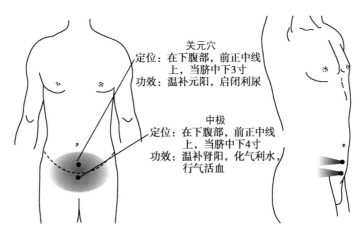

关元穴
定位：在下腹部，前正中线
上，当脐中下3寸
功效：温补元阳，启闭利尿

中极
定位：在下腹部，前正中线
上，当脐中下4寸
功效：温补肾阳，化气利水，
行气活血

图 4-6-1　中极穴或关元穴单点灸

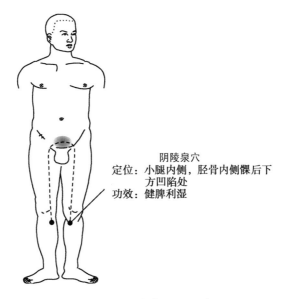

阴陵泉穴
定位：小腿内侧，胫骨内侧髁后下
方凹陷处
功效：健脾利湿

图 4-6-2　阴陵泉穴双点灸

3. 命门穴单点灸　保健者可自觉热感透向深部甚至腹腔，或向四周扩散，或表面不（微）热深部热等，灸至热敏灸感消失（图4-6-3）。

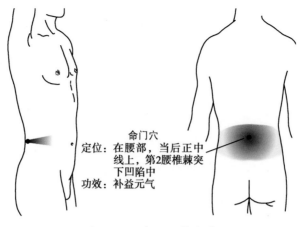

命门穴
定位：在腰部，当后正中
线上，第2腰椎棘突
下凹陷中
功效：补益元气

图 4-6-3　命门穴单点灸

【建议灸量】

每次选取上述 1~2 组穴位，每穴施灸时间以热敏灸感消失为度，每周 2~3 次，每月不少于 10 次。

【灸后防护】

1. 热敏灸能激发经气，使气至病所，改善前列腺血液循环。

2. 调节情志，性生活适度。保证充足睡眠，避免过度劳累、酗酒和进食辛辣食物，保持大便通畅。

【验案举例】

周先生，35 岁，会阴部有不适感 1 年余，近 1 个月来尿频、腰部酸胀，性欲减退，阳物不举。在关元穴、命门穴探及穴位热敏，于关元穴施单点灸，数分钟后感热流徐徐入里，并向小腹深部扩散，10 分钟后感小腹温热，并出现明显酸胀感，灸感持续约 45 分钟后热流渐回缩至关元穴，并感皮肤灼热，乃停灸关元穴。继续命门穴施灸，感扩热，自觉腰背部温热舒适，15 分钟后热感透向腹腔深部，该灸感持续约 40 分钟回缩至命门穴，感传消失，并感皮肤灼热，遂停灸，完成 1 次热敏灸保健。次日，感精神好转，食欲增加，晨起阳物能举数分钟。继续按该法保健 15 次，精力旺盛，会阴部不适等症状消失。6 个月后随访已无不适。

第七节 男性性功能保健

【保健对象】

因工作、生活压力过大，劳累过度、烟酒过量等引起性生活质量下降的中年男性人群。

【自我判断】

1. 性欲障碍，包括性欲低落，对性生活无要求，无性冲动等。
2. 阴茎勃起障碍，包括阴茎勃起不坚或勃而不久等。
3. 射精障碍，包括早泄、遗精等。

【热敏探查】

对本病的穴位热敏高发部位关元、气冲、肾俞、腰阳关、血海等穴区进行穴位热敏探查，标记热敏穴位。

【施灸手法】

1. 关元、气冲穴温和灸 保健者可自觉热感深透至腹腔，灸至热敏灸感消失（图4-7-1）。

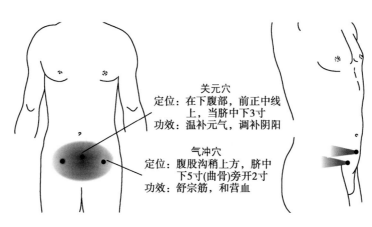

关元穴
定位：在下腹部，前正中线
上，当脐中下3寸
功效：温补元气，调补阴阳

气冲穴
定位：腹股沟稍上方，脐中
下5寸(曲骨)旁开2寸
功效：舒宗筋，和营血

图 4-7-1 关元、气冲穴温和灸

2．**肾俞穴双点灸**　保健者可自觉热感深透至腹腔，或扩散至腰骶部，或向下肢传导，灸至热敏灸感消失（图4-7-2）。

3．**腰阳关穴单点灸**　保健者可自觉热感深透至腹腔，或扩散至腰骶部，或向下肢传导，灸至热敏灸感消失（图4-7-2）。

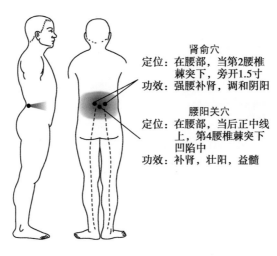

肾俞穴
定位：在腰部，当第2腰椎棘突下，旁开1.5寸
功效：强腰补肾，调和阴阳

腰阳关穴
定位：在腰部，当后正中线上，第4腰椎棘突下凹陷中
功效：补肾，壮阳，益髓

图 4-7-2　肾俞、腰阳关穴温和灸

4．**血海穴双点灸**　保健者可自觉热感沿大腿向上传导；部分保健者的感传可直接到达下腹部；如感传仍不能上至下腹部者，再取一支点燃的艾条放置于感传所达部位的近心端点，进行接力灸，使感传到达下腹部，最后将两支艾条分别固定于血海和下腹部进行温和灸，灸至热敏灸感消失（图4-7-3）。

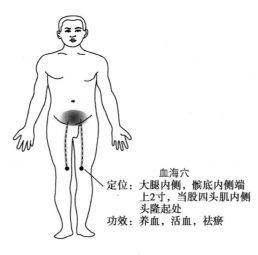

血海穴
定位：大腿内侧，髌底内侧端上2寸，当股四头肌内侧头隆起处
功效：养血，活血，祛瘀

图 4-7-3　血海穴双点灸

【建议灸量】

每次选取上述 1～2 组穴位，每穴施灸时间以热敏灸感消失为度，每周 2～3 次，每月不少于 10 次。

【灸后防护】

1. 调节情志，养成良好的生活习惯，适量参加户外运动，保持积极的生活态度。

2. 应多食优质蛋白质，适当摄入脂肪，补充维生素和微量元素。

3. 保证足够的睡眠与休息时间，养成睡前温水洗脚的习惯，平时少穿紧身三角裤，性生活适度。

4. 可经常进行性功能保健操如双掌推腹，搓摩腹股沟部，搓揉强肾穴等。

【验案举例】

王先生，42 岁，已婚，8 个月前因工作劳累出现阳物举而不坚，失眠、心悸，精神疲乏，食欲差。在关元穴、左肾俞穴探及穴位热敏，于左肾俞穴、关元穴施双点灸，数分钟后左肾俞穴出现透热、扩热现象，感热流徐徐入里，5 分钟后热流呈片状扩散至左腰背部，感温热舒适，并向左腰外侧扩散至左腹部，10 分钟后感整个左腹部温热舒适。同时关元穴出现透热现象，热流渗透入里，并感两股热流于腹部深处汇合成片，感整个小腹滚热，自觉小腹热感明显高于左腰背部，灸感持续约 50 分钟后热流回缩至关元穴，并感皮肤灼热，遂停灸关元穴。左肾俞穴仍有透热现象，继灸左肾俞穴 5 分钟，感传消失，完成 1 次热敏灸保健。按上述方法保健 3 次后精神、食欲明显好转，继续按该法行保健热敏灸 10 次，性生活恢复正常。半年后随访，无复发。

第八节　卵巢保健

【保健对象】

适宜于生活节奏紧张，工作压力大，健康状态不佳，更年期或有卵巢功能早衰征象的女性。

【自我判断】

1. 月经提前或错后，或经期前后不定，经前腹痛，月经量过多或过少。
2. 性功能减退。
3. 面部黄褐斑，皮肤老化早衰，更年期提前等。

【热敏探查】

对本病的穴位热敏高发部位关元、归来、肾俞、三阴交等穴区进行穴位热敏探查，标记热敏穴位。

【施灸手法】

1. 关元穴单点灸　保健者可自觉热感深透至腹腔，或出现表面不（微）热深部热现象，灸至热敏灸感消失（图 4-8-1）。
2. 归来穴双点灸　保健者可自觉热感深透至腹腔，或出现表面不（微）热深部热现象，灸至热敏灸感消失（图 4-8-1）。
3. 肾俞穴双点灸　保健者可自觉热感深透至腹腔，或出现表面不（微）热深部热现象，灸至热敏灸感消失（图 4-8-2）。
4. 三阴交穴双点灸　保健者可出现深部热或热流向上传导至腹部，部分保健者的感传可直接到达腹部；如感传仍不能上至腹部者，再取一支点燃的艾条放置于感传所达部位的近心端点，进行接力灸，依次接力使感传到达腹部，最后将两支艾条分别固定于三阴交和腹部进行温和灸，灸至热敏灸感消失（图 4-8-3）。

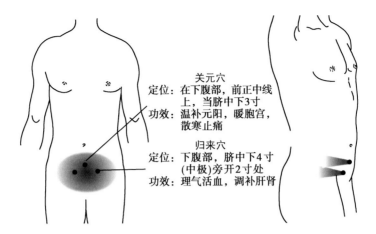

关元穴
定位：在下腹部，前正中线
上，当脐中下3寸
功效：温补元阳，暖胞宫，
散寒止痛

归来穴
定位：下腹部，脐中下4寸
(中极)旁开2寸处
功效：理气活血，调补肝肾

图 4-8-1 关元穴、归来穴温和灸

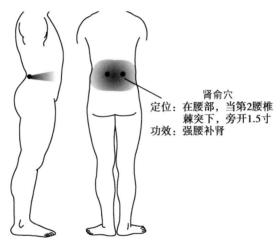

肾俞穴
定位：在腰部，当第2腰椎
棘突下，旁开1.5寸
功效：强腰补肾

图 4-8-2 肾俞穴双点灸

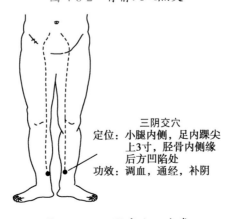

三阴交穴
定位：小腿内侧，足内踝尖
上3寸，胫骨内侧缘
后方凹陷处
功效：调血，通经，补阴

图 4-8-3 三阴交穴双点灸

每次选取上述 1 ~ 2 组穴位，每穴施灸时间以热敏灸感消失为度，每月不少于 4 次。

【灸后防护】

1. 热敏灸能调节内分泌及卵巢功能，已有临床报道。同时保持健康和谐的性生活，可使精神愉快，缓解心理压力，增强对生活的信心，对卵巢功能和内分泌均有助益。

2. 不可服用促排卵药，以防卵巢功能早衰。

【验案举例】

付女士，35 岁，已婚，月经无定期、性欲减退 2 年余，伴入睡困难、多梦，甚是苦恼。在左归来、右三阴交两穴查及穴位热敏，于左归来穴施单点灸，感热流徐徐入里，15 分钟后热流传向下腹部深部，热流团团涌动，下腹轻松感，灸感持续约 30 分钟后渐回缩至左归来穴，并感此处皮肤灼热，遂停灸。改灸右三阴交穴，有温热感沿大腿内侧向上传导，施接力灸，热流一直上传于右下腹，感右下腹酸胀舒适，灸感持续约 30 分钟后渐回缩至右三阴交穴，并感皮肤灼热，乃停灸，完成 1 次热敏灸保健。按上述方法热敏灸保健 15 次，睡眠改善，性欲增加，继续每月热敏灸保健 4 次，共 5 个月经周期后，月经基本正常，性生活和谐。

第九节　乳房保健

【保健对象】

适宜于生活节奏紧张、工作压力大的经前乳房胀痛，或乳房发育不佳，或有乳腺增生的女性。

【自我判断】

1. 经前乳房胀痛，经后减轻，或可扪及包块。
2. 乳房下垂，乳头内陷，乳房发育不佳等。

【热敏探查】

对本病的穴位热敏高发部位膻中、天池、中脘、膈俞、肝俞、肩贞等穴区进行穴位热敏探查，标记热敏穴位。

【施灸手法】

1. 膻中、天池（患侧）穴双点灸　保健者可自觉热感透入深部，或热感扩至整个乳房，或出现表面不（微）热深部热现象，灸至热敏灸感消失（图4-9-1）。

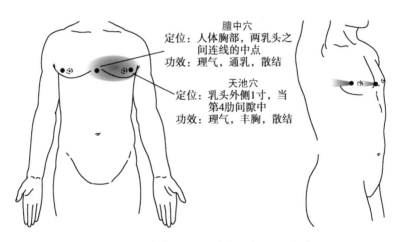

膻中穴
定位：人体胸部，两乳头之间连线的中点
功效：理气，通乳，散结

天池穴
定位：乳头外侧1寸，当第4肋间隙中
功效：理气，丰胸，散结

图 4-9-1　膻中、天池（患侧）穴双点灸

2. 中脘穴单点灸　保健者可自觉热感透入上腹深部，或出现表面不（微）热深部热现象，灸至热敏灸感消失（图4-9-2）。

3. 膈俞穴双点灸　保健者可自觉热感深透或沿两侧扩散至胸部，灸至热敏灸感消失（图4-9-3）。

4. 肝俞穴双点灸　保健者可自觉热感深透至腹腔或扩散至背腰部，灸至热敏灸感消失（图4-9-3）。

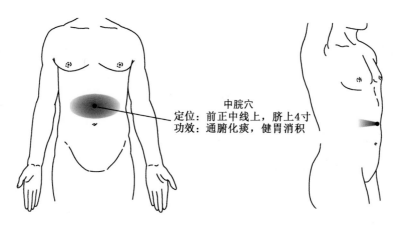

图 4-9-2　中脘穴单点灸

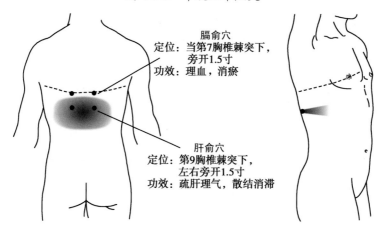

图 4-9-3　膈俞穴、肝俞穴温和灸

5. **肩贞穴双点灸**　保健者可自觉深部热或酸胀，或热流向上肢传导等，灸至热敏灸感消失（图 4-9-4）。

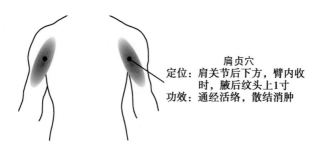

图 4-9-4　肩贞穴双点灸

【建议灸量】

每次选取上述 1~2 组穴位，每穴施灸时间以热敏灸感消失为度，每月不少于 4 次。

【灸后防护】

1. 热敏灸能疏肝理气，化痰通络，因此对乳房保健有较好作用。
2. 定期找专科医生做乳房的体格检查，发现问题，及时就诊。

【验案举例】

张女士，35 岁，6 个月前开始出现月经来潮前乳房轻微胀痛，经后胀痛消失，未予重视，后因胀痛加重，要求热敏灸保健。经查中脘、肝俞穴存在穴位热敏，于中脘穴行单点灸，自觉热感透入上腹深部，灸感持续约 20 分钟后，向上传至胸部，感胸部温热舒适，乳房胀痛有所减轻，灸感持续约 30 分钟后退缩至上腹部，10 分钟后回缩至中脘穴，并感皮肤灼热，乃停灸。继续行肝俞穴双点灸，自觉热感扩散至背腰部，15 分钟后深透至腹腔，感腹腔深部温热舒适，25 分钟后回缩至双侧肝俞穴，并感皮肤灼热，乃停灸，完成 1 次热敏灸保健，即感乳房胀痛有所减轻。按上述方法每月月经前热敏灸保健 4 次，连续 3 个月经周期，共 12 次，症状消失，6 个月后随访，未见复发。

第十节　胃动力保健

【保健对象】

素体瘦弱、饮食不节、工作压力大及疲于应酬的人群。

【自我判断】

1. 纳谷不香，食欲缺乏，食量减少，稍多食即上腹饱胀。

2．常有嗳气、反酸、刷牙时恶心等表现。

【热敏探查】

对本病的穴位热敏高发部位天枢、中脘、关元、胃俞、足三里等穴区进行穴位热敏探查，标记热敏穴位。

【施灸手法】

1．天枢穴双点灸　保健者可自觉热感深透至腹腔或沿两侧扩散至腰部，灸至热敏灸感消失（图4-10-1）。

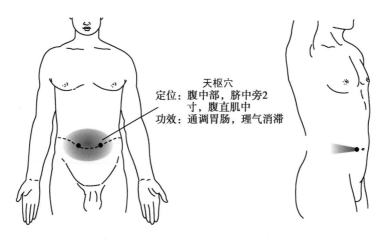

天枢穴
定位：腹中部，脐中旁2
寸，腹直肌中
功效：通调胃肠，理气消滞

图 4-10-1　天枢穴双点灸

2．中脘、关元穴双点灸　保健者可自觉热感透至腹腔内，灸至热敏灸感消失（图4-10-2）。

3．胃俞穴双点灸　保健者可自觉热感深透至腹腔或扩散至背腰部，灸至热敏灸感消失（图4-10-3）。

4．足三里穴双点灸　保健者可自觉热感深透，或向上或向下沿足阳明胃经传导，灸至热敏灸感消失（图4-10-4）。

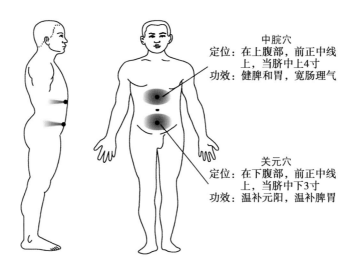

中脘穴
定位：在上腹部，前正中线
上，当脐中上4寸
功效：健脾和胃，宽肠理气

关元穴
定位：在下腹部，前正中线
上，当脐中下3寸
功效：温补元阳，温补脾胃

图 4-10-2　中脘、关元穴双点灸

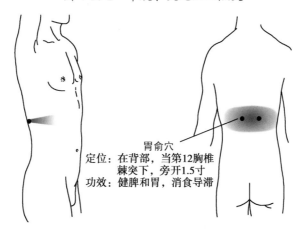

胃俞穴
定位：在背部，当第12胸椎
棘突下，旁开1.5寸
功效：健脾和胃，消食导滞

图 4-10-3　胃俞穴双点灸

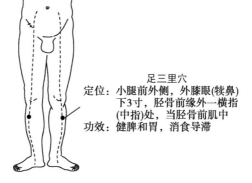

足三里穴
定位：小腿前外侧，外膝眼(犊鼻)
下3寸，胫骨前缘外一横指
(中指)处，当胫骨前肌中
功效：健脾和胃，消食导滞

图 4-10-4　足三里穴双点灸

【建议灸量】

每次选取上述 1~2 组穴位，每穴施灸时间以热敏灸感消失为度，每周 2~3 次，每月不少于 10 次。

【灸后防护】

1. 热敏灸能温胃散寒、调节胃动力，保健效果明显，无任何毒副作用。
2. 加强体育锻炼，调畅情志。保持良好的饮食习惯，避免进食肥甘厚腻及刺激性食物。

【验案举例】

高女士，38 岁，自感进餐后上腹部胀满不适 2 年余，时好时坏，且感恶心、反酸，因工作原因，不能按时进餐，故反复发作。在双胃俞穴探及穴位热敏，于双胃俞穴施双点灸，几分钟后自感热流向内传入，并慢慢扩散汇合在一起，15 分钟后热流由腰背部渐渐深透至上腹部，热流在上腹部团团涌动，整个上腹部温热、舒适，灸感持续约 40 分钟后热流渐回缩至双胃俞穴，仍感透热，数分钟后，左、右胃俞穴先后感皮肤灼热，遂停灸，完成 1 次热敏灸保健，自觉上腹部胀满不适减轻。按上述方法热敏灸保健 10 次，症状消失，嘱其注意饮食，防寒保暖，平时可自灸中脘、天枢等穴强身保健。随访半年未见复发。

第十一节　肠道保健

【保健对象】

素体瘦弱、饮食不节、工作压力大及疲于应酬的人群。

【自我判断】

1. 经常腹部胀气。

2．大便经常秘结。

3．大便不成形，易腹泻，腹泻多与饮食刺激相关，常在进食生冷、油腻食物后发生或加重。

【热敏探查】

对本病的穴位热敏高发部位天枢、关元、大肠俞、足三里等穴区进行穴位热敏探查，标记热敏穴位。

【施灸手法】

1．天枢穴双点灸　保健者可自觉热感深透至腹腔或沿两侧扩散至腰部，灸至热敏灸感消失（图4-11-1）。

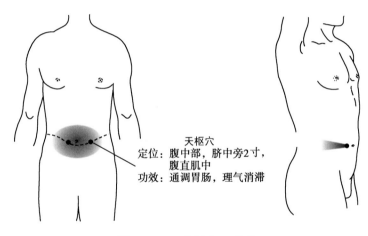

天枢穴
定位：腹中部，脐中旁2寸，
　　　腹直肌中
功效：通调胃肠，理气消滞

图 4-11-1　天枢穴双点灸

2．关元穴单点灸　保健者可自觉热感透至腹腔内，灸至热敏灸感消失（图4-11-2）。

3．大肠俞穴双点灸　保健者可自觉热感深透至腹腔，或扩散至腰骶部，或向下肢传导，灸至热敏灸感消失（图4-11-3）。

4．足三里穴双点灸　保健者可自觉热感深透，或向上或向下沿足阳明胃经传导，灸至热敏灸感消失（图4-11-4）。

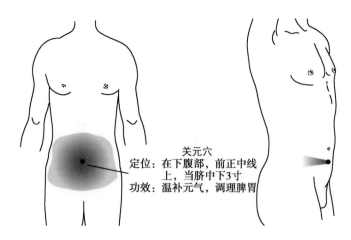

关元穴
定位：在下腹部，前正中线
上，当脐中下3寸
功效：温补元气，调理脾胃

图 4-11-2　关元穴单点灸

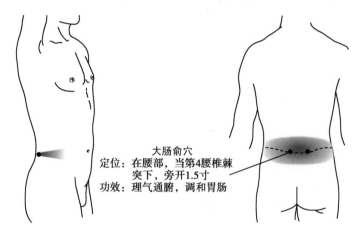

大肠俞穴
定位：在腰部，当第4腰椎棘
突下，旁开1.5寸
功效：理气通腑，调和胃肠

图 4-11-3　大肠俞穴双点灸

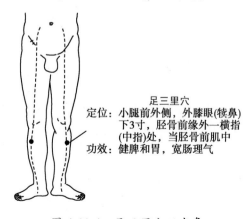

足三里穴
定位：小腿前外侧，外膝眼(犊鼻)
下3寸，胫骨前缘外一横指
(中指)处，当胫骨前肌中
功效：健脾和胃，宽肠理气

图 4-11-4　足三里穴双点灸

【建议灸量】

每次选取上述 1～2 组穴位，每穴施灸时间以热敏灸感消失为度，每周 2～3 次，每月不少于 10 次。

【灸后防护】

1. 热敏灸对肠道保健效果显著，且避免了服用药物可能对肠道产生的不良反应，可作为肠道保健的首选方法。

2. 保持膳食结构的平衡合理，讲究饮食卫生，注意生活规律，保持平和的情绪等均有利于肠道保健。

【验案举例】

董先生，34 岁，腹胀、大便不成形反复发作 1 年。近 1 周来不适加重，左下腹胀闷不适，每天大便 1～2 次，呈稀糊状。在关元穴处探及穴位热敏，即对关元穴施单点灸，于数分钟后感热流如"水注"向腹腔深部灌注，并向左下腹涌动，整个左下腹部感到滚烫温热，自觉左下腹热感明显高于施灸点，灸感持续约 20 分钟后左下腹热流均回缩至关元穴并感皮肤灼热，遂停灸。次日即觉精神好，睡眠佳，腹胀减轻。按上述方法进行热敏灸保健 20 次，精神佳，睡眠好，无腹胀，大便每日 1 次，黄软成形。嘱调情志，睡前自灸双天枢穴，每穴 30 分钟，每日 1 次，连续 1 个月，以巩固疗效，6 个月后未复发。

第十二节　心脏保健

【保健对象】

1. 心电图检查示曾有心肌缺血改变的中老年人群。

2. 既往有心绞痛发作史的中老年人群。

3. 有动脉粥样硬化、冠心病、高血压及糖尿病史的中老年人群。

【自我判断】

1. 曾出现一过性胸闷气短、胸前区隐痛，心悸心慌，倦怠乏力。
2. 无明显临床症状，但心电图检查示曾有心肌缺血改变。
3. 血脂、血糖、血压检查高于正常。

【热敏探查】

对本病的穴位热敏高发部位至阳、心俞、内关等穴区进行穴位热敏探查，标记热敏穴位。

【施灸手法】

1. 至阳穴单点灸　保健者可自觉热感深透至胸腔或向四周扩散，或出现表面不（微）热深部热现象，灸至热敏灸感消失（图 4-12-1）。

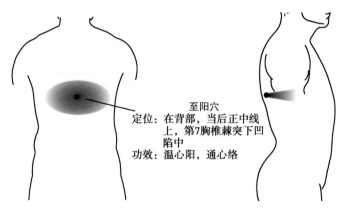

至阳穴
定位：在背部，当后正中线上，第7胸椎棘突下凹陷中
功效：温心阳，通心络

图 4-12-1　至阳穴单点灸

2. 心俞穴双点灸　保健者可自觉热感深透至胸腔，或向四周扩散，或向上肢传导，或出现表面不（微）热深部热现象，灸至热敏灸感消失（图 4-12-2）。
3. 内关穴双点灸　保健者可自觉热感深透，或向上或向下沿手厥阴心包经传导，灸至热敏灸感消失（图 4-12-3）。

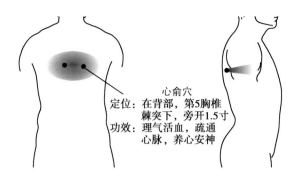

心俞穴
定位：在背部，第5胸椎
棘突下，旁开1.5寸
功效：理气活血，疏通
心脉，养心安神

图 4-12-2 心俞穴双点灸

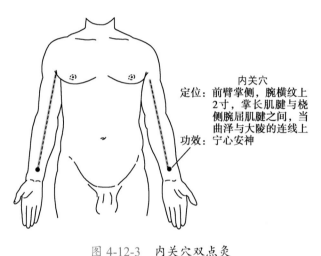

内关穴
定位：前臂掌侧，腕横纹上
2寸，掌长肌腱与桡
侧腕屈肌腱之间，当
曲泽与大陵的连线上
功效：宁心安神

图 4-12-3 内关穴双点灸

【建议灸量】

每次选取上述 1~2 组穴位，每穴施灸时间以热敏灸感消失为度，每月不少于 4 次。

【灸后防护】

1. 热敏灸可通经活络，开胸理气，能改善冠脉血流，有较好的心脏保健功能。

2. 注意劳逸结合，消除紧张、焦虑、恐惧情绪，适当参加户外体育锻炼。清淡饮食，少量多餐，忌冷饮，避免过饱、刺激性食物，限烟酒，多吃蔬菜、水果。

【验案举例】

李先生，62岁，近6个月来常感胸闷心慌，上楼气喘，精神乏力，易醒多梦，心电图检查示有心肌缺血改变。在至阳穴探及穴位热敏，对至阳穴施单点灸，感明显扩热并深透至胸腔，5分钟后自觉整个胸腔温热舒适，该灸感持续约30分钟后消失，并感皮肤灼热，遂停灸，完成1次热敏灸保健。灸后，感觉精神好，胸闷心慌明显好转。按上述方法进行热敏灸保健20次，白天精神佳，无胸闷心慌。嘱自灸膻中穴，每晚1次，每次40分钟，每月由医生保健灸4次，以巩固效果。

第十三节　血脂保健

【保健对象】

素体肥胖，有家族性高脂血症或喜食、常食肥甘厚味或血脂边缘性升高的人群。

【自我判断】

一般成年人空腹血清中总胆固醇超5.72mmol/L、甘油三酯超1.70mmol/L，可诊断为高脂血症，而总胆固醇在5.2~5.7mmol/L者称为边缘性升高。

【热敏探查】

对本病的穴位热敏高发部位天枢、胃俞、内关、阴陵泉、丰隆等穴区进行穴位热敏探查，标记热敏穴位。

【施灸手法】

1. 天枢穴双点灸　保健者可自觉热感深透至腹腔或沿两侧扩散至腰部，灸至热敏灸感消失（图4-13-1）。

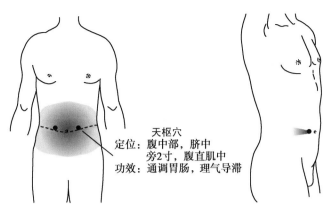

天枢穴
定位：腹中部，脐中
　　　旁2寸，腹直肌中
功效：通调胃肠，理气导滞

图 4-13-1　天枢穴双点灸

2. **胃俞穴双点灸**　保健者可自觉热感深透至腹腔或扩散至背腰部，灸至热敏灸感消失（图 4-13-2）。

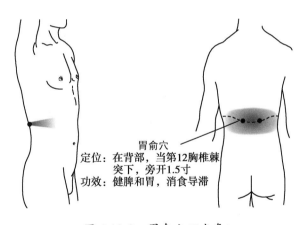

胃俞穴
定位：在背部，当第12胸椎棘
　　　突下，旁开1.5寸
功效：健脾和胃，消食导滞

图 4-13-2　胃俞穴双点灸

3. **内关穴双点灸**　保健者可自觉热感深透，或向上或向下沿手厥阴心包经传导，灸至热敏灸感消失（图 4-13-3）。

4. **阴陵泉穴双点灸**　保健者可自觉热感深透，或向上或向下沿足太阴脾经传导，灸至热敏灸感消失（图 4-13-4）。、

5. **丰隆穴双点灸**　保健者可自觉热感深透，或向上或向下沿足阳明胃经传导，灸至热敏灸感消失（图 4-13-5）。

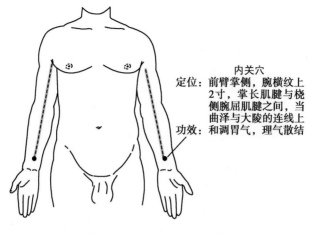

内关穴
定位：前臂掌侧，腕横纹上2寸，掌长肌腱与桡侧腕屈肌腱之间，当曲泽与大陵的连线上
功效：和调胃气，理气散结

图 4-13-3　内关穴双点灸

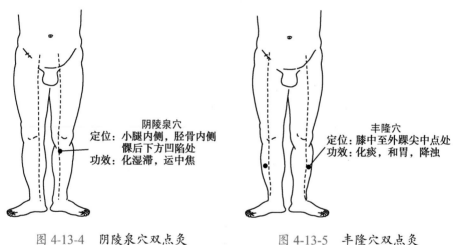

阴陵泉穴
定位：小腿内侧，胫骨内侧髁后下方凹陷处
功效：化湿滞，运中焦

图 4-13-4　阴陵泉穴双点灸

丰隆穴
定位：膝中至外踝尖中点处
功效：化痰，和胃，降浊

图 4-13-5　丰隆穴双点灸

【建议灸量】

每次选取上述 1～2 组穴位，每穴施灸时间以热敏灸感消失为度，每周 2～3 次，每月不少于 10 次。

【灸后防护】

1. 热敏灸并不能直接产生燃烧脂肪降低血脂水平的作用，而是通过增强机体对血脂的调节能力，在中枢和局部的双重作用下，有效调节人体血脂水平。

2. 合理进行饮食调养：饥饱适度，提倡清淡饮食，限制高脂肪、高胆固醇类、糖类食品，少吃甜食和零食，多吃蔬菜和水果，定期进行血脂监测。

【验案举例】

付先生，40 岁，工作压力大，近 1 年来体重明显增加（就诊时身高 171cm，体重 92kg），就诊前半月，单位体检，总胆固醇在 7.1mmol/L，甘油三酯 1.8mmol/L。在右天枢穴探及穴位热敏，即对右天枢穴施单点灸，数分钟后感热流向右腹腔深部灌注，并向右下腹涌动，整个右下腹部感到滚烫温热，自觉右下腹热明显高于施灸点，灸感持续约 35 分钟后右下腹热流均回缩至右天枢穴并感皮肤灼热，遂停灸。按上述方法进行热敏灸保健 20 次，体重 84kg，精神好，睡眠佳。3 个月后随访，总胆固醇 5.1mmol/L，甘油三酯 1.61mmol/L，体重 78kg，精神好。

第十四节　血压保健

【保健对象】

临界性高血压的人群。

【自我判断】

1. 正常成人血压：静息时收缩压≤135mmHg，静息时舒张压≤85mmHg。
2. 高血压（成人）：收缩压≥140mmHg 和（或）舒张压≥90mmHg。
3. 临界性高血压：血压值在上述正常与高血压之间。
4. 临界性高血压状态时偶可见头痛、头晕、耳鸣、心悸、眼花、注意力不集中、记忆力减退、疲乏无力、易烦躁等症状。

【热敏探查】

对本病的穴位热敏高发部位气海、人迎、足三里、内关、涌泉等穴区进行穴位热敏探查，标记热敏穴位。

【施灸手法】

1. **气海穴单点灸**　保健者可自觉热感深透至腹腔或沿两侧扩散至腰部，灸至热敏灸感消失（图 4-14-1）。

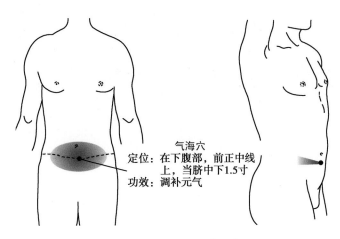

气海穴
定位：在下腹部，前正中线
上，当脐中下1.5寸
功效：调补元气

图 4-14-1　气海穴单点灸

2. **人迎穴双点灸**　可出现深部热、扩热或热感向上肢传导等现象，灸至热敏灸感消失（图 4-14-2）。

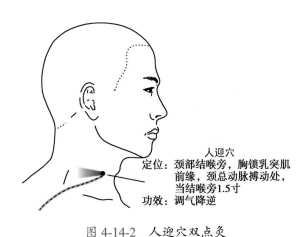

人迎穴
定位：颈部结喉旁，胸锁乳突肌
前缘，颈总动脉搏动处，
当结喉旁1.5寸
功效：调气降逆

图 4-14-2　人迎穴双点灸

3. 足三里穴双点灸　保健者可自觉热感深透，或向上或向下沿足阳明胃经传导，灸至热敏灸感消失（图4-14-3）。

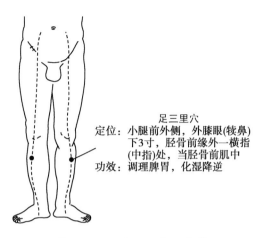

足三里穴
定位：小腿前外侧，外膝眼(犊鼻)
下3寸，胫骨前缘外一横指
(中指)处，当胫骨前肌中
功效：调理脾胃，化湿降逆

图4-14-3　足三里穴双点灸

4. 内关穴双点灸　保健者可自觉热感深透，或向上或向下沿手厥阴心包经传导，灸至热敏灸感消失（图4-14-4）。

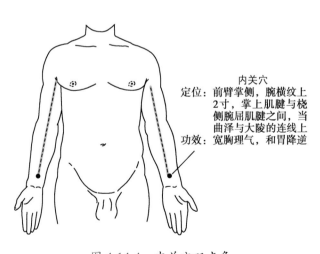

内关穴
定位：前臂掌侧，腕横纹上
2寸，掌上肌腱与桡
侧腕屈肌腱之间，当
曲泽与大陵的连线上
功效：宽胸理气，和胃降逆

图4-14-4　内关穴双点灸

5. 涌泉穴双点灸　保健者多自觉透热或扩热等现象，灸至热敏灸感消失（图4-14-5）。

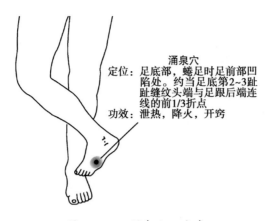

涌泉穴

定位：足底部，蜷足时足前部凹
陷处。约当足底第2~3趾
趾缝纹头端与足跟后端连
线的前1/3折点

功效：泄热，降火，开窍

图 4-14-5　涌泉穴双点灸

【建议灸量】

每次选取上述 1~2 组穴位，每穴施灸时间以热敏灸感消失为度，每
周 2~3 次，每月不少于 10 次。

【灸后防护】

1. 热敏灸降压，用之得当则降压迅速，有时比药物降压见效更快，
且不致使血压降至过低。因艾灸具有双向调节作用，可使高血压下降，使
低血压升高，无药物的不良反应及耐受现象。

2. 保持充足睡眠，劳逸结合，心情舒畅，清淡饮食，戒烟、限酒，
定期进行血压监测。

【验案举例】

高女士，58 岁，疲倦乏力、易烦躁，常感手脚麻木，头晕、耳鸣
等。收缩压多在 130~140mmHg，舒张压多在 85~90mmHg，未服药。
在气海穴探及穴位热敏，即对气海穴施单点灸，立感温热舒适，10 分钟
后感热流向腹腔深部渗透，整个腹部感到滚烫温热，15 分钟后热流向腰
部流动，自觉腰部温热舒适，全身有温热放松感，灸感持续约 40 分钟后
热流渐回缩至气海穴，并感皮肤灼热，遂停灸。次日，即感精神好，睡
眠佳，头晕、耳鸣等症状发作次数明显减少，血压 130/85mmHg。按上
述方法进行热敏灸保健 20 次，上述不适反应均消失，血压基本维持在

120～130mmHg/70～85mmHg。嘱清淡饮食，定期监测血压。6个月后随访，血压恢复正常。

第十五节 血糖保健

【保健对象】

适宜于因工作紧张、进食过量、疲于应酬、烟酒摄入量较大及糖耐量减低的人群。

【自我判断】

1. 正常人的血糖浓度空腹波动 3.9～6.1mmol/L，餐后 2 小时血糖略高，但应该＜7.8mmol/L。

2. 血糖轻度升高，虽已超过正常范围，但仍未达到糖尿病的诊断标准，如空腹血糖在 6.2～7.0mmol/L，餐后 2 小时血糖在 7.8～11.1mmol/L 时，即为一种过渡状态，称之为糖耐量减低（impaired glucose tolerance，IGT），某种意义上讲，是一种糖尿病的危险信号。

3. 当血糖明显升高到某种程度（如空腹血糖超过 7.0mmol/L 或餐后 2 小时血糖超过 11.1mmol/L），即达到糖尿病的诊断标准，称之为糖尿病。

【热敏探查】

对本病的穴位热敏高发部位神阙、脾俞、胰俞、三阴交等穴区进行穴位热敏探查，标记热敏穴位。

【施灸手法】

1. **神阙穴单点灸** 保健者可自觉热感深透至腹腔或沿两侧扩散至腰部，灸至热敏灸感消失（图 4-15-1）。

2. **脾俞穴双点灸** 保健者可自觉热感深透至腹腔或扩散至背腰部，灸至热敏灸感消失（图 4-15-2）。

3．胰俞穴双点灸　保健者可自觉热感深透至腹腔或扩散至背腰部，灸至热敏灸感消失（图 4-15-2）。

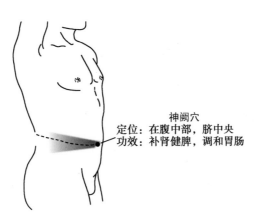

神阙穴
定位：在腹中部，脐中央
功效：补肾健脾，调和胃肠

图 4-15-1　神阙穴单点灸

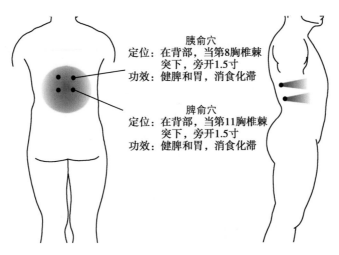

胰俞穴
定位：在背部，当第8胸椎棘突下，旁开1.5寸
功效：健脾和胃，消食化滞

脾俞穴
定位：在背部，当第11胸椎棘突下，旁开1.5寸
功效：健脾和胃，消食化滞

图 4-15-2　脾俞、胰俞穴双点灸

4．三阴交穴双点灸　保健者可自觉热感深透，或向上或向下沿足太阴脾经传导，灸至热敏灸感消失（图 4-15-3）。

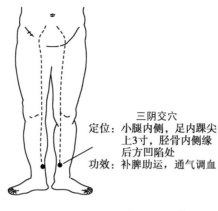

三阴交穴
定位：小腿内侧，足内踝尖
上3寸，胫骨内侧缘
后方凹陷处
功效：补脾助运，通气调血

图 4-15-3 三阴交穴双点灸

【建议灸量】

每次选取上述 1～2 组穴位，每穴施灸时间以热敏灸感消失为度，每周 2～3 次，每月不少于 10 次。

【灸后防护】

1. 热敏灸降血糖效果明显，且不致使血糖降至过低。因艾灸具有双向调节作用，可使高血糖下降，使低血糖升高，无药物的不良反应及耐受现象。

2. 合理饮食，戒烟限酒，适度运动，保持心情愉快，定期进行血糖监测。

【验案举例】

吴先生，44 岁，常在外面餐馆进食，近日感口干，精神差，1 个月前工作单位体检，餐前血糖 6.9mmol/L，餐后 2 小时血糖 7.8mmol/L，前来我院行热敏灸保健。在神阙穴探及穴位热敏，即对神阙穴施单点灸，自觉热感透至腹腔内，并向上腹部传导，整个上腹部感到滚烫温热，灸感持续约 30 分钟后施灸点皮肤灼热，遂停灸。次日即感精神好，睡眠佳。按上述方法进行艾灸保健 20 次，并嘱清淡饮食，控制食量，1 个月后复查血糖，餐前血糖 5.2mmol/L，餐后 2 小时血糖 6.7mmol/L。嘱自灸双侧三阴交穴，每晚 1 次，以巩固疗效。并嘱清淡饮食，控制食量，适量运动。半年后随访，复查血糖，餐前血糖 4.9mmol/L，餐后 2 小时血糖 6.5mmol/L。

第五章

抗疫篇

第一节　热敏灸参与抗击新冠疫情概况

2020 年初，我国遇到了新冠病毒的袭击，全国上下抗击疫情，热敏灸积极参与了这场战斗。临床数据证明，热敏灸治疗新冠肺炎能够发挥很好的作用。

疫情发生后，我们在想，新冠肺炎是不是热敏灸的适应证？热敏灸在治疗新冠肺炎中能不能发挥作用？于是我们通过热敏灸团队医生在一线隔离病房采集新冠肺炎患者中医信息的方式，了解其中医证候特点，以判断新冠肺炎是不是热敏灸的适应证，热敏灸能不能发挥作用。通过分析新冠肺炎患者的临床特点与舌象，发现不管患者是白苔还是黄苔，都是腻苔，结合 2020 年 1 月 23 日国家卫健委发布的《新型冠状病毒感染的肺炎诊疗方案（试行第三版）》，认识到这次新冠肺炎属中医的湿毒疫病。而热敏灸恰恰具有温阳益气、芳香化湿的功效，与此次疫情的中医病因病机相符，因此，我们认为新冠肺炎是热敏灸的适应证。由于现代医学对这次新冠病毒无特效药，而自古就有中医艾灸防治疫病的记载，使我们坚定了要让灸法发挥作用的信心。

于是，我们立即进行讨论与反复论证，制定了居家预防新冠肺炎的一艾三用方，并发布在江西省中医药管理局印发的《江西省新型冠状病毒感染的肺炎中医药防治方案（试行第二版）》中。一艾三用方是指一支热敏灸艾条三种用法，即闻艾香，艾泡脚，施艾灸。之后，我们针对新冠肺炎的病因病机反复讨论，制定了热敏灸治疗新冠肺炎的方案。这个治疗方案包括"理、法、方、穴、具、剂、量"七大要素，并发布在江西省中医药管理局印发的《江西省新型冠状病毒肺炎中医药防治方案（试行第三版）》中。

由于隔离病房施灸有特殊要求：第一要求尽量减少近距离和患者接触的时间；第二是病房不开空调，温度偏低，在此环境下要快速得气；第三，要及时把艾烟艾味消掉，因此，我们研制了能够满足要求的高效激发艾灸得气及净化艾烟艾味的专用热敏灸设备。同时我们制备了专用艾条，其直径是 2.5cm，长度是 4.0cm。艾条不是越大越好，也不是越粗越好，关键是要发挥穴位的小刺激、大反应。每次施灸使用两小段艾条，它足够燃烧 30～40 分钟，高效激发得气，产生透热、扩热、传热，甚至一身烘热。

在隔离病房施灸，医生的操作与平时的治疗操作有很大的不同。他们穿着防护服，戴着护目镜，要求他们不允许出现任何的误操作；调节艾热强度，要求方便，要求迅速，要求稳定。因此，我们的医生开始反复训练，严格操作，即使穿着防护服，戴着护目镜，也能够非常熟练地完成施灸过程，达到进入隔离病房的要求。

经过上述的充分准备，2 月 13 日，热敏灸医生进入隔离病房参与治疗普通型新冠肺炎患者，一共治疗新冠肺炎患者 42 例（272 人次），取得显著效果。由于疗效好，2 月 24 日湖北蕲春县新冠肺炎疫情防控指挥部向江西省中医药管理局发出邀请函，邀请热敏灸团队支持蕲春县新冠肺炎医疗救治工作。2 月 27 日我们派出热敏灸医生（包括热敏灸专用设备）赴蕲春县人民医院支援。到 3 月 10 日，江西省中医院抚生院区定点医院和蕲春定点医院最后一位患者相继出院，清零。

在此期间，许多媒体相继报道。在世界针灸学会联合会主席刘保延教授指导下，我们在中文核心期刊《中国针灸》杂志发表了论文《热敏灸治疗新型冠状病毒肺炎临床观察》，供大家交流。同时又收到加拿大北美中医药发展促进中心、加拿大热敏灸分院关于联合抗击加拿大新冠肺炎疫情支援请求函，开始国际合作抗疫。

在这次抗击新冠疫情的战斗中，我们有以下四点很深的体会：

1. 热敏灸是一种安全、有效的外治法，新冠肺炎患者普遍乐于接受。

2. 热敏灸对于寒湿致病是有效的，即使湿蕴化热，湿遏热伏，亦能化湿透热。

3. 患者艾灸得气率达到 100%，说明该类患者的相关穴位需要外界艾热的帮助，提示热敏灸适合新冠肺炎的中医病机，能够发挥较好的作用。

4. 我们观察到，每次热敏灸治疗后，大部分患者感到体内温暖舒适，身体轻松，心情舒畅，负性情绪减轻，增强了战胜疾病的信心。热敏灸得气时产生的一身烘热、一身轻松、心情舒畅，都是热敏灸调神的具体表现，也是热敏灸的独特优势。

第二节 热敏灸治疗新冠肺炎临床思路

通过分析新冠肺炎患者的临床表现，结合 2020 年 1 月 23 日国家卫健委发布的《新型冠状病毒感染的肺炎诊疗方案（试行第三版）》，我们认识到这次新冠肺炎属中医的湿毒疫病，病因以湿邪为主，早期病机是湿遏热伏，后期病机是湿毒伤阳，病位主要涉及肺、脾上中两焦。由此可知，热敏灸温阳益气、芳香化湿的功效与此次疫情的中医病因病机是符合的，而且自古就有中医艾灸防治疫病的记载。因此，我们肯定热敏灸在新冠肺炎的治疗中可发挥作用。湿性黏腻缠绵，是六淫邪气中最棘手的病邪。根据 30 年的热敏灸研究成果及临床经验，艾灸祛除湿邪非"小刺激大反应"不可，也就是"非敏不除湿"，而热敏穴位恰恰有这种小刺激、大反应的特点，所以就形成了采用热敏灸法治疗新冠肺炎的思路，而不是常规的辨证施灸。这个思路概括起来，就是以辨敏施灸为理论指导，制定了辨敏选穴、灸敏得气、消敏定量、依敏制具的"四敏"治疗方案。

1. **辨敏选穴** 穴位是艾灸的施灸部位，穴位的精准定位很重要。热敏灸的前期研究表明穴位有状态之别，有静息态与敏化态的区别。当人体在疾病状态时，穴位会从静息态转化为敏化态，敏化态穴位对针灸刺激发生小刺激大反应，能够显著提高临床疗效。新冠肺炎以湿邪为主，病位在上、中二焦。湿在三阳，可郁而化热，湿遏热伏；湿入三阴，湿邪伤阳。艾灸可温阳、可化湿、可透热。神阙穴具有温阳益气、温脾化湿、肺脾同治作用，因此推断神阙区域应该是新冠肺炎的热敏穴区，肺脾同病从神阙施灸，也是我们过去长期的临床经验。天枢穴是足阳明胃经穴位，又是大肠募穴，肺与大肠相表里，通腑宣肺，也应该是新冠肺炎的热敏穴区。因此本治疗方案确定选穴为神阙、天枢穴区，在此基础上探敏定位。

2. **灸敏得气** 艾灸强调得气，气至而有效。艾灸得气是艾灸疗法的精髓，是机体内源性抗病功能充分调动的标志，能够显著提高灸疗效果，这是以往热敏灸研究揭示的临床规律。艾灸得气的表现是透热、扩热、传热、深部热、远部热、身烘热、舒适、轻松、心情舒畅等。古人使用灸法也强调"必火足气到，始能求愈"，如何才能艾灸得气呢？艾灸热敏穴位是艾灸得气的关键之一，上面第一个环节辨敏选穴已奠定了基础。艾热强度也很重要，按照我们既往研究揭示的临床规律，选定艾灸得气的较佳艾热强度参数为 42℃ 左右。

3．消敏定量　艾灸量既要保证充分发挥疗效，又不致过量施灸是热敏灸治疗疾病的关键要素。笔者团队制定了标准化中个体化、个体化中标准化的消敏灸量标准，即以得气消退为度。这是既往大样本、多中心、中央随机对照试验证明的可以显著提高艾灸疗效的灸量标准，平均时间约 45 分钟。

4．依敏制具　工欲善其事，必先利其器。要艾灸得气，施灸工具很重要。进入隔离病房施灸，有 3 个特殊要求：①尽量减少近距离与患者接触的时间；②在病房内温度较低的情况下能快速得气；③要及时消除艾灸带来的艾烟。于是本团队研制了对艾热强度可方便单元调节的、艾热辐射可形成特定梯度的灸具，缩短了艾灸激发得气的潜伏期及医生与患者近距离接触的时间。由于隔离病房不能有艾燃烧产生的烟与味，故采用便携式消烟器，可消除空气中艾灸产生的 99% 的艾烟。

第三节　热敏灸防治新冠肺炎临床方案

一、热敏灸治疗新冠肺炎的方案

2020 年 2 月 21 日江西省中医药管理局正式发布《江西省新型冠状病毒肺炎中医药防治方案（试行第三版）》，公布了我们制定的热敏灸治疗新冠肺炎方案，并明确指出其适用于轻型、普通型及恢复期的肺脾气虚证。

1．灸位　神阙、天枢（双）、大横（双）。神阙穴位于前正中线上，脐中（如图 5-3-1），天枢穴位于人体腹部，脐中旁开 2 寸处（图 5-3-2），大横穴位于腹中部，脐中旁开 4 寸处（图 5-3-3）。

2．体位　取舒适仰卧位，全身放松。

3．灸具　如图 5-3-4。

4．操作　被灸者仰卧，分别点燃两段直径 2.5cm、长 4cm 的热敏灸艾柱，插入内有艾热反射腔、能够调节单元热度的专用灸具中。灸具长 22cm、宽 16cm，将灸具以肚脐为中心横向放置，灸具的出烟口与便携式消烟器相连。施灸过程中可通过调整每个施灸单元手柄来调节艾热强度，使施灸的腹部穴区感到热而均匀、舒适、不灼痛为宜。通过灸具在肚脐上下左右移动，找到出现有渗透、远传、扩散、舒适等艾灸得气热感的位置，静置施灸。整个施灸过程中务必保证热而均匀、舒适、不灼痛，灸至深部热、远部热、身烘热、额汗出等热敏感应消退为度（见图 5-3-5）。

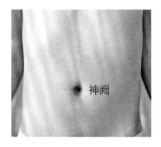

图 5-3-1　神阙穴

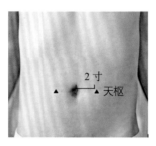

图 5-3-2　天枢穴

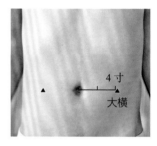

图 5-3-3　大横穴

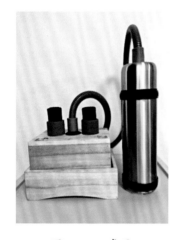

图 5-3-4　灸具

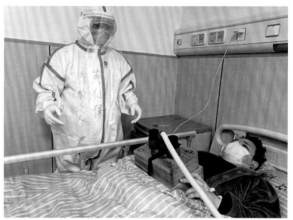

图 5-3-5　新冠肺炎患者正在做热敏灸

5．灸量　每日 1 次，40～60 分钟，每次施灸一般不超过 60 分钟。

6．方案解说　通过对新冠肺炎患者的临床观察，可知本病病因以湿邪为主，早中期病位在上、中二焦，主要涉及肺脾两脏。同时湿邪可郁而化热，造成湿热蒸腾弥漫三阳，湿遏热伏；后期则湿入三阴，湿邪伤阳。热敏灸可以温阳益气，化湿透热，散寒通络，对新冠肺炎可发挥重要治疗作用。治疗方案中神阙是温阳益气的重要腧穴，灸之则可以温阳益气，散寒化湿。天枢既是足阳明胃经的穴位，又是大肠募穴，灸之可以强健脾胃，通调肠腑，同时可扶土生金增强肺的宣发肃降功能。肺与大肠相表里，艾灸天枢通调腑气亦可以助肺气的通降功能。大横乃足太阴脾经穴位，可以强健脾胃的功能，增强脾胃的升降功能，助力中焦气血生化及疏布。诸穴共享，共奏益气温阳、温脾益肺、芳香化湿、通调腑气的作用。在采用上述方案施灸过程中，要求得气，即出现一身烘热、一身汗出、温暖、舒适等特殊感应，灸后身体轻松，心情舒畅，焦虑、紧张的情绪明显减轻。

二、热敏灸预防新冠肺炎的方案

2020 年 2 月 3 日江西省中医药管理局正式发布《江西省新型冠状病毒感染的肺炎中医药防治方案（试行第二版）》，并在全省医疗机构推广使用，公布了我们制定的热敏灸预防新冠肺炎方案——"一艾三用方"，即一根热敏灸艾条三种用法。

（一）闻艾香

芳香舒怡的嗅觉感受可以明显提高人体免疫力。热敏灸艾条中纯净艾绒的芳香成分及羌活、独活、细辛、川芎中芳香药性具有很好的芳香醒脑，敏化嗅觉，净化鼻咽内环境，提高鼻咽部免疫力的作用，特别适用于宣化上焦湿邪。具体操作为：将热敏灸艾条的药艾绒，放入具有密封功能的小盒内，盖好备用。闻艾香时将备好的小盒盖子打开，放置于鼻前，每次自然地深吸气 5~8 吸，每次吸气后停留 2~3 秒，再缓缓呼气，其目的是保证吸入的艾香在鼻咽部尽可能保留一段时间，更好地发挥作用，每天可反复闻艾香数次。

（二）艾泡脚

人体经络具有联系脏腑、沟通内外，运行气血、营养全身，抵御病邪、保卫机体的作用。足部分布有足三阴三阳、阴阳跷、阴阳维等多条经脉，尤其是足太阳膀胱经脉，用适宜温度的艾叶水泡脚可温助足太阳经脉的卫阳功能，与闻艾香、施艾灸并用，可达到温阳益气、芳香化湿、宣通三焦的功效。具体操作为：取热敏灸艾条半支，撕开外包装纸，将艾绒均匀揉散，放入纱布袋中，封口后放入盆中，倒入约 1000ml 热水，泡脚 30 分钟，泡脚过程中可以分次少量的加入热水，并用脚反复多次踩压装有艾绒的纱布袋，帮助药汁渗入水中。每日 1 次，以额头或者腰背部微微汗出为佳。建议水量能浸泡到脚踝上 3 寸处，尽可能保持全程水温恒定，有助于微微汗出。

（三）施艾灸

热敏腧穴对艾热刺激特别敏感，通过特定艾灸手法将艾热作用于热敏腧穴可以高效激发得气，调动人体自身抗病功能，防病治病，强身健体。中脘、神阙、关元是温运中焦要穴。通过特定动灸手法艾灸以上三穴，可以起到扶阳益气、温脾化湿的作用。具体操作为：被灸者仰卧，充分暴露中脘、神阙、关元穴区。中脘在肚脐与剑突连线的中点；神阙即是肚脐；关元在肚脐下一横掌的位置。取两根点燃的艾条，两根艾条间隔 0.5cm 左右，在以上三个穴位分布区，以温热而无灼痛的艾热强度进行循经往返灸。在出现热感有渗透、远传、扩散、舒适等灸感的位置，进行重点施灸，灸出阵阵深部热、远部热的得气感。每日 1 次，每次 40～60 分钟。如果自灸，也可选用聚热效果好、能够调节单元热度的热敏灸具进行施灸。施灸过程中，被施灸者应注意防寒保暖，室温保持在 25℃左右；注意用火安全，及时处理艾灰，避免火星灼伤皮肤等；施灸后 2 小时内不宜洗澡。

在上述基础上，能够接受麦粒灸者，对足三里穴加用麦粒灸，效果更佳。足三里是强健脾胃、增强抵抗力的重要穴位，自古就有"若要安，三里常不干"的记载。将麦粒大小的艾绒直接置于足三里穴施灸，具有非常好的强身健体效果。具体操作为：将艾绒搓成麦粒大小，一粒即为一壮，放置被灸者足三里穴位上。足三里在小腿前外侧，当犊鼻下 3 寸，距胫骨前缘一横指处。用点燃的线香点燃艾粒顶部，当被灸者感觉足三里穴灼痛难忍时用手按灭，即完成一壮，每次每侧 12～15 壮，隔日 1 次。施灸过程中有热感远传、渗透、扩散或灸后身体温热、舒适、轻松者效果尤佳。第 1 次施灸时，艾粒可由小至大施灸，逐渐加大灸量。每壮施灸时在能够忍受程度下，最好灼痛时间能够持续 3 秒钟，保证刺激强度。第二次施灸时，仍在原位置施灸。麦粒灸属于直接灸法，施灸过程中会出现不同程度的灼痛感，施灸后多数人会留有灸印，可酌情选择。糖尿病患者不宜应用。

第四节　热敏灸治疗新冠肺炎临床疗效

2020 年 2 月 11 日，江西省新冠肺炎疫情防控应急指挥部下发通知，江西中医药大学附属医院抚生院区（江西热敏灸医院）为江西省新冠肺炎医疗救治省级中西医结合定点医院。2 月 13 日热敏灸团队成员正式进入隔离病房开展热敏灸治疗新冠肺炎工作。2 月 24 日应湖北省蕲春县新冠肺炎疫情防控指挥部邀请，同时选派热敏灸团队成员前往蕲春县人民医院支援，助力当地开展热敏灸治疗新冠肺炎工作，均取得显著成效。

（一）临床资料

1．一般资料　病例来源于 2020 年 2 月 13 日至 2020 年 3 月 9 日江西中医药大学附属医院抚生院区与蕲春县人民医院收治的新冠肺炎（普通型）患者。共纳入新冠肺炎（普通型）患者 42 例，其中江西中医药大学附属医院抚生院区 28 例，蕲春县人民医院 14 例；男 28 例，女 14 例；年龄 29～76（47±11）岁，60 岁以下患者 35 例；30 例有明确疫区史或与新冠肺炎患者接触史；11 例患有基础疾病，其中高血压 5 例，糖尿病 2 例，合并高血压、糖尿病者 2 例，合并糖尿病、冠状动脉粥样硬化性心脏病者 1 例，哮喘 1 例。本研究通过江西中医药大学附属医院的伦理审批（伦理批准号：JZFYKYLL20200210002）。

2．诊断标准　诊断标准与临床分型依据国家卫生健康委员会于 2020 年 1 月 27 日公布的《新型冠状病毒感染的肺炎诊疗方案（试行第四版）》。

3．纳入标准　①符合新冠肺炎诊断标准，其临床分型属于普通型。②年龄 18～80 岁。③能配合艾灸治疗、能正确表达灸感。④自愿加入本试验并签署知情同意书。

4．排除标准　①体温超过 38.0℃者。②具有严重全身性疾病（心、肝、肺、肾、血液病等），精神病患者。③晕灸者或惧怕艾灸者。④施灸部位具有溃疡、皮损等影响灸感者。

（二）治疗方法

在常规对症治疗的基础上，参照《江西省新型冠状病毒肺炎中医药防治方案（试行第三版）》，对患者施以热敏灸治疗。

1．灸位　神阙、天枢（双）、大横（双）。

2．体位　取舒适仰卧位，全身放松。

3．操作　被灸者仰卧，分别点燃两段直径 2.5cm、长 4cm 的热敏灸艾柱，插入内有艾热反射腔、能够调节单元热度的专用灸具中。灸具长 22cm、宽 16cm，将灸具以肚脐为中心横向放置，灸具的出烟口与便携式消烟器相连。施灸过程中可通过调整每个施灸单元手柄来调节艾热强度，使施灸的腹部穴区感到热而均匀、舒适、不灼痛为宜。通过在肚脐上下左右移动灸具，找到出现热感且有渗透、远传、扩散、舒适等艾灸得气热感的位置，静置施灸。整个施灸过程中务必保证热而均匀、舒适、不灼痛，灸至深部热、远部热、身烘热、额汗出等热敏感应消退为度。

4．灸量　每日 1 次，每次施灸以患者热敏灸感消退为度，约 40～60 分钟，不超过 60 分钟。

（三）疗效观察

1．观察指标

（1）**艾灸得气率**:《黄帝内经》上说"气至而有效"，得气是疗效的一个非常好的预测指标。艾灸得气率为艾灸得气病例数占总病例数的百分比。患者艾灸得气分别在首次施灸 20 分钟、40 分钟、1 小时进行评估。艾灸得气的标准是：被施灸者产生透热、扩热、传热、非热觉、身烘热、额汗出、肢端热、胃肠蠕动反应等热敏灸感中的 1 种或 1 种以上，则判定为艾灸得气。

（2）**胸闷、纳差症状改善情况**：参考《中药新药临床研究指导原则（试行）》的中医证候量表，评价艾灸前后患者胸闷、纳差等中医证候变化。胸闷或纳差症状（评分为 0～3 分）的发生率为胸闷或纳差病例数占总病例数的百分比。分别于治疗前及治疗第 1 次、治疗第 2 次、治疗第 3 次结束后进行胸闷、纳差症状评估。

（3）**负性情绪减轻情况**：这是一个艾灸调神的指标。采用正负性情绪量表（the positive and negative affect scale，PANAS）评估患者的负性情绪，包含 20 个条目，其中第 2、4、6、7、8、11、13、15、18、20 等 10 项条目为负性情绪评估项，以 1～5 级计分，1 分表示完全没有，5 分表示极其多，全部为正向计分，其总分在 10～50 分。10～20 分患者负性情绪较少，表明身体舒适和心情舒畅；21～50 分则负性情绪较多，表明身体存在较多不舒适和心情不舒畅。身体舒适和心情舒畅的发生率为评估 10～20 分的病例数占总病例数的百分比。分别于治疗前及治疗第 1 次、治疗第 2 次、治疗第 3 次结束后进行负性情绪评估，见表 5-4-1。

表 5-4-1　正负性情绪量表（PANAS）

		完全没有	比较少	中等程度	比较多	极其多
1	感兴趣的	1	2	3	4	5
2	心烦的	1	2	3	4	5
3	精神活力高的	1	2	3	4	5
4	心神不宁的	1	2	3	4	5
5	劲头足的	1	2	3	4	5
6	内疚的	1	2	3	4	5
7	恐惧的	1	2	3	4	5
8	敌意的	1	2	3	4	5
9	热情的	1	2	3	4	5
10	自豪的	1	2	3	4	5
11	易怒的	1	2	3	4	5
12	警觉性高的	1	2	3	4	5
13	害羞的	1	2	3	4	5
14	备受鼓舞的	1	2	3	4	5
15	紧张的	1	2	3	4	5
16	意志坚定的	1	2	3	4	5
17	注意力集中的	1	2	3	4	5
18	坐立不安的	1	2	3	4	5
19	有活力的	1	2	3	4	5
20	害怕的	1	2	3	4	5

（4）**热敏灸的主动接受率**：这也是一个艾灸调神的指标。热敏灸的接受度与认可度分为不接受（拒绝艾灸治疗）、被动接受（由医生推荐艾灸治疗，患者表示愿意尝试治疗）及主动接受（患者自己主动要求艾

灸治疗）3 种情况。热敏灸的主动接受率为主动接受病例数占总病例数的百分比。患者于治疗前和第 1 次治疗结束后进行热敏灸主动接受率的调查。

2．统计学处理　数据采用 SPSS19.0 统计软件进行分析。计量资料以均数 ± 标准差（$\bar{x} \pm s$）表示；计数资料采用例数（%）的形式表示，组内比较采用 χ^2 检验。以 $P<0.05$ 为差异有统计学意义。

3．治疗结果

（1）**艾灸得气率**：热敏灸治疗新冠肺炎（普通型）患者 42 例，共施灸 272 人次。热敏灸治疗在病区覆盖率100%。热敏灸 20 分钟，艾灸得气率达 52.4%（22/42）；热敏灸 30 分钟，艾灸得气率达 78.6%（33/42）；热敏灸 40 分钟，艾灸得气率达 90.5%（38/42）；热敏灸 1 小时，艾灸得气率达 100%。患者在施灸过程中出现舒适、透热、扩热、传热、四肢末端热、深部热、远部热、身烘热等反应。施灸后部分患者感到身体轻松、心情舒畅。说明该类患者的相关穴位普遍发出了对艾热的需求信号，表明热敏灸非常适合新冠肺炎患者的治疗，并能发挥较好的作用。

（2）**胸闷、纳差症状改善情况**：患者胸闷症状在第 1 次、第 2 次、第 3 次热敏灸得气后的发生率分别为 23.8%（10/42）、16.7%（7/42）、9.5%（4/42），低于热敏灸治疗前的 50.0%（21/42，$P<0.05$）。表明热敏灸治疗可以改善新冠肺炎（普通型）患者的胸闷症状。患者纳差症状在第 1 次、第 2 次、第 3 次热敏灸得气后的发生率分别为 26.2%（11/42）、19.0%（8/42）、9.5%（4/42），低于热敏灸治疗前的 57.1%（24/42，$P<0.05$），表明热敏灸治疗可以改善新冠肺炎（普通型）患者的纳差症状。

（3）**负性情绪减轻情况**：患者第 1 次、第 2 次、第 3 次热敏灸得气后立即感到身体轻松与心情舒畅的发生率分别为 61.9%（26/42）、73.8%（31/42）、92.9%（39/42），高于热敏灸治疗前的 42.9%（18/42，$P<0.05$）。表明热敏灸能有效减轻负性情绪，增强患者战胜疾病的信心。

（4）**患者热敏灸的主动接受率的变化**：第 1 次治疗后，患者对热敏灸治疗的主动接受率为 100%（42/42），高于热敏灸治疗前的 11.9%（5/42），表明热敏灸对于新冠肺炎患者来说是一种舒适、易于接受的治疗方法。

（5）**不良反应情况**：42 例接受热敏灸治疗的新冠肺炎患者，均未出现晕灸、皮肤烫伤、症状加重等不良反应。

（四）临床体会

应用上述灸疗方案治疗新型冠状病毒肺炎，是一次有益的探索，有以下体会：

1. **艾灸得气** 得气的概念，源于《灵枢·九针十二原》："刺之要，气至而有效。效之信，若风之吹云，明乎若见苍天。"说明得气很重要。但是艾灸需不需要得气，黄帝内经未提及。直到《医宗金鉴》："凡灸诸病，必火足气到，始能求愈。"明确说明灸法也要得气，但是灸法得气的表现是什么？仍未明确。2008年《中国针灸》杂志发表了我们的研究成果《灸之要，气至而有效》，在这篇文章里明确提出透热、扩热、传热、深部热、远部热才是得气的表现，而不是皮肤局部热、表面热。2018年，我们的研究成果再次在《中国针灸》杂志发表，论述了完整的艾灸得气的十大条目，即透热、扩热、传热、喜热、肢端热、身烘热、非热觉、额汗出、胃肠蠕动反应、皮肤扩散性潮红。2019年，《中国针灸》杂志发表了我们关于艾灸得气的理论研究文章，这篇文章给艾灸得气下了一个明确的定义，即：艾灸得气是指与疗效相关的舒适的一组躯体感应。在这个定义中，"躯体感应"是表现；舒适的、疗效相关的两个定语才是艾灸得气的本质。艾灸得气能够提高疗效，在我们过去的研究中已经揭示。我们做了三个病症，支气管哮喘（慢性持续期）、膝关节骨性关节炎、腰椎间盘突出症，都是采用大样本、多中心、中央随机对照临床试验方法，取得了高级别的证据。因此，艾灸得气很重要，要充分重视艾灸过程中激发艾灸得气。这次热敏灸治疗新冠肺炎我们就采用了"灸敏得气"的技术方案，取得显著疗效。

2. **艾灸化湿** 湿邪是六淫邪气中最棘手的病邪。根据我们的临床经验，艾灸祛除湿邪，非"小刺激大反应"不能除之，即"非敏不除湿"，热敏穴位恰恰具有这种功能。湿性黏滞，病程缠绵难愈；湿为阴邪，易损伤阳气；湿聚为饮，阻滞气机；湿蕴化热，湿遏热伏。灸法非常适合湿邪为病的上述主证与变化证候，具有温脾化湿、温阳益气、温利水饮、温透郁热的作用。临床中反复证明，一些湿阻中焦的患者舌苔厚腻，食欲不佳，大便黏腻不成形，如果艾灸中脘、水分等穴激发得气，每次施灸1小时，经过2~3次治疗，患者舌苔明显变薄，食欲改善，大便成形。因此，湿邪为病，选择艾灸应大力倡导。

3. 艾灸调神　《灵枢·本神》云："凡刺之法，必先本于神。"又《灵枢·官能》说："用针之要，无忘其神。"中医治病强调治人，治人先治神，神安则体安，心神不安必然影响神经 – 内分泌 – 免疫网络功能。热敏灸得气时产生的一身烘热、一身轻松、心情舒畅，这就是艾灸调神的具体表现，也是热敏灸的独特优势。现代医学已证明，疾病过程中的负性情绪会严重影响人体抗病机能的发挥。因此，充分重视与发挥热敏灸的调神作用，减轻患者负性情绪，增强抗病机能，是值得重视和应用的。在这次疫情中，患者普遍存在忧郁、低落、焦虑、恐慌心理状态，患者热敏灸得气后，身体烘热、身体舒适、心情舒畅，显著提高了患者对疾病治疗的信心。因此，针灸疗法非常重视治神，艾灸调神是艾灸瑰宝，要推广应用。

本次热敏灸参与治疗新型冠状病毒肺炎，是一个灸法亮剑意义的尝试。虽然样本量小，无法随机分组对照，但是上述四个指标都是热敏灸干预的即时效应，能够独立反映热敏灸疗效，具有独立评估价值。上述结果提示了灸法治疗新冠肺炎的可行性与有效性，开启了灸法治疗疫病的新思路。

第五节　病案举例

●【探敏施灸案】

屈某，男，31 岁，因咳嗽 10 余天入院。患者于 2020 年 2 月 4 日出现发热、咳嗽，测体温为 38.6℃，自诉有新冠肺炎患者接触史，遂至当地医院就诊，拟"疑似新型冠状病毒肺炎"收治入院。经咽拭子新型冠状病毒核酸检测示阳性，行肺部 CT 示双肺炎性改变，遂确诊为"新型冠状病毒肺炎"，予以对症支持治疗，后患者体温恢复正常，但咳嗽未见明显缓解，于 2 月 14 日转入我院抚生院区治疗。入院症见：患者神志清，精神可，咳嗽咳痰，痰白量少，咽中异物感，言语频繁时较为明显，无恶寒发热，食纳尚可，睡眠一般，大便平，小便正常。舌质暗红，苔白腻，脉细滑。中医诊断：疫毒证（痰湿郁肺）；治法：健脾宣肺，理气化痰。

于2020年2月15日开始热敏灸治疗。分别点燃两段直径2.5cm、长4cm的艾柱插入专用灸具中，将灸具以神阙穴为中心横向放置。第1次施灸至5分钟时患者诉仅感局部、表面灼热，遂调整两个施灸单元手柄，调节艾热强度，使施灸的腹部穴区感到热而均匀、舒适、不灼痛，并通过灸具在神阙穴上下左右移动探感定位，当灸具移动至神阙穴偏上位置时，患者诉腹中有透热感，施灸约15分钟后患者一身烘热，灸至30分钟，灸感减弱，遂停灸。感全身轻松、心情舒畅。按上法继续施灸，次日患者诉施灸时腹中透热感较前明显，双足心微热，灸后全身轻松、心情舒畅，咽中异物感较前减轻，咳嗽缓解。第3次施灸时患者诉小腹内透热甚，全身烘热明显，灸后自诉全身舒适感，咳嗽较前明显减轻，咽中异物感基本消失。按上述方案继续施灸4天，患者诉咽中异物感基本消除，偶尔咳嗽，无咳痰。行胸部CT示：两肺病灶较前有所吸收、减淡。但2月21日行咽拭子及痰液新冠病毒核酸检测示阳性，遂继续按照以上方法予以热敏灸治疗，每日1次，患者诉腹部透热感渐渐增强，且双侧足心、腰部逐渐出现烘热，全身感觉轻松舒适，心情渐渐舒畅，咽中异物感、咳嗽基本消失。无咳嗽，纳寐尚可，二便平。舌质暗红，舌苔薄白，脉滑。分别于2月28日、3月1日行痰与咽拭子新型冠状病毒核酸检测均为阴性，且连续3天以上无发热，遂于3月2日出院。

按语：探敏施灸，即探查热敏穴位施灸，是以经穴部位作为热敏穴位的高发区域，采用热敏灸具在该穴区缓慢上下左右移动探查，当移动至某一部位出现一种或一种以上的"透热、扩热、传热"等热敏现象时，该部位就是热敏穴位的准确位置。以此为灸位施灸，而不拘其是否在准确的经穴位置上，是保证艾灸治疗新冠肺炎发挥疗效的首要环节。

●【消敏定量案】

吴某，男，67岁，因咳嗽胸闷10余天入院。患者于2020年1月下旬开始无明显诱因出现咳嗽，无咳痰，伴胸闷、发热，测体温38.5℃，午后发热为主，无畏寒。1月31日在当地县中医院住院治疗，后转入当地县人民医院住院，2月9日行胸部CT示双肺多发炎症，行咽拭子新型冠状病毒核酸检测为阳性，诊断为"新型冠状病毒肺炎"。入院后予对症治疗，发热、咳嗽基本消失，但仍胸闷、气喘，遂于2020年2月15日转入我院抚生院区治疗。入院症见：精神一般，面色少华，胸闷不适，活动后气喘，无咳嗽咳痰，声低懒言，乏力，食纳差，夜寐欠安，难以入睡，大便1次每日，小便略黄，无烧灼感。舌质暗红，苔薄黄腻，脉弦滑。中医诊断：疫毒证（湿郁肺脾，湿遏热伏）；治法：温脾益气，温阳化湿。

于2020年2月16日开始热敏灸治疗。分别点燃两段直径2.5cm、长4cm的艾柱插入专用灸具中，将灸具以神阙穴为中心横向放置。第1次施灸至约10分钟时患者诉仅感局部、表面灼热，遂调整两个施灸单元手柄，降低艾热强度至七分，使施灸的腹部穴区感到热而均匀、舒适、温热，并通过灸具在神阙穴上下左右移动探感定位，当灸具移动至神阙穴偏左上位置时患者感腹部微微透热，施灸约20分钟后腹部透热感渐渐增强，且腰部、双足底微热，全身轻微汗出，施灸约50分钟后透热感减弱，遂停灸。第1次施灸后患者一身轻松，心情舒畅，乏力、胸闷缓解约30%。第2次施灸时患者自诉腹腔内透热增强，腰部、双足底微热，且全身有轻微汗出，诉乏力、胸闷不适缓解约50%，食欲增加。第3次施灸时患者腹腔透热及腰部、双足底热感均较前明显，全身烘热舒适，灸后乏力、胸闷不适缓解约60%，活动后气喘明显改善，食欲、睡眠改善。第4次施灸时患者自诉腹腔透热及腰部、双足底热感明显增强，灸后全身微汗出，一身轻松，乏力、胸闷缓解约80%，纳寐改善。按上述方案继续施灸4次，患者乏力、胸闷等症状基本消除，食欲明显增加。患者分别于2月17日、19日、21日、23日行新型冠状病毒咽拭子新型冠状病毒核酸检测，均为阴性，连续3天无发热，遂于2月24日出院。

按语：消敏定量，是指以热敏灸感（艾灸得气）消失为度来确定个体化的施灸时间，这是根据患者机体自身表达出来的需求灸量确定的灸量标准，是最佳的个体化充足灸量。由于灸量与施灸强度、面积、时间相关，强度、面积在施灸过程中是相对不变的常量，而施灸时间是个体化的变量，如何把敏化的穴位灸满、灸透、灸足，是使灸疗疗效潜力充分发挥的又一个关键因素。按照灸感－灸时－灸效的研究成果，"以热敏灸感消失为度"可作为充足灸疗时间的标准，突破了灸疗临床长期以来每穴

10～15min 固定灸时的固有观念，为临床充分发挥灸疗疗效提供了灸疗时间的量学标准，实现了灸疗时间标准化与个体化的有机统一。

●【证感相关案】

陈某，男，29 岁，因咳嗽 18 天入院。患者于 2020 年 1 月 31 日无明显诱因出现咳嗽咳痰，痰黄脓，咽痛、恶寒发热，测体温最高达 39℃，全身乏力，于 2 月 4 日至当地医院住院治疗。行胸部 CT 示：左肺上叶前段磨玻璃样结节影，考虑少量炎性病变；左肺下叶背段少量陈旧性病灶。2 月 5 日行咽拭子新型冠状病毒核酸检测阳性，遂确诊为"新冠肺炎"，经对症治疗后患者无发热，但仍咳嗽，怕冷，大便稀。于 2020 年 2 月 18 日转入我院抚生院区治疗。入院症见：咳嗽，以干咳为主，咽痒，无咽痛，无发热，怕冷，无恶风，喜温饮，无潮热盗汗，纳食差，夜寐安，大便偏稀，2 次每日，小便偏黄。舌质红，苔薄白，脉细。

中医诊断：疫毒证（脾肺气虚）；治法：健脾益肺，培土生金。

于 2020 年 2 月 19 日开始热敏灸治疗。分别点燃两段直径 2.5cm、长 4cm 的艾柱插入专用灸具中，将灸具以神阙穴为中心横向放置。第 1 次施灸至约 8 分钟时患者诉仅仅感局部、表面灼热，遂调整两个施灸单元手柄调节艾热强度，使施灸的腹部穴区感到热而均匀、舒适、不灼痛，并通过灸具在神阙穴上下左右移动探感定位，当灸具移动至神阙穴偏右上位置时患者感艾热徐徐向腹腔内渗透，施灸约 20 分钟后患者渐渐感艾热向上传导至胸腔，并感双足心烘热感明显，施灸约 40 分钟后透热感减弱，遂停灸。第 1 次施灸后感觉全身轻松。次日患者诉胸腹腔、双足心烘热感较明显，灸后全身轻松感觉，咳嗽稍缓解，纳食改善。第 3 次患者诉胸腹腔、双足心热感较前明显，灸后全身轻松感觉，咳嗽减轻，大便成形，怕冷减轻，纳食明显改善。继续施灸 6 天，患者诉腹部有透热感，胸腔、腰部及双足底有热感，全身微汗，轻松舒适。分别于 2 月 24 日、26 日行咽拭子新型冠状病毒核酸检测阴性，连续 3 天以上无发热，患者已达出院标准，遂于 2 月 27 日出院。

按语：新冠肺炎患者在不同的发病阶段，表现为不同的证候，而施灸过程中出现的灸感类型也各不相同。临床研究表明：不同热敏灸感携带着不同的艾灸信息，有首选与候选、主选与次选之分，需要进一步分析、辨别。分析新冠肺炎患者不同证型表现的不同热敏灸感蕴含的信息对提高灸疗疗效有重要作用，如湿邪束表，以一身烘热、微汗出灸感为宜；寒湿直中脾胃，以腹腔内透热、深部热灸感为宜；脾肺气虚，湿阻三焦，以腹腔透热、传热至胸腔、身烘热等灸感为佳。

●【痰湿宜和案】

康某，男，42 岁，因咳嗽胸闷 2 天入院。患者于 2020 年 2 月 5 日无明显诱因出现发热，体温最高 38.5℃，轻微胸背部疼痛，无恶寒，无咳嗽咳痰，自行在家休养症状未见缓解，遂于 2020 年 2 月 8 日至当地医院就诊，行胸部 CT 示双肺感染，2 月 10 日行新型冠状病毒核酸检测示阳性，遂诊断为"新冠肺炎"。于 2020 年 2 月 14 日转入我院抚生院区治疗，入院症见：咳嗽，咳少量灰色痰，胸闷，活动后气喘，口干不欲饮，平素喜温饮，少气懒言，无发热恶寒，四肢酸痛，食纳可，睡眠一般，大便质软，小便黄。舌质淡红，苔白腻，脉缓。中医诊断：疫毒证（痰湿蕴肺证）；治法：健脾，化痰，宣肺。

于 2020 年 2 月 15 日开始热敏灸治疗。分别点燃两段直径 2.5cm、长 4cm 的艾柱插入专用灸具中，将灸具以神阙穴为中心横向放置。第 1 次施灸至约 8 分钟时患者诉仅仅感局部、表面温热，遂调整两个施灸单元手柄改变艾热强度，使施灸的腹部穴区感到温热而均匀、舒适、不灼痛，并通过灸具在神阙穴上下左右移动探感定位，当灸具移动至神阙穴偏右上位置时患者觉腹部有透热感，施灸约 25 分钟后患者渐渐感腰部温热，双足心有微热感，施灸约 45 分钟后透热感减弱，遂停灸。第 1 次施灸后自诉全身微微汗出，感觉舒适轻松。第 2 次施灸时腹部透热感稍增强，腰部热甚，双足心有热微汗，灸后舒适轻松感觉，咳嗽减轻，胸闷缓解 30% 左右。第 3 次施灸时患者诉腹部透热感较前明显增强，腰部、双足心热感较前明显，灸后自诉全身烘热舒适感，咳嗽缓解 50%，胸闷缓解 50% 左右，活动后气喘缓解。第 4 次施灸时患者腹腔内透热明显，腰部、双足心热甚，灸后咳嗽缓解 70%，胸闷缓解 80% 左右。按上述方案继续施灸 5 天，施灸时患者腹腔内透热感不断增强，腰部、双足心热感也渐渐明显，且双足心微汗出，全身烘热，灸后全身轻松舒适，无明显咳嗽、胸闷，活动尚可。患者分别于 2 月 17 日、19 日行咽拭子新型冠状病毒核酸检测阴性，且连续 3 天无发热，遂于 2 月 24 日出院。

按语：湿属阴邪，黏腻缠绵，易聚成痰成饮，阻遏气机，损伤阳气。张仲景所著《金匮要略·痰饮咳嗽病脉证并治》篇明确提出治痰饮之大法："病痰饮者，当以温药和之。"即治痰饮宜用平和的温性之品振奋阳气，温化痰饮，而不可过用大辛燥烈之品，以防伤阴耗气。同理，湿聚痰饮者，当以灸法和之。热敏灸温化痰湿，每次施灸的灸热强度不宜过大，灸时稍长为宜，通过灸量的不断累积，机体阳气渐充，痰饮阴邪渐渐温化，从而达到治疗目的。

●【湿热可灸案】

杜某，男，67 岁，因咳嗽 5 天，伴胸闷气促 4 天入院。患者于 2020 年 2 月 2 日无明显诱因出现发热，无恶寒，体温最高 37.3℃，无明显咳嗽咳痰，在当地诊所予口服药物（具体不详）治疗，体温未见缓解，遂至当地医院就诊。胸部 CT 示：考虑双肺感染，建议结合临床及相关排查。2020 年 2 月 13 日新型冠状病毒核酸检测阳性，诊断为"新型冠状病毒肺炎"，因咳嗽、胸闷等症状加重，遂于 2020 年 2 月 15 日转入我院。刻下症见：咳嗽无痰，活动后胸闷气促，无胸前区疼痛，无发热恶寒，无鼻塞流涕，无恶心呕吐，纳可，寐一般，二便可。舌质淡红，苔黄，脉滑数。中医诊断：疫毒证（湿热蕴肺）；治法：宣肺、化湿、透热。

于 2020 年 2 月 16 日开始热敏灸治疗。分别点燃两段直径 2.5cm、长 4cm 的艾柱插入专用灸具中，将灸具以神阙穴为中心横向放置。第 1 次施灸至约 10 分钟时患者诉仅仅感局部、表面灼热，遂调整两个施灸单元手柄，降低艾热强度，使施灸的腹部穴区感到温热而均匀、舒适、不灼痛，并通过灸具在神阙穴上下左右移动探感定位，当灸具移动至神阙穴偏向上位置时患者感艾热徐徐向腹腔内渗透，施灸约 20 分钟后患者渐渐感艾热向上传导至胸腔、后背，并觉双足心烘热感明显，施灸约 40 分钟后透热感减弱，遂停灸。第 1 次施灸后咳嗽、胸闷缓解约 30%，全身稍轻松；第 2 次施灸时患者自诉腹中透热较前增强，且背部烘热，双足底温热，额部微汗，咳嗽、胸闷气促缓解约 40%，全身较轻松。第 3 次施灸时患者自诉腹中透热明显，背部烘热，足心微热且全身汗出，咳嗽、胸闷气促缓解约 50%，全身轻松感较前明显。第 4 次施灸时患者自诉腹部有透热感，腰背部烘热，足心热甚，且全身汗出，咳嗽、胸闷气促缓解约 80%，全身轻松感较前明显，且心情舒畅。第 5 次施灸时，患者感当天灸感最佳，腹部出现明显透热感，且从背部至足热感明显，额部微汗出，灸后全身烘热舒适，咳嗽明显减轻，胸闷消失，活动量明显增加，全身非常轻松，且心情舒畅，患者诉抗病信心倍增。继续予以热敏灸巩固治疗 1 周。患者于 2020 年 2 月 28 日及 2020 年 3 月 1 日行新型冠状病毒核酸检测示阴性。遂于 3 月 2 日出院。

　　按语：湿邪为病，蕴而化热，湿遏热伏。热敏灸能温阳益气、宣达三焦、宣化湿浊，能达到温阳化湿而透热的目的，湿除则热散，故湿热亦可灸。但施灸过程中要掌握适宜的刺激强度。由于部分患者因湿伏热蕴、湿热熏蒸，施灸初期常常表现为拒热、不耐热，此时，艾热强度宜由小到大、灸量宜由少到多，以温热强度（灸热七分）为佳。待湿邪渐去、湿化热透后，逐渐增加艾热强度。对改善因湿蕴肺脾引起的低热或不发热，微恶寒、乏力，头身困重，肌肉酸痛，咳嗽少痰或有黄痰，咽痛，憋闷气促，腹胀，便秘不畅等湿热证能起到意想不到的效果。

●【灸可调神案】

　　罗某，43 岁，因乏力、发热 5 周，盗汗 4 周入院。患者于 2020 年 1 月下旬在武汉居住及湖北多地旅游后开始出现神疲乏力，难以完成日常体力活动，有低热，多出现于夜间，体温波动于 37～38℃，伴纳差厌油，饥饿不欲食，口干口苦口黏，至当地医院住院治疗，行胸部 CT 示双肺下叶炎症。当地疾控中心新型冠状病毒核酸检测呈阳性，遂诊断为"新型冠状病毒肺炎"，予以药物对症治疗 1 周后体温恢复正常，精神食欲改善，开始出现夜间盗汗，入睡即汗出，一夜需更换 3～4 次睡衣，睡眠差，自觉心慌气短，伴便溏，开始为水样便后为糊状，日解 2 次，间断服用中药（不详）未缓解，多次复查胸部 CT，示胸部病灶吸收较好，但当地疾控中心先后 4 次行新型冠状病毒核酸检测均提示阳性。2 月 26 日转入我院抚生院区治疗。入院症见：夜间盗汗，寐差，乏力、心慌气短，便溏，日解 2 次，纳差厌油，饥饿不欲食，口干、口苦、口黏，心情焦虑，舌质红苔薄，舌根稍黄腻，脉滑数。中医诊断：疫毒证（湿遏热伏）；治法：温脾益胃，化湿透热，温养心神。

于 2020 年 2 月 26 日开始热敏灸治疗。分别点燃两段直径 2.5cm、长 4cm 的艾柱插入专用灸具中，将灸具以神阙穴为中心横向放置。第 1 次施灸至约 8 分钟时患者诉仅仅感局部表面灼热，遂调整两个施灸单元手柄降低艾热强度，使施灸的腹部穴区感到温热而均匀、舒适、不灼痛，并通过灸具在神阙穴上下左右移动探感定位，当灸具移动至神阙穴偏右上位置时患者感腹部表面温热舒适，施灸约 20 分钟后患者渐渐感艾热向四周扩散，施灸约 40 分钟后扩热感减弱，遂停灸。第 1 次施灸后乏力感稍缓解。按上述方法继续施灸，次日施灸时患者诉腹部有热感向上传至胸腔，施灸后全身烘热，一身轻松，心情舒畅，乏力感缓解约 50%。第 3 次施灸时患者诉腹部有热感，并渐渐向下传至双足心，灸后全身烘热，一身轻松，心情舒畅，乏力感缓解约 70%，大便好转成形，日 1 次，食欲增强，睡眠改善。按上述方法连续施灸 5 日，施灸时患者均觉腹部有透热感，腰部、足心烘热，全身微汗，一身轻松，心情舒畅。施灸后患者盗汗、乏力明显改善，纳食正常，二便平。分别于 3 月 2 日、3 月 4 日行咽拭子新型冠状病毒核酸检测阴性，连续 3 天无发热，影像学提示肺部感染病灶吸收。患者遂于 3 月 5 日出院。

按语：新冠肺炎患者普遍存在紧张、焦虑、恐慌、心慌、失眠、精神萎靡、情绪低落或烦躁不安等心理状态。热敏灸得气后，身体烘热、舒适、心情舒畅，显著提高了患者战胜疾病的信心。因此，充分重视与发挥热敏灸的调神作用，减轻患者负性情绪，增强抗病机能，是值得重视和应用的。

附 录

一、热敏灸研究系列重要成果证书

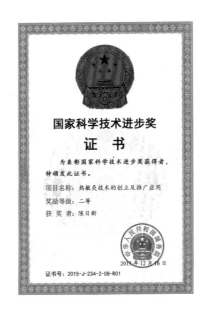

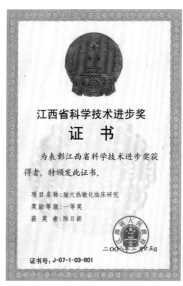

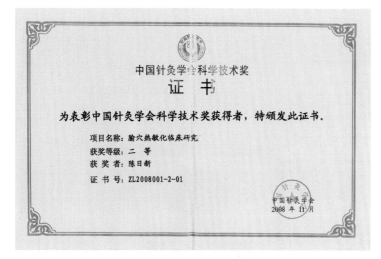

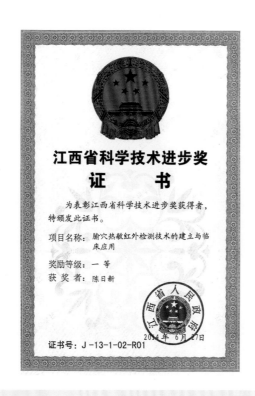

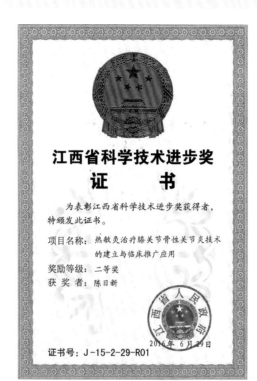

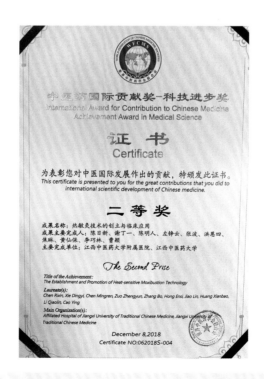

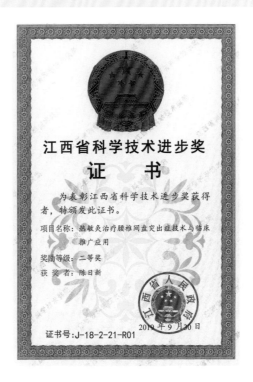

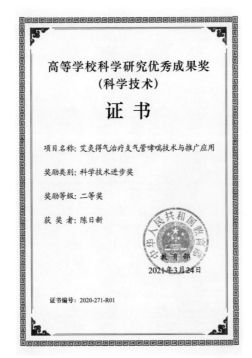

二、热敏灸技术操作规范（世界中联国际组织标准，2018 年发布）

ICS 11.040.11

SCM

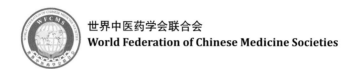

世界中医药学会联合会
World Federation of Chinese Medicine Societies

SCM0023-2018

热敏灸技术操作规范

Standardized Manipulations of Heat-sensitive Moxibustion Therapy

世界中联国际组织标准
International Standard of WFCMS

2018-06-24发布实施
Issued & implemented on June 24th, 2018

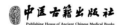

中医古籍出版社
Publishing House of Ancient Chinese Medical Books

三、热敏灸安全操作规范（江西省地方标准，2022 年发布）

ICS 11.020
C 05

DB36

江 西 省 地 方 标 准

DB36/T 1637—2022

热敏灸安全操作规范

Safety operation specification of heat-sensitive moxibustion

2022－09－26 发布   2022－09－26 实施

江西省市场监督管理局   发 布

四、热敏灸红外热成像图示例

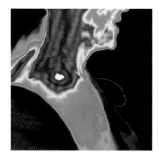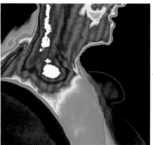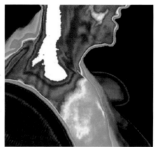

传热

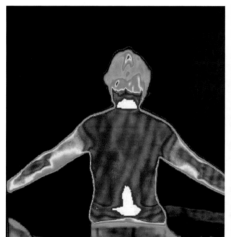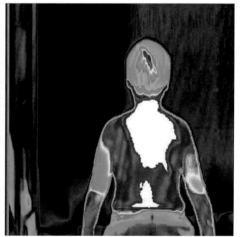

扩热

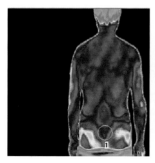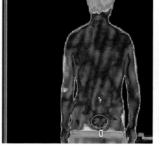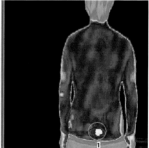

透热

五、热敏灸研究部分 SCI 收录论文

Neuroscience Letters 503 (2011) 131–135

Contents lists available at SciVerse ScienceDirect

Neuroscience Letters

journal homepage: www.elsevier.com/locate/neulet

Stroke treatment in rats with tail temperature increase by 40-min moxibustion

Ri-Xin Chen[a],[*],[1], Zhi-Mai Lv[b],[1], Ming-Ren Chen[a], Fan Yi[c], Xin An[a], Ding-Yi Xie[a]

[a] Affiliated Hospital of Jiangxi University of TCM, Nanchang 330006, PR China
[b] The First Affiliated Hospital of Gannan Medical University, Ganzhou, PR China
[c] Department of Health of Jiangxi Province, Nanchang, PR China

ARTICLE INFO

Article history:
Received 11 April 2011
Received in revised form 23 June 2011
Accepted 12 August 2011

Keywords:
Moxibustion
Cerebral ischemia
Inflammation
Apoptosis

ABSTRACT

The distant heat induced by suspended moxibustion (SM) for 40 min is confirmed to have a favorable effect in treating diseases such as ischemic brain injury in the clinical setting, but its precise mechanism remains to be explained. Since a similar reaction to the phenomenon of distant heat is found in some transient middle cerebral artery occlusion (tMCAO) rats treated by a 40-min SM session with tail temperature increase (TTI), we hereby study its mechanism by comparing the neuroprotective effect of 40 min's SM with TTI to those without. The experimental results show that 40 min's SM with TTI can significantly reduce the infarct volume and neurological deficit score in tMCAO rats. Western blot demonstrates that a reduction in the levels of cyclooxygenase-2 (COX-2), inducible nitric oxide synthase (iNOS) expression in tMCAO rats with TTI is more striking than that of the rats without TTI. The expression of caspase-3 protein is inhibited in tMCAO rats with TTI. The results suggest that the efficacy of SM for 40 min with TTI is higher than that without. Although neuroprotective effects present in tMCAO rats with and without TTI, those with TTI revealed a higher level of anti-inflammation effect and exhibited an anti-apoptosis effect.

1. Introduction

Ischemic stroke is universally acknowledged as a common cause of long-term disability or even death [7]. It is widely known that cerebral inflammation and neural apoptosis after cerebral infarction contribute largely to ischemic brain injury. Inhibiting the above pathological process is effective in reducing brain injury and can ward off neurological impairment in patients [6].

SM (suspended moxibustion), being one of the indirect moxibustions, is moxibustion placed superficially over the skin without making contact. Some researchers have used this method to treat stroke patients, but strong evidence of its therapeutic effectiveness is lacking [9]. We have studied SM for 20 years in the clinical setting and observed an important phenomenon in SM treatment. Moxibustion placed above certain acupoints can often induce a phenomenon of distant heat which is the sensation felt and physically detectable away from the SM acupoint. There is a substantial increase in moxibustion's efficacy when distant heat occurs [2]. The phenomenon is evidenced by two major aspects: (a) moxibustion heat penetrates deep into the tissues or internal organs of the body;

(b) moxibustion heat is transferred from the original moxibustion acupoint to the other areas of the body [3]. Distant heat first appears on the patient at about 15 min time point in the SM treatment session. After the 15 min time point, a rapid increase in distant heat is exhibited in the patients and maintained until the end of the treatment [4].

Our previous studies showed that there was a higher efficacy of SM for 40 min than that for 15 min in treating tMCAO rats, and some tMCAO rats with SM for 40 min exhibited a definite TTI, while SM for 15 min did not result in TTI [5]. These studies suggest that SM for 40 min with TTI was more efficient than that without, but the exact process had not been investigated.

We hereby propose a hypothesis that the reaction of TTI is similar to the phenomenon (b) described above, so the greater efficacy of SM for 40 min with TTI is directly related to the phenomenon of TTI. In order to confirm this hypothesis, we treated the tMCAO rat by SM for 40 min to observe the TTI, determine the efficacy of SM, and investigate the expression of the inflammatory and apoptosis-associated agents to gain a clearer understanding of the molecular biological mechanisms.

2. Materials and methods

2.1. Animal preparation

Adult male Sprague-Dawley rats (220–250 g) were purchased from a commercial source (Shanghai Lab. Animal Resources

Abbreviations: SM, suspended moxibustion; TTI, tail temperature increase.
* Corresponding author. Tel.: +86 791 6362712; fax: +86 791 6363357.
E-mail address: jxchenrixin@yahoo.com.cn (R.-X. Chen).
[1] These authors contributed equally to this work.

132   R.-X. Chen et al. / Neuroscience Letters 503 (2011) 131–135

Center, Shanghai, China), and were divided randomly into 3 groups. (1) Sham-operated group (sham, $n = 20$), (2) ischemic control group (C, $n = 20$), (3) ischemia with SM for 40 min group (M, $n = 40$). According to the tail temperature change, the M group was further divided into two subgroups, including a non-increasing subgroup ($\leq 1\,°C$ an average of 7 days, M1 group) and an increasing subgroup ($> 1\,°C$ an average of 7 days, M2 group). All experimental procedures involving the use of animals were conducted in accordance with NIH Guidelines and approved by the Animal Use and Care Committee for Jiangxi University of TCM.

2.2. Experimental stroke in rats

The rats were anesthetized with an intraperitoneal injection of sodium pentobarbital (3%) at a dose of 30 mg/kg. Core body temperature was monitored using a rectal probe and maintained at $37 \pm 0.5\,°C$ by a heating lamp and a heating pad. The arterial blood gases of pH, PaO_2, $PaCO_2$, and blood pressure were closely monitored via catheterizing the right femoral artery. The middle cerebral artery occlusion (MCAO) was achieved by the Intraluminal Filament method as previously described [5]. A fishing line (Simago Fishing Tackle Company) of 0.205 mm in diameter and 5 cm in length with a rounded tip was inserted through the common carotid artery and gently advanced to the origin of the middle cerebral artery. After 2 h of occlusion, the fishing line was withdrawn to allow for reperfusion. Sham-operated rats were manipulated in the same way, but the MCA was not occluded. Adequacy of vascular occlusion and reperfusion was assessed by Laser Doppler Monitoring of cerebral cortical perfusion.

The exclusion criteria were as follows:

(a) Death within 24 h after tMCAO
(b) Neurological severity score (see below) = 0 (24 h after tMCAO)
(c) Subarachnoid hemorrhage (SAH; as macroscopically assessed during brain biopsy)

2 out of the 20 ischemic control rats (2 deaths) and 3 out of the 40 ischemic rats with SM (2 deaths and 1 non-fatal SAH) met at least one of the exclusion criteria. In total, 75 out of 80 rats were included for final analysis.

2.3. Suspended moxibustion

A special cage in which the rat can maintain a comfortable position and the rat's motion is restricted was used while testing. The cage was convenient to the operation of SM. Room temperature was maintained at $25 \pm 2\,°C$ for the entire experimental process. The acupoint dà zhuī (DU 14), which is considered very important for brain functions [11], was heated by SM using a moxa (exclusively used on animals, length 12 cm, diameter 0.6 cm, made by the Affiliated Hospital of Jiangxi University of TCM, China) at approximately 3 cm high over the hairless skin once a day for 7 days. Stimulation of moxibustion was performed 6 h after reperfusion on the first day. We performed SM for 40 min on the test subjects.

2.4. Tail temperature measurement

Thermal texture mapping (TTM, Bioyear Medical Intl. Co. Ltd.) was used for detecting the infrared warmth information on the dorsal axis of the rat before and after each 40-min SM treatment session. Temperature differences of less than $0.05\,°C$ were registered with TTM. As the temperature detected by TTM was of relative value, the rat's midpoint tail temperature was recorded precisely by an electro-digital thermometer (Shanghai Medical Instrument Factory, Shanghai, China). The testing environment was kept quiet,

and the room temperature was maintained at $25 \pm 2\,°C$. The rats were placed in a cage for 30 min before the experiment started.

2.5. Neurological assessment

Neurological assessment was performed 0 h, 1d, 3d and 7d after tMCAO by a researcher who was unaware of the experimental groups, using a modified neurological severity score, as described previously [5].

2.6. Assessment of infarct size

Cerebral infarction was determined at 24.5 h after reperfusion by 2,3,5-triphenyltetrazolium chloride (TTC) histology in thick (2-mm) coronal sections. Slices were photographed, and images were analyzed with image-analysis software (IPP6.0). Infarct volume in all slices was expressed as a percentage of the bilateral hemisphere after correcting for edema as previously described [12].

2.7. Western blot

This procedure was performed the same as described previously [5]. The membranes were probed with primary antibodies against caspase-3 (1:500, sc-7148, Santa Cruz), iNOS (1:500, sc-651, Santa Cruz), COX-2 (1:500, sc-7951, Santa Cruz), GAPDH (1:1000, sc-25778, Santa Cruz). GAPDH was used as a loading control. The proteins were detected using HRP-conjugated anti-rabbit secondary antibodies and visualized using chemiluminescence reagents provided with the ECL kit (Amersham Pharmacia Biotech, Piscataway, NJ) and exposed to film. The intensity of blots was quantified with densitometry (Quantity one, Bio-Rad).

2.8. Statistic analysis

Data were analyzed with a t test for two groups and one-way analysis of variance (ANOVA) with post hoc Newman–Keuls multiple range test for multiple groups. SPSS 10.0 was used for analysis. $P < 0.05$ was considered statistically significant. All values were expressed as the mean $\pm$ SD.

3. Results

3.1. Physiological parameters and cerebral blood flow

The physiological parameters before, during, and after stroke surgery are provided in Table 1. There was no significant difference in physiological parameters including mean arterial blood pressure, blood gas parameters (including pH, $PaCO_2$ and PaO_2) or rectal temperature among sham, C and M groups. Regional cerebral blood flow (rCBF) was reduced to <20% of baseline and similar between C and M groups ($17.5\% \pm 3.5\%$, $18.2\% \pm 3.2\%$; $P > 0.05$) after advancing the fishing line to the origin of the MCA. After removal of the fishing line, rCBF in the MCA territory was reconstituted to >60% of baseline levels and again did not significantly differ between the two groups ($61\% \pm 6\%$, $62\% \pm 7.5\%$; $P > 0.05$).

3.2. Moxibustion-induced TTI in some tMCAO rats

After 40 min of SM treatment, there were some tMCAO rats exhibiting TTI (more than $2\,°C$ on average) in M group (Table 2 and Fig. 1). The occurrence rate of TTI is 20 out of 37 (54.1%). Furthermore, the temperature increased at about 15 min and the peak temperature was maintained until the end of the treatment at 40 min. There was no change in the tail temperature of tMCAO rats without treatment (Fig. 1).

Table 1
Physiological parameters.

Group	MABP (mmHg)	pH	PaCO$_2$ (mmHg)	PaO$_2$ (mmHg)	Rectal temperature
Before ischemia					
Sham	96.0 ± 4.0	7.34 ± 0.05	45.4 ± 2.9	95.8 ± 4.6	36.9 ± 0.1
C	99.0 ± 5.0	7.35 ± 0.06	44.7 ± 3.5	95.3 ± 5.4	36.4 ± 0.3
M	98.0 ± 3.0	7.36 ± 0.03	45.6 ± 2.4	94.5 ± 4.5	36.6 ± 0.4
During ischemia					
Sham	98.0 ± 5.0	7.35 ± 0.04	45.2 ± 3.9	94.2 ± 4.0	37.1 ± 0.2
C	105.0 ± 3.0	7.31 ± 0.06	46.4 ± 4.9	93.8 ± 4.5	37.0 ± 0.3
M	104.0 ± 6.0	7.30 ± 0.03	46.8 ± 3.2	93.6 ± 5.3	37.2 ± 0.1
After ischemia					
Sham	99.0 ± 6.0	7.32 ± 0.03	44.4 ± 2.8	93.8 ± 3.4	36.8 ± 0.2
C	99.0 ± 4.0	7.32 ± 0.05	46.7 ± 3.9	94.5 ± 4.2	36.5 ± 0.5
M	98.0 ± 5.0	7.30 ± 0.06	46.5 ± 4.7	95.6 ± 4.8	36.7 ± 0.3

Table 2
The tail temperature change in tMCAO rats with SM.

Subgroups	Tail temperature increase (M group)			
	≤1°C M1		>1°C M2	
	0.67 ± 0.21	0.76 ± 0.16	2.13 ± 0.32	2.87 ± 0.22
	0.75 ± 0.19	0.87 ± 0.23	2.78 ± 0.31	2.65 ± 0.24
	0.92 ± 0.23	0.92 ± 0.12	2.85 ± 0.29	2.82 ± 0.22
	0.85 ± 0.16	0.75 ± 0.25	2.84 ± 0.26	2.67 ± 0.26
	0.84 ± 0.37	0.88 ± 0.22	2.45 ± 0.28	2.58 ± 0.19
	0.83 ± 0.21	0.94 ± 0.16	2.57 ± 0.27	2.76 ± 0.25
	0.91 ± 0.24	0.79 ± 0.18	2.12 ± 0.22	2.45 ± 0.21
	0.78 ± 0.32		2.65 ± 0.21	2.75 ± 0.30
	0.76 ± 0.26		2.86 ± 0.34	2.48 ± 0.26
	0.68 ± 0.18		2.44 ± 0.25	2.18 ± 0.17
Total	17		20	

3.3. Infarct volume and neurological deficits score

To confirm the efficacy of SM for 40 min in tMCAO rats, we examined the infarct size for 24.5 h and the neurological deficit score for 0 h, 1d, 3d and 7d after tMCAO. The results showed that SM for 40 min with TTI significantly decreased the infarct size compared to the C and M1 groups. There were no differences between C and M1 group's infarct size at 1d (Fig. 2A and B). M2 group ameliorated the neurological deficits score significantly at 3d and 7d compared to the C and M1 groups, while the M1 group reduced neurological deficits score markedly at 7d compared to the C group (Fig. 2C).

3.4. Suppression of COX-2 and iNOS protein expression

To investigate the level of inflammation in the rat's brain during the 40-min SM treatment session with TTI, COX-2 and iNOS proteins were measured by Western Blot at the inflammatory peak. The data showed that SM for 40 min with TTI decreased COX-2 and iNOS protein levels significantly at 1d compared to the C and M1 groups, while the expression in M1 group was not impacted at this point compared to the C group (Fig. 3A and B). Those proteins were suppressed in M1 group at 3d time point relative to the C group, at which time point the expression of proteins in M2 groups were lower than that in the M1 group (Fig. 3A and C). Low expressions of COX-2 and iNOS were detected in the sham-operated group. The experiments were performed at least three times.

3.5. Inhibition of caspases-3 protein expression

To study SM for 40 min with TTI on apoptosis, the activity of the most important downstream effective caspase in apoptosis, caspase-3 (cleaved caspase-3 p20) was assayed at apoptotic peak time. Caspase-3 was suppressed in M2 group at the 1d and 3d time points compared to C and M1 groups. There was no difference between C and M1 groups at any testing point (Fig. 3). A low expression of caspase-3 protein was detected in the sham-operated group. All assays were performed in three independent experiments.

4. Discussion

The major findings of this study: (a) SM for 40 min on the acupoint DU 14 could induce TTI in some of the tMCAO rats; (b) SM for 40 min with TTI protected the ischemic brain significantly more than those without TTI; (c) SM for 40 min with TTI reduced the levels of COX-2 and iNOS earlier and more substantially than those without TTI of the tMCAO rats; (d) SM for 40 min with TTI inhibited the level of caspase-3 of the tMCAO rat' brain.

SM is an important treatment method in Traditional Chinese Medicine. However, recent studies have shown that the effects of SM treatment remain elusive [10]. Through observing the patients' reactions during SM treatment, we surprisingly found that SM on certain acupoints often induces a phenomenon of distant heat in patients. The duration of the treatment process lasts 40 min on average. SM efficacy was greatly improved with these distant heat reactions [2]. However, we have not yet detected distant heat reactions after conducting 15 min moxibustion treatment, which is the traditional moxibustion treatment duration. Furthermore, the acupoints that can be stimulated to produce the phenomenon of distant heat may vary between patients who suffer from the same disease. In order to induce the phenomenon of distant heat in the clinic, we can adjust the heating point according to the patients' verbal and physical responses [3].

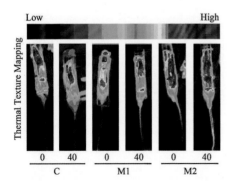

Fig. 1. The tail temperature was measured by TTM. The first image was taken before SM. The second was taken at 40 min after SM. The tail temperature increased significantly in the M2 group, but slightly in the M1 group. There was no change in the C group.

R.-X. Chen et al. / Neuroscience Letters 503 (2011) 131–135

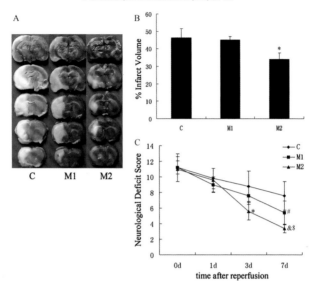

Fig. 2. SM for 40 min on infarct volume and neurological deficit score in the tMCAO rat. (A) Coronal sections from ischemic rat brain stained with TTC, sections shown are 24.5 h after reperfusion; (B) infarct volume was compared between the control and treated groups; and (C) neurological deficit scores in the control and treated groups. *$P < 0.05$ vs. C and M1 groups; #$P < 0.05$ vs. C group; &$P < 0.05$ vs. M1 group; $$P < 0.01$ vs. C group.

Our previous studies showed a higher efficacy of SM for 40 min than that for 15 min in treating tMCAO rats. We have also found a similar reaction to the phenomenon of distant heat in the clinic when observing a TTI during 40 min of SM in some of the tMCAO rats [5].

In order to prove TTI is similar to the distant heat effect in patients, we compared the efficacy of SM for 40 min with TTI to those without. The results showed that SM for 40 min with TTI protected the ischemic brain substantially more than those that exhibited no TTI.

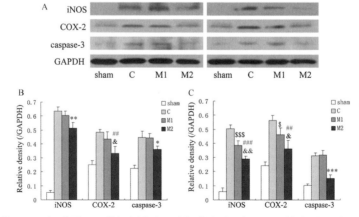

Fig. 3. A 40-min SM treatment session with TTI suppressed ischemia-induced upregulation of iNOS, COX-2 and caspase-3 protein in the tMCAO rat. The upper panel represents Western blot (left strips are at 1d after reperfusion and right strips are at 3d after reperfusion), and the lower panel is a summary graph of the above protein levels relative to GAPDH (B represents 1d and C represents 3d after reperfusion). *$P < 0.05$ vs. C and M1 groups; **$P < 0.01$ vs. C and M1 groups; ***$P < 0.001$ vs. C and M1 groups; ##$P < 0.01$ vs. C group; ###$P < 0.001$ vs. C group; &$P < 0.05$ vs. M1 group; &&$P < 0.01$ vs. M1 group; $$P < 0.05$ vs. C group; $$$$P < 0.001$ vs. C group.

R.-X. Chen et al. / Neuroscience Letters 503 (2011) 131–135

In our preliminary studies, we also treated the sham-operated rats with SM for 40 min, but did not find TTI in any of the subjects (data not shown). This is consistent with the fact that distant heat induced by SM is highly relevant to the pathological process of diseases [2]. Therefore, we did not treat another sham-operated group with SM for 40 min in this experiment. Furthermore, the tail is far from the heating acupoint. Thermal radiation from the igniting moxa does not contribute to TTI following SM. Otherwise, the tail temperature in sham-operated rats would also show a similar increase with SM for 40 min. However, in the traditional Chinese channel theory, DU 14 and the tail are both on the DU channel (Governor Vessel) [11] and stimulating the DU14 provides heat for the tail through the channel. This is how TTI is understood in Traditional Chinese Medicine theory. Why did not the other tMCAO subjects exhibit a marked TTI? As previously mentioned, acupoints that can be stimulated to cause distant heat may have different locations in subjects who are afflicted with the same disease. Acupoints other than DU 14 were stimulated in the tMCAO rats in order to produce TTI. Our previous test showed 40–60% of the rats that received SM on DU 14 exhibited a TTI. The result also showed that the occurrence rate of TTI was 54.1% in M group. Therefore, the number of M1 or M2 test subjects selected from the M group is almost the same as the other groups.

Following ischemia, several inflammatory factors in the brain increased and exacerbated cerebral ischemic injury, such as COX-2 and iNOS [8]. SM for 40 min with TTI reduced their expression levels early in the 1d testing point, while SM for 40 min without TTI inhibited expression in the 3d testing point. Further more, the inhibition of them with TTI is more striking than that without TTI in the 3d testing point. This result indicated that SM for 40 min on the acupoint DU 14 with TTI has a more powerful anti-inflammatory effect.

Neuron apoptosis, as the other important pathological mechanism of cerebral infarction, is activated by exogenous and endogenous approaches following ischemic cerebral injury. Apoptotic executive protein caspase-3 is considered as the most important marker reflecting cell apoptosis [1]. The data showed that SM with TTI inhibited the expression level of caspase-3. However, SM without TTI had no impact on it. This indicated that the former exhibited an anti-apoptosis effect.

As a powerful anti-inflammatory and anti-apoptosis effect, a 40-min SM session on DU 14 with TTI drastically reduced the infarct size and neurological deficits score in this experiment, compared to those without TTI. In view of this, TTI may be comparable to the phenomenon of distant heat in patients. Other regulation mechanisms of stroke may also contribute to the neuroprotective effects

in this treatment, which we will investigate further. Full attention paid to distant heat resulting from SM can help us treat diseases more effectively.

In conclusion, this study confirms the efficacy of a 40-min SM session on the acupoint DU 14 with TTI is higher than that without. Although neuroprotective effects present in tMCAO rats with and without TTI, those with TTI revealed a higher level of anti-inflammation effect and exhibited an anti-apoptosis effect.

Acknowledgments

We would like to thank the Major State Basic Research Development Program of People's Republic of China (2009CB522902), the National Natural Science Foundation of China (30760320), Jiangxi Key R&D Project, Natural Science Foundation of Jiangxi Province (2010Gzy0126) and Traditional Chinese Medicine Research Fund of Health Department of Jiangxi Province (2009Z05) for their support.

References

[1] P.H. Chan, Mitochondria and neuronal death/survival signaling pathways in cerebral ischemia, Neurochem. Res. 29 (2004) 1943–1949.

[2] R.X. Chen, M.R. Chen, J. Xiong, F. Yi, Z.H. Chi, B. Zhang, Comparison of heat-sensitive moxibustion versus fluticasone/salmeterol (seretide) combination in the treatment of chronic persistent asthma: design of a multicenter randomized controlled trial, Trials 11 (2010) 121.

[3] R.X. Chen, M.R. Chen, M.F. Kang, Practical Reading of Heat-sensitization Moxibustion, 1st ed., People's Medical Publishing Press, Beijing, 2009.

[4] R.X. Chen, M.R. Chen, M.F. Kang, J. Xiong, Z.H. Chi, B. Zhang, Y. Fu, The design and protocol of heat-sensitive moxibustion for knee osteoarthritis: a multicenter randomized controlled trial on the rules of selecting moxibustion location, BMC Complement. Altern. Med. 10 (2010) 32.

[5] R.X. Chen, Z.M. Lv, M.R. Chen, X. An, D.Y. Xie, J. Yi, Neuronal apoptosis and inflammatory reaction in rat models of focal cerebral ischemia following 40-min suspended moxibustion, Neural Regen. Res. 6 (2011) 1180–1184.

[6] C. Culmsee, J. Krieglstein, Ischaemic brain damage after stroke: new insights into efficient therapeutic strategies. International symposium on neurodegeneration and neuroprotection, EMBO Rep. 8 (2007) 129–133.

[7] A. Durukan, T. Tatlisumak, Acute ischemic stroke: overview of major experimental rodent models, pathophysiology, and therapy of focal cerebral ischemia, Pharmacol. Biochem. Behav. 87 (2007) 179–197.

[8] J. Huang, U.M. Upadhyay, R.J. Tamargo, Inflammation in stroke and focal cerebral ischemia, Surg. Neurol. 66 (2006) 232–245.

[9] M.S. Lee, B.C. Shin, J.I. Kim, C.H. Han, E. Ernst, Moxibustion for stroke rehabilitation: systematic review, Stroke 41 (2010) 817–820.

[10] M.S. Lee, J.W. Kang, E. Ernst, Does moxibustion work? An overview of systematic reviews, BMC Res. Notes 3 (2010) 284.

[11] Y.F. Luo, Subject of Acupoint, 1st ed., Shanghai Science And Technology Publishing House, Shanghai, 2000.

[12] W. Zhang, I.P. Koerner, R. Noppens, M. Grafe, H.J. Tsai, C. Morisseau, A. Luria, B.D. Hammock, J.R. Falck, N.J. Alkayed, Soluble epoxide hydrolase: a novel therapeutic target in stroke, J. Cereb. Blood Flow Metab. 27 (2007) 1931–1940.

NEURAL REGENERATION RESEARCH
Volume 6, Issue 15, May 2011

www.nrronline.org

Cite this article as: Neural Regen Res. 2011;6(15):1180-1184.

Neuronal apoptosis and inflammatory reaction in rat models of focal cerebral ischemia following 40-minute suspended moxibustion*****★

Rixin Chen[1], Zhimai Lv[2], Mingren Chen[1], Xin An[1], Dingyi Xie[1], Jing Yi[1]

1Affiliated Hospital of Jiangxi University of Traditional Chinese Medicine, Nanchang 330006, Jiangxi Province, China
2The First Affiliated Hospital of Gannan Medical University, Ganzhou 341000, Jiangxi Province, China

Abstract

The treatment duration of heat-sensitive moxibustion (approximately 40 minutes on average) is longer than that of traditional suspended moxibustion. The present study investigated expression changes of three inflammatory and apoptosis-associated proteins (inducible nitric oxide synthase, cyclooxygenase-2 and caspase-3) in transient middle cerebral artery occlusion model rats following suspended moxibustion for 40 minutes, to explore the mechanisms underlying neuroprotective action of suspended moxibustion. The results indicated that suspended moxibustion at acupoint Dazhui (DU 14) for 40 minutes reduced the cortical expression of caspase-3, cyclooxygenase-2 and inducible nitric oxide synthase proteins of transient middle cerebral artery occlusion model rats, as well as decreasing infarct volume and ameliorating the neurological deficit score. Outcomes with 40 minutes of moxibustion were superior to the outcomes after suspended moxibustion for 15 minutes.
Key Words: moxibustion; cerebral ischemia; caspase-3; cyclooxygenase-2; inducible nitric oxide synthase; neural regeneration

Rixin Chen★, Master, Professor, Affiliated Hospital of Jiangxi University of Traditional Chinese Medicine, Nanchang 330006, Jiangxi Province, China

Corresponding author: Rixin Chen, Affiliated Hospital of Jiangxi University of Traditional Chinese Medicine, Nanchang 330006, Jiangxi Province, China
jxchenrixin@yahoo.com.cn

Supported by: the Major State Basic Research Development Program of China, No. 2009CB522902*; the National Natural Science Foundation of China, No. 30760320*; the Jiangxi Key R&D Project*; the Natural Science Foundation of Jiangxi Province, No. 2010Gzy0126*

Received: 2011-01-15
Accepted: 2011-03-12
(N20101129004/ZW)

Chen RX, Lv ZM, Chen MR, An X, Xie DY, Yi J. Neuronal apoptosis and inflammatory reaction in rat models of focal cerebral ischemia following 40-minute suspended moxibustion. Neural Regen Res. 2011;6(15):1180-1184.

www.crter.cn
www.nrronline.org

doi:10.3969/j.issn.1673-5374.
2011.15.011

INTRODUCTION

Suspended moxibustion, an indirect form of moxibustion, is moxibustion placed superficially over the skin without contact with the skin. The application of suspended moxibustion for 15 minutes is considered the stage of meridian-Qi excitation. An extended period of suspended moxibustion may provide an effective treatment stage, but traditional suspended moxibustion is usually stopped at this time point. The effect of traditional suspended moxibustion has recently been greatly improved by the development of "heat-sensitive" suspended moxibustion. The most important feature of heat-sensitive moxibustion is that the duration (about 40 minutes on average) is longer than that of traditional suspended moxibustion, which is one of the reasons for its high efficiency[1-2]. Clinical practice has shown that heat-sensitive moxibustion has a positive effect on cerebral infarction[1]. However, little is known about the mechanisms underlying the neuroprotective action of this new treatment.

It is well known that inflammation and apoptosis are important pathological mechanisms of cerebral infarction[3-5]. A previous study reported that proinflammatory enzymes including inducible nitric oxide synthase (iNOS) and cyclooxygenase-2 (COX-2) play important roles in inflammatory responses to cerebral infarction, and may contribute to ischemic injury[6]. Iadecola et al [7] demonstrated that cerebral ischemia leads to enhanced expression of iNOS mRNA, which can result in the development of ischemic brain injury. Selective iNOS inhibitors have been found to inhibit iNOS activity and reduce infarct volume in middle cerebral artery occlusion (MCAO)[8]. Nogawa et al [9] suggested that COX-2 mRNA is significantly expressed in MCAO model rats. Inhibiting COX-2 activity ameliorates cerebral ischemia injury[10], and cerebral ischemia-induced apoptotic neuronal death in ischemic hemispheres also plays an important role in the pathological mechanisms involved in stroke[11-12].

To verify whether the mechanism underlying neuroprotective action of heat-sensitive moxibustion is associated with inflammation and apoptosis after cerebral ischemia, the present study measured the effects of suspended moxibustion for 40 minutes (the average treatment time of clinical heat-sensitive moxibustion) in transient middle cerebral artery occlusion (tMCAO) model rats. We investigated expression changes of inflammatory and apoptosis-associated proteins (iNOS, COX-2 and caspase-3) to explore the

Chen RX, et al. / Neural Regeneration Research. 2011;6(15):1180-1184.

mechanisms underlying the neuroprotective effects of heat-sensitive moxibustion.

RESULTS

Quantitative analysis of experimental animals

A total of 50 rats were randomly divided into four groups: a sham-operated group (n = 12), an ischemia control group (n = 12), an ischemia with 15-minute moxibustion group (n = 13), and an ischemia with 40-minute moxibustion group (n = 13). One of the 12 sham-operated rats (one death), one of the 12 ischemic control rats (one death), two of the 13 ischemia with 15-minute moxibustion rats (one death, one non-fatal subarachnoid hemorrhage), and two of the 13 ischemia with 40-minute moxibustion rats (two non-fatal subarachnoid hemorrhages) met at least one of the exclusion criteria. Thus 44 rats were included in the final analysis.

Infarct volume of brain and neurological deficits score

To investigate the efficacy of 40 minutes of suspended moxibustion, we examined infarct size and neurological deficit score following tMCAO in rats. The results revealed that moxibustion for 40 minutes significantly reduced infarct size at 1 or 3 days after reperfusion and ameliorated the neurological deficit score at 3 days after reperfusion, compared with the ischemia control group (P < 0.05). The neurological deficit score (normal score, 0; maximal deficit score, 18) was clearly reduced at 7 days after reperfusion in the ischemia with 40-minute moxibustion group, compared with the ischemia control group (P < 0.01) and the ischemia with 15-minute moxibustion group (P < 0.05). In contrast, traditional moxibustion for 15 minutes did not have any significant neuroprotective effects (P > 0.05), as shown in Figure 1.

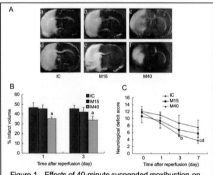

Figure 1 Effects of 40-minute suspended moxibustion on infarct volume and neurological deficit score in transient middle cerebral artery occlusion rats. (A) Coronal sections from ischemic rat brain stained with 2, 3, 5-triphenyltetrazolium chloride, sections shown are 1 day (a, b, c) and 3 days (d, e, f) after reperfusion; (B) infarct volume; and (C) neurological deficit scores. Data are expressed as mean ± SEM. [a]P < 0.05, vs. ischemia control (IC) and M15 groups; [b]P < 0.05, [c]P < 0.01, vs. IC group; [d]P < 0.05, vs. M15 group. M15: ischemia with 15-minute moxibustion group; M40: ischemia with 40-minute moxibustion group.

Expression changes of COX-2, iNOS and caspase-3 proteins in the ipsilateral hemisphere of moxibustion-treated or non-treated rats

To determine whether suspended moxibustion for 40 minutes could inhibit inflammation of cerebral infarction, two important mediators of inflammation (COX-2 and iNOS) were tested with western blot assay. In the ischemia with 40-minute moxibustion group, expressions of COX-2 and iNOS were significantly decreased at 1 day (P < 0.05) and 3 days (P < 0.001) after reperfusion (inflammatory peak), compared with the ischemia control and ischemia with 15-minute moxibustion groups. There was no significant difference between ischemia control and ischemia with 15-minute moxibustion groups at any time point (P > 0.05). Low expression of COX-2 and iNOS proteins was detected in the sham-operated group (Figures 2A, B).

Activity of the most important downstream effective caspase in apoptosis, caspase-3 (cleaved caspase-3 p20) was assayed[12]. The ischemia with 40-minute moxibustion group exhibited significant suppression of caspase-3 expression induced by cerebral ischemia at 1 and 3 days (P < 0.01) after reperfusion (apoptotic peak), compared with the ischemia control group and the ischemia with 15-minute moxibustion group. The ischemia with 15-minute moxibustion group exhibited no effect on caspase-3 expression, compared with the ischemia control group (P > 0.05). A low level of expression of caspase-3 protein was detected in the sham-operated group (Figures 2A, C).

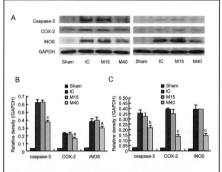

Figure 2 Suspended moxibustion at the point Dazhui (DU 14) for 40 minutes suppressed ischemia-induced upregulation of caspase-3, cyclooxygenase-2 (COX-2) and inducible nitric oxide synthase (iNOS) protein in transient middle cerebral artery occlusion rats. Western blot (left strips are at 1 day after reperfusion and right strips are at 3 days after reperfusion) is shown in A, and the above proteins levels (relative densities) at 1 day and 3 days after reperfusion are shown in B and C. Data are expressed as mean ± SEM. [a]P < 0.05, [b]P < 0.01, [c]P < 0.001, vs. control and M15 groups. Sham: sham-operated group; IC: ischemia control group; M15: ischemia with 15-minute moxibustion group; M40: ischemia with 40-minute moxibustion group.

Chen RX, et al. / Neural Regeneration Research. 2011;6(15):1180-1184.

DISCUSSION

The traditional duration of a moxibustion treatment is 15 minutes, and is focused on fixed acupoints. Although some randomized, controlled trials confirmed the efficiency of traditional moxibustion[13-14], strong evidence for therapeutic effectiveness is currently lacking. However, there is a substantial difference in treatment time and procedure between traditional moxibustion and heat-sensitive moxibustion. The latter is focused on the effects of distant heat. This type of distant heat includes two major aspects: moxibustion heat that penetrates deeply into the tissues or internal organs of the body, and moxibustion heat that is transferred from the original moxibustion acupoint to other areas of the body. The phenomenon of distant heat is an important marker for predicting the heat-sensitive moxibustion[1]. The application of heat-sensitive moxibustion for a sufficient duration may provide method of inducing the phenomenon of distant heat, while treatment with the traditional duration of suspended moxibustion does not. Therefore, the duration of treatment appears to be critical for improving the efficacy of moxibustion. Since moxibustion duration is an important factor affecting the occurrence of this phenomenon, the duration of heat-sensitive moxibustion treatment is often longer than that of traditional moxibustion[1]. Therefore, this experiment employed a 40-minute moxibustion period, representing the heat-sensitive moxibustion time, and applied 15 minutes as the traditional moxibustion time. The present data revealed that the application of suspended moxibustion for 40 minutes significantly reduced the infarction area at 1 and 3 days after reperfusion and significantly attenuated the neurological deficit score at 7 days after reperfusion, relative to ischemia control and ischemia with 15-minute moxibustion group. In addition, suspended moxibustion for 15 minutes had no effect on reducing infarction area or neurological deficit score, compared with the ischemia control group. These results suggest that prolonging the duration of moxibustion for 40 minutes improves its efficacy.

The pathological mechanism of ischemic cerebral injury is extremely complicated, involving disruption of cellular metabolism in the brain, excitability amino acid toxicity, intracellular calcium overload, oxidative stress injuries and nerve cell apoptosis. Inflammation plays a key role in ischemic injury[15], and iNOS and COX-2 are the main mediators of inflammatory effects in the brain. Both of these proteins exert important effects in inflammatory injury and cerebral edema following cerebral ischemia. Inhibiting these two types of inflammatory mediators would thus be expected to have neuroprotective effects[6]. Our results indicate that levels of COX-2 and iNOS were significantly reduced in the ischemia with 40-minute moxibustion group at 1 and 3 days, compared with the ischemia control or ischemia with 15-minute moxibustion

groups. This suggests that suspended moxibustion for 40 minutes may reduce inflammation by inhibiting proinflammatory mediators such as iNOS and COX-2 after cerebral infarction, and that the efficacy of suspended moxibustion for 40 minutes may be related to the suppression of inflammation.

Apoptosis, another key pathological mechanism in cerebral infarction, has an important effect on neurological recovery and the magnitude of cerebral infarctions. After ischemic cerebral injury, apoptosis-related proteins are gradually activated by exogenous and endogenous factors of neurons. When the final apoptotic executive protein caspase-3 is activated, cellular apoptosis occurs[16]. This event tends to peak after 24 to 48 hours of reperfusion[17]. Apoptotic executive protein caspase-3 is considered to be the most important marker of cellular apoptosis. Therefore, we employed the expression of caspase-3 protein as a measure of the effects of heat-sensitive moxibustion treatment on neural cell apoptosis. Our results revealed that the expression of caspase-3 protein was significantly reduced at 1 and 3 days in the ischemia with 40-minute moxibustion group, compared with the ischemia control or ischemia with 15-minute moxibustion groups. This result indicates that early intervention of heat-sensitive moxibustion in cerebral infarction may help to inhibit neural apoptosis, exerting neuroprotective effects.

It should be noted that suspended moxibustion at the Dazhui point (DU 14) for 40 minutes in the present study caused the tail temperature to rise (> 2°C) in some tMCAO rats (six of 11), while suspended moxibustion for 15 minutes did not have the same effect (data not shown). However, the Dazhui point is located far from the tail, meaning that thermal radiation from the ignited moxa is unable to explain the increase in tail temperature following suspended moxibustion. Otherwise, the temperature of the tail during ischemia in the 15-minute moxibustion group would be expected to show a similar increase to that during ischemia in the 40-minute moxibustion group. In traditional Chinese channel theory, Dazhui and the tail are both on the Du channel (Governor Vessel)[18], and stimulating the acupoint Dazhui provides heat to the tail through the channel. Therefore, the increase in tail temperature induced by heating the Dazhui acupoint appears to be consistent with the transferral of moxibustion heat from the original moxibustion acupoint to other areas of the body. This result suggests that the beneficial effects of moxibustion for 40 minutes we abserved in tMCAO rats were related to the increase in tail temperature. Further investigation of tail temperature in tMCAO rats is required to determine whether suspended moxibustion for 40 minutes contributes to the mechanism of heat-sensitive moxibustion.

In summary, this study is the first demonstration that heat-sensitive moxibustion can exert neuroprotective effects in tMCAO model rats. The results revealed that suspended moxibustion for 40 minutes significantly

Chen RX, et al. / Neural Regeneration Research. 2011;6(15):1180-1184.

reduced neurological deficit scores and cerebral infarct volume produced by tMCAO. In contrast, no significant effect was observed following treatment with suspended moxibustion for 15 minutes. Suspended moxibustion for 40 minutes inhibited the expression of iNOS, COX-2 and caspase-3 proteins, whereas suspended moxibustion for 15 minutes had no effect on these proteins. These results provide a scientific basis for the use of heat-sensitive moxibustion in treatment of stroke.

MATERIALS AND METHODS

Design
A randomized, controlled, animal experiment.
Time and setting
This experiment was performed at the Experimental Animal Center of Jiangxi University of Traditional Chinese Medicine in China, from May to June 2010.
Materials
A total of 50 clean, adult, male, Sprague-Dawley rats, weighing 220–250 g, were purchased from the Shanghai Lab Animal Resources Center (SCXK (Hu) 2003-0002, Shanghai, China).
Methods
Preparation of MCAO rat model
Transient focal cerebral ischemia was induced in spontaneously breathing rats. All animals were anesthetized with an intraperitoneal injection of sodium pentobarbital (3%) at a dose of 30 mg/kg. Body temperature was maintained at 37 ± 0.5°C by a heating lamp and heating pad. tMCAO was achieved using intraluminal filament methods, as described previously[19], with minor modifications. Briefly, a midline neck incision was made, and the right common carotid artery, internal carotid artery, and external carotid artery were isolated. The external carotid artery was ligated with 4-0 silk suture distal from carotid bifurcation and the common carotid artery was ligated with 4-0 silk suture at the proximal end. Another 4-0 silk suture was tied loosely around the common carotid artery close to the carotid bifurcation. A piece of fishing line (Simago Fishing Tackle Company, Hangzhou, Zhejiang Province, China) 0.205 mm in diameter and 5 cm in length with a rounded tip was introduced into a small incision in the common carotid artery and gently advanced to the origin of the middle cerebral artery (18 mm from carotid bifurcation). The silk suture around the common carotid artery stump was tied tightly to prevent bleeding and secure the fishing line. After 2 hours of occlusion, the fishing line was withdrawn to allow for reperfusion. Sham-operated rats were manipulated in the same way, but the middle cerebral artery was not occluded.
The following exclusion criteria were applied: (1) death within 24 hours after tMCAO; (2) neurological severity score (see below) = 0 (24 hours after tMCAO); and (3) subarachnoid hemorrhage (as macroscopically

assessed during brain biopsy).
Suspended moxibustion treatment
The *Dazhui* points (region in C_7–T_1), considered to be important for brain function[18], were heated by suspended moxibustion using an moxibustion-cigar produced from mugwort (custom made for use with animals, length 12 cm, diameter 0.6 cm, in the Affiliated Hospital of Jiangxi University of Traditional Chinese Medicine, China) at 3 cm high approximately over a hairless area of skin once a day for 7 days. Stimulation of moxibustion was performed at 6 hours after reperfusion on the day 1. Since the time of heat-sensitive moxibustion ranges from 30 minutes to 1 hour and is usually longer than conventional moxibustion (usually around 15 minutes). This study used an average duration of 40 minutes as the treatment time and 15 minutes as the control treatment time.
Assessment of infarct size
Cerebral infarction of each group was determined at 1 or 3 days reperfusion using 2, 3, 5-triphenyltetrazolium chloride histology in thick (2-mm) coronal sections[20]. Slices were photographed with a Nikon COOLPIX L1 camera (Nikon Corporation, Tokyo, Japan), and images were analyzed using IPP6.0 image-analysis software (Media Cybernetics, Bethesda, MD, USA). Infarct volume in all slices was expressed as a percentage of the bilateral hemisphere volume after correcting for edema, as previously described[21]. To account for the effects of edema, the infarct area was estimated indirectly by subtracting the non-infarct area in the ipsilateral hemisphere from the contralateral hemisphere, and expressing infarct volume as a percentage of the bilateral hemispheres.
Neurological assessment
Neurological assessment was performed at 0 hour, 1, 3 and 7 days after tMCAO by an investigator who was blinded to the experimental groups, using a modified neurological severity scale, as described previously[22]. In brief, scores on this scale are derived by evaluating animals for hemiparesis (response to raising the rat by the tail or placing the rat on a flat surface), sensory deficits (placing, proprioception), beam balance tests (response to placement and posture on a narrow beam and time before falling), absent reflexes (pinna, corneal, startle), and abnormal movement (seizure, myoclonus, myodystony). Neurological deficit scores were graded on a scale of 0 to 18 (normal score, 0; maximal deficit score, 18). One point is awarded for the inability to perform a task or the lack of a reflex.
Western blot assay
Cortical tissue was dissected from ipsilateral hemisphere of moxibustion-treated or non-treated rats subjected to 2 hours of MCAO followed by 1 or 3 days of reperfusion, and stored at −80°C. Frozen brain tissue was thawed in lysis buffer, supplemented with 250 mmol/L sucrose, 1 mmol/L ethylenediamine tetraacetic acid, 10 mmol/L KPO_4, 0.1 mmol/L phenylmethylsulfonyl fluoride (pH 7.7), in the presence of protease inhibitors, and the

1183

Chen RX, et al. / Neural Regeneration Research. 2011;6(15):1180-1184.

homogenate was sonicated, incubated on ice for 30 minutes, and centrifuged at 14 000 × g for 15 minutes at 4°C. The protein concentration was measured in the supernatant, and samples of 100 μg were loaded on 10–20% Tris/Ntris(hydroxymethyl)methylglycine/peptide gel, separated, and transferred for 1.5–2.0 hours at 4°C to a polyvinylidene fluoride membrane. Blots were blocked for 1 hour with PBS containing 5% nonfat dry milk and 0.1% Tween 20 at room temperature and incubated overnight with rabbit anti polyclonal antibodies against caspase-3 (1: 500; sc-7148; Santa Cruz Biotechnology, Santa Cruz, CA, USA), iNOS (1: 500; sc-651; Santa Cruz Biotechnology), COX-2 (1: 500; sc-7951; Santa Cruz Biotechnology), glyceraldehyde 3-phosphate dehydrogenase (GAPDH; 1: 1 000; sc-25778; Santa Cruz Biotechnology) in 5% milk in PBS with Tween 20. GAPDH was used as a loading control. Membranes were washed with PBS with Tween 20 and then incubated with horseradish peroxidase-conjugated goat anti-rabbit second antibody (1: 2 000; ZB-2301; ZSGB-BIO, Beijing, China) for 1.5 hours. The signal was detected using enhanced chemiluminescence (Amersham Pharmacia Biotech, Piscataway, NJ, USA) and film autoradiography. Films were scanned and densitometric analysis of the bands was performed using Quantity One 4.4 Analysis System (Bio-Rad, San Francisco, CA, USA). The experiments were performed at least 3 times.

Statistical analysis

Data were expressed as mean ± SEM and analyzed using one-way analyses of variance with *post hoc* Newman-Keuls multiple range tests for multiple groups. SPSS 13.0 (SPSS, Chicago, IL, USA) was used for analysis. A value of $P < 0.05$ was considered statistically significant, and $P < 0.01$ was considered very statistically significant.

Author contributions: Rixin Chen designed and carried out the study. Mingren Chen supervised the project. Zhimai Lv and Dingyi Xie generated the models. Zhimai Lv carried out the 2, 3, 5-triphenyltetrazolium chloride histological observation and western blot assay. Xin An, Dingyi Xie and Jing Yi performed the moxibustion and neurological assessment. Rixin Chen and Zhimai Lv collected and analyzed data, discussed the interpretation of the results, and wrote the manuscript. All authors read and approved the final manuscript.

Conflicts of interest: None declared.

Funding: This study was supported by the Major State Basic Research Development Program of China, No. 2009CB522902; the National Natural Science Foundation of China, No. 30760320; the Jiangxi Key R&D Project; and the Natural Science Foundation of Jiangxi Province, No. 2010Gzy0126.

Ethical approval: All experimental procedures involving the use of animals were approved by the Animal Use and Care Committee for Jiangxi University of Traditional Chinese Medicine.

REFERENCES

[1] Chen RX, Chen MR, Kang MF. Practical Reading of Heat-sensitization Moxibustion. Beijing: People's Medical Publishing House. 2009.

[2] Jing F, Xu B, Wang LL. Discussion of moxibustion time. Zhenjiu Linchuang Zazhi. 2010;26(3):13-16.

[3] Durukan A, Tatlisumak T. Acute ischemic stroke: overview of major experimental rodent models, pathophysiology, and therapy of focal cerebral ischemia. Pharmacol Biochem Behav. 2007; 87(1):179-197.

[4] Lapchak PA, Araujo DM. Advances in ischemic stroke treatment: neuroprotective and combination therapies. Expert Opin Emerg Drugs. 2007;12(1):97-112.

[5] Culmsee C, Krieglstein J. Ischaemic brain damage after stroke: new insights into efficient therapeutic strategies. International Symposium on Neurodegeneration and Neuroprotection. EMBO Rep. 2007;8(2):129-33.

[6] Wang Q, Tang XN, Yenari MA. The inflammatory response in stroke. J Neuroimmunol. 2007;184(1-2):53-68.

[7] Iadecola C, Zhang F, Casey R, et al. Delayed reduction of ischemic brain injury and neurological deficits in mice lacking the iNOS gene. J Neurosci. 1997;17(23):9157-9164

[8] Iadecola C, Zhang F, Xu X. Inhibition of inducible nitric oxide synthase ameliorates cerebral ischemic damage. Am J Physiol Regul Integr Comp Physiol. 1995;268(1 Pt 2):286-292.

[9] Nogawa S, Zhang F, Ross ME, et al. Cyclo-oxygenase-2 gene expression in neurons contributes to ischemic brain damage. J Neurosci. 1997;17(8):2746-2755.

[10] Candelario-Jalil E, Gonza´lez-Falco´n A, Garci´a-Cabrera M, et al. Wide therapeutic time window for nimesulide neuroprotection in a model of transient focal cerebral ischemia in the rat. Brain Res. 2004;1007(1-2):98-108.

[11] Mehta SL, Manhas N, Raghubir R. Molecular targets in cerebral ischemia for developing novel therapeutics. Brain Res Rev. 2007; 54(1):34-66.

[12] Broughton BR, Reutens DC, Sobey CG. Apoptotic mechanisms after cerebral ischemia. Stroke. 2009;40(5):e331-339.

[13] Rao P, Zhou L, Mao M, et al. A randomized controlled trial of acupuncture treatment of acute ischemic stroke. Zhongguo Zhenjiu. 2006;26(10):694-696.

[14] Zhang SH, Liu M, Asplund K, et al. Acupuncture for acute stroke. Cochrane Database Syst Rev. 2005;(2):CD003317.

[15] Huang J, Upadhyay UM, Tamargo RJ. Inflammation in stroke and focal cerebral ischemia. Surg Neurol. 2006;66(3):232-245.

[16] Chan PH. Mitochondria and neuronal death/survival signaling pathways in cerebral ischemia. Neurochem Res. 2004;29(11): 1943-1949.

[17] Mehta SL, Manhas N, Raghubir R. Molecular targets in cerebral ischemia for developing novel therapeutics. Brain Res Rev. 2007;54(1):34-66.

[18] Luo YF. Subject of Acupoint. 5th ed. Shanghai: Shanghai Science and Technology Publishing House. 2000.

[19] Longa EZ, Weinstein PR, Carlson S, et al. Reversible middle cerebral artery occlusion without craniectomy in rats. Stroke. 1989;20(1):84-91.

[20] Bederson JB, Pitts LH, Germano SM, et al. Evaluation of 2,3,5-triphenyltetrazolium chloride as a stain for detection and quantification of experimental cerebral infarction in rats. Stroke. 1986;17(6):1304-1308.

[21] Zhang W, Koerner IP, Noppens R, et al. Soluble epoxide hydrolase: a novel therapeutic target in stroke. J Cereb Blood Flow Metab. 2007;27(12):1931-1940.

[22] Chen J, Sanberg PR, Li Y, et al. Intravenous administration of human umbilical cord blood reduces behavioral deficits after stroke in rats. Stroke. 2001;32(11):2682-2688.

(Edited by Ma J, Mei ZG/Qiu Y/Song LP)

NEURAL REGENERATION RESEARCH
Volume 8, Issue 12, April 2013

www.nrronline.org

doi:10.3969/j.issn.1673-5374.2013.12.008   [http://www.nrronline.org; http://www.sjzsyj.org]
Chen RX, Lv ZM, Huang DD, Chen MR, Yi F. Efficacy of suspended moxibustion in stroke rats is associated with a change in tail temperature. Neural Regen Res. 2013;8(12):1132-1138.

Efficacy of suspended moxibustion in stroke rats is associated with a change in tail temperature***

Rixin Chen[1], Zhimai Lv[2], Dangdang Huang[3], Mingren Chen[1], Fan Yi[4]

1 Affiliated Hospital of Jiangxi University of Traditional Chinese Medicine, Nanchang 330006, Jiangxi Province, China
2 The First Affiliated Hospital of Gannan Medical University, Ganzhou 341000, Jiangxi Province, China
3 Gannan Medical University, Ganzhou 341000, Jiangxi Province, China
4 Department of Health of Jiangxi Province, Nanchang 330006, Jiangxi Province, China

Abstract

Suspended moxibustion-produced heat can transfer from the acupoint to other sites of the body. The suspended moxibustion should be terminated when clinical propagated sensation disappears, because this implies that the quantity of moxibustion is sufficient. We wanted to investigate if this phenomenon also occurs in experimental animals. In the present study, a rat model of stroke was established and treated with suspended moxibustion at *Dazhui* (DU14) for 60 minutes. Results showed that the increase in tail temperature began at 15 minutes after suspended moxibustion and decreased gradually at 40 minutes. In addition, neurological function was significantly improved in stroke rats with tail temperature increase following suspended moxibustion, and this effect was associated with significantly reduced tumor necrosis factor α and interleukin 1β mRNA. However, there was no significant difference between 40- and 60-minute suspended moxibustion. The findings indicate that elevated tail temperature began to decrease at 40 minutes after suspended moxibustion, and further suspended moxibustion was not useful in the recovery of stroke rats.

Rixin Chen and Zhimai Lv contributed equally to this work.

Corresponding author: Rixin Chen, Professor, Doctoral supervisor, Affiliated Hospital of Jiangxi University of Traditional Chinese Medicine, Nanchang 330006, Jiangxi Province, China, jxchenrixin@yahoo.com.cn.

Received: 2012-06-28
Accepted: 2013-01-24
(N20120413002)

Key Words

neural regeneration; traditional Chinese medicine; acupuncture and moxibustion; suspended moxibustion; stroke; tail temperature; tumor necrosis factor-alpha; interleukin-1 beta; grants-supported paper; neuroregeneration

Research Highlights

(1) Tail temperature increased after 15-minute suspended moxibustion, but decreased after 40 minutes in stroke rats.
(2) Suspended moxibustion with tail temperature increase improved neurological deficit better than did moxibustion without tail temperature increase.
(3) Continuing suspended moxibustion could not further strengthen its efficacy when tail temperature began to decrease.
(4) This finding is in accordance with the rules of heat-sensitive moxibustion, which states that moxibustion should be terminated when the propagated sensation disappears, as this implies that the quantity of moxibustion is sufficient.

Chen RX, et al. / Neural Regeneration Research. 2013;8(12):1132-1138.

INTRODUCTION

Suspended moxibustion is an important treatment method in traditional Chinese medicine in which moxibustion is placed superficially over the skin but does not make contact. It has been widely used to treat various diseases, such as stroke. Although strong evidence regarding its therapeutic efficacy is lacking[1], it has been suggested that if the duration of the suspended moxibustion is appropriately extended and a phenomenon called "distant heat" is produced, then the efficacy of the suspended moxibustion is significantly strengthened[2]. The phenomenon of distant heat has been demonstrated in a clinical setting, where moxibustion heat is transferred from the original moxibustion acupoint to other areas of the body[3]. We have also found a similar reaction to the phenomenon of distant heat when observing tail temperature increase during 40-minute suspended moxibustion on the *Dazhui* (DU14) acupoint in a rat model of transient middle cerebral artery occlusion[4]. In traditional Chinese channel theory, *Dazhui* and the tail are both on the *DU* channel (Governor Vessel) and stimulating *Dazhui* could provide heat for the tail through the channel[5]. Transient middle cerebral artery occlusion rats with tail temperature increase were found to recover better than those without. Furthermore, temperature increased at about 15 minutes, and peak temperature was maintained until the end of the 40-minute treatment[4]. However, two issues remained: how long will tail temperature increase last if the duration of suspended moxibustion is increased, and is it useful for recovery of transient middle cerebral artery occlusion rats if suspended moxibustion continues after tail temperature increase begins to decrease. The present study was designed to resolve these issues, and investigated the mRNA expression of two important inflammatory mediators, tumor necrosis factor-α and interleukin-1β in the cortex of stroke rats. The study could help deepen the understanding of the underlying biological mechanisms of this moxibustion technique.

RESULTS

Quantitative analysis of experimental animals

Of 120 rats used, 30 were randomly assigned to the sham-surgery (n = 10) and ischemia (n = 20) groups, both of which underwent suspended moxibustion for 3 days. The ischemia group was subdivided into non-tail temperature increase (temperature change less than 1°C)

and tail temperature increase (temperature change more than 1°C) according to tail temperature changes. The remaining 90 rats were used to establish transient middle cerebral artery occlusion models and assigned to the ischemic control (n = 15), suspended moxibustion for 15 (M15; n = 15), 40 (M40; n = 30) and 60 minutes (M60; n = 30) groups. The M40 and M60 groups were further divided into two subgroups according to tail temperature changes in 7 days, a non-tail temperature increase subgroup (temperature change ≤ 1°C in 7 days: M40-non-tail temperature increase group, n = 13; M60-non-tail temperature increase group, n = 14) and a tail temperature increase subgroup (temperature change > 1°C in 7 days: M40-tail temperature increase group, n = 14; M60-tail temperature increase group, n = 15). In the first part of experiments, two rats were excluded (one died and one failed in establishing the model). In the second part of experiments, two rats from the ischemic control group died, two from the M15 group failed to establish the model, one from the M40 group died, two failed in model establishment, and 1 from M60 died. Finally, 28 rats in the first part of the experiment and 82 in the second part of the experiment were included in the final analysis.

Tail temperature change following suspended moxibustion

In the first part of experiments, tail temperature began to quickly increase immediately after suspended moxibustion. At about 5–10 minutes, the temperature reached a relatively stable level, but was an increase of less than 1°C on average. The tail temperature remained unchanged in nine rats from the ischemia group and all the control rats (non-tail temperature increase) throughout the treatment session. However, the other nine transient middle cerebral artery occlusion rats exhibited tail temperature increase (more than 2°C on average). Furthermore, the tail temperature in the rats with tail temperature increase increased to a peak value at around 15 minutes, and peak temperature was maintained until 40 minutes. Up to 50 minutes, tail temperature decreased to a level similar to that of the non-tail temperature increase or sham-surgery rats. Results were similar during the next 3 consecutive days (Figure 1). According to the change in tail temperature, we selected 15, 40 and 60 minutes as the suspended moxibustion duration in subsequent experiments. In the second part of the experiments, no rats exhibited tail temperature increase in the ischemic control or M15 groups. There were 15 rats from the M40 and 16 from M60 groups which exhibited tail temperature increase.

1133

Chen RX, et al. / Neural Regeneration Research. 2013;8(12):1132-1138.

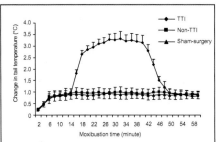

Figure 1　Change in tail temperature induced by 60-minute suspended moxibustion in the first part of the experiments.

Because the changes in tail temperature were similar across the three consecutive testing days, data from the first day were presented as representative findings. Data are expressed as mean ± SD. TTI: Tail temperature increase.

Suspended moxibustion significantly improved the neurological function of rats

To investigate the efficacy of suspended moxibustion of different durations, we examined the neurological deficit scores following transient middle cerebral artery occlusion in the second part of the experiment. Results revealed that the neurological deficit scores were significantly reduced in the M40-tail temperature increase group and the M60-tail temperature increase group at 3 days after reperfusion compared with the ischemic control and the M15 groups ($P < 0.05$). The neurological deficit scores were further ameliorated in the M40-tail temperature increase and M60-tail temperature increase groups at 7 days after reperfusion, compared with the ischemic control, M15, M40-non-tail temperature increase and M60-non-tail temperature increase groups ($P < 0.05$). However, there was no significant difference between M40-tail temperature increase and M60-tail temperature increase groups at 1, 3 or 7 days. The neurological deficit scores at 7 days were significantly reduced in the M40-non-tail temperature increase and M60-non-tail temperature increase groups compared to the ischemic control and M15 groups ($P < 0.05$), but scores were similar between the M40-non-tail temperature increase and M60-non-tail temperature increase groups. The M15 group did not exhibit any protective effect compared to the ischemic control (Figure 2).

Suspended moxibustion suppressed cortical tumor necrosis factor-α and interleukin-1β mRNA expression in tail temperature increase rats

To investigate the level of inflammation in the cortex

following transient middle cerebral artery occlusion, tumor necrosis factor-α and interleukin-1β mRNA was measured using real time PCR at the inflammatory peak (the 1 or 3 days testing point)[6]. Results showed that the M40-tail temperature increase ($P < 0.01$) or M60-tail temperature increase ($P < 0.01$) group attenuated the increase of tumor necrosis factor-α and interleukin-1β mRNA caused by transient middle cerebral artery occlusion at 1 day post ischemia, while other treatment groups had no effect on these inflammatory mediators compared to the ischemic control group. At 3 days post ischemia, both tumor necrosis factor-α and interleukin-1β mRNA levels were reduced in M40-non-tail temperature increase, M60-non-tail temperature increase, M40-tail temperature increase and M60-tail temperature increase groups, while M15 had no effect on tumor necrosis factor-α and interleukin-1β mRNA compared to ischemic control group. The suppression of tumor necrosis factor-α and interleukin-1β mRNA in the M40-tail temperature increase and M60-tail temperature increase groups was more evident than in the M40-non-tail temperature increase or M60-non-tail temperature increase groups at 3 days post ischemia. In addition, there was no significant difference in tumor necrosis factor-α and interleukin-1β mRNA expression between M40-tail temperature increase and M60-tail temperature increase groups at 1 or 3 days. Low expression of tumor necrosis factor-α and interleukin-1β mRNA was detected in the sham-surgery group (Figure 3).

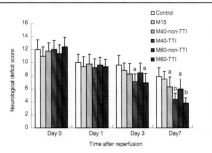

Figure 2　Effect of suspended moxibustion on neurological deficit scores in rats undergoing transient middle cerebral artery occlusion.

Neurological deficit scores were graded on a scale of 0 to 18 (normal score, 0; maximal deficit score, 18). Data are presented as mean ± SD. [a]$P < 0.05$, vs. ischemic control and M15 groups; [b]$P < 0.05$, vs. ischemic control, M15, M40-non-TTI and M60-non-TTI groups using one-way analysis of variance.

M15, M40, M60: Suspended moxibustion for 15, 40 and 60 minutes; TTI: tail temperature increase.

Chen RX, et al. / Neural Regeneration Research. 2013;8(12):1132-1138.

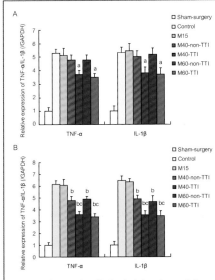

Figure 3 Suppression of ischemia-induced upregulation of tumor necrosis factor (TNF)-α and interleukin (IL)-1β mRNA in rats undergoing transient middle cerebral artery occlusion.

Expression of TNF-α and IL-1β mRNA at 1 (A) and 3 days post ischemia (B). [a]$P < 0.01$, vs. ischemic control, M15, M40-non-TTI and M60-non-TTI groups; [b]$P < 0.01$, vs. ischemic control and M15 groups; [c]$P < 0.01$, vs. M40-non-TTI and M60-non-TTI groups using one-way analysis of variance. Data are presented as mean ± SD.

M15, M40, M60: Suspended moxibustion for 15, 40 and 60 minutes; TTI: tail temperature increase.

DISCUSSION

In the first part of experiments, we selected 60 minutes as the suspended moxibustion duration so that the observing time was long enough to study the regular pattern of tail temperature variation. Results showed that the tail temperature of the sham-surgery rats and nine transient middle cerebral artery occlusion rats reached a relatively stable level but less than 1°C on average at about 5–10 minutes. Stable temperature was maintained until the end of the 60-minute suspended moxibustion treatment. However, the other nine transient middle cerebral artery occlusion rats exhibited tail temperature increase. It was revealed that tail temperature increase did not appear in sham-surgery rats. This indicates that tail temperature increase is relevant to stroke. This seems to be consistent with the fact in clinical settings

that distant heat induced by suspended moxibustion is highly relevant to the pathological process of diseases[2]. However, why did the nine transient middle cerebral artery occlusion animals not exhibit a marked tail temperature increase? As we discussed previously[2, 4], acupoint stimulation can cause distant heat at different locations in subjects who are afflicted with the same disease. Acupoints other than *Dazhui* were stimulated in the nine transient middle cerebral artery occlusion rats in order to produce tail temperature increase. Our previous study showed that 40–60% of the stroke rats that received suspended moxibustion on *Dazhui* exhibited a tail temperature increase[4]. Therefore, we utilized double the number of transient middle cerebral artery occlusion rats than the sham-surgery group so that the number of non-tail temperature increase subjects or tail temperature increase subjects selected from the suspended moxibustion group was almost the same as the sham-surgery group. The above explanations can also be applied to the second part of the experiments.

Prior to the second part of experiments, we had carefully studied the variation of tail temperature in rats with tail temperature increase. Tail temperature increased quickly at about 15 minutes but declined after 40 minutes. Hence, we selected 15, 40 and 60 minutes as the suspended moxibustion duration in the second part of studies, in which we confirmed the key role of tail temperature increase in improving suspended moxibustion efficacy. The application of suspended moxibustion for 15 minutes is considered the stage of meridian-*Qi* excitation[2], so it is not enough to induce tail temperature increase. This is exactly the reason why 15-minute suspended moxibustion has no effect on the recovery of rats. Although the efficacy of M40-non-tail temperature increase or M60-non-tail temperature increase was not as strong as the M40-tail temperature increase or M60-tail temperature increase group, a therapeutic effect was still observed compared to the M15 group. These findings revealed that the duration of suspended moxibustion was important to therapeutic efficacy. However, this does not show that the longer duration of suspended moxibustion session, the better the effects, because the effects also depend on whether tail temperature increase appears. Our data showed that the efficacy of suspended moxibustion without tail temperature increase for 40 or 60 minutes seemed to be limited, while suspended moxibustion with tail temperature increase significantly strengthened the efficacy of suspended moxibustion. In addition, there was no difference in efficacy of suspended moxibustion with tail temperature increase between 40 and 60 minutes. This

Chen RX, et al. / Neural Regeneration Research. 2013;8(12):1132-1138.

suggests that continuing suspended moxibustion after 40 minutes of treatment was useless for recovery from transient middle cerebral artery occlusion when tail temperature began to decline. It seemed that suspended moxibustion for 40 minutes was more suitable for recovery from transient middle cerebral artery occlusion because it took less curative time and achieved a similar effect as 60-minute treatment. These observations are useful for guiding the use of clinical suspended moxibustion.

It is widely known that tumor necrosis factor-α and interleukin-1β in the brain increase and exacerbate ischemic brain injury following ischemia[7]. This study showed that suspended moxibustion for 40 or 60 minutes with tail temperature increase significantly reduced the expression levels of tumor necrosis factor-α and interleukin-1β mRNA induced by transient middle cerebral artery occlusion compared with the other treatment groups. Furthermore, there was no difference in tumor necrosis factor-α and interleukin-1β mRNA between M40-tail temperature increase and M60-tail temperature increase groups at 1 or 3 days. This result indicates that suspended moxibustion at the Dazhui acu-point for 40 or 60 minutes with tail temperature increase can create an anti-inflammatory effect.

In summary, after suspended moxibustion at Dazhui in transient middle cerebral artery occlusion rats, the tail temperature began to increase significantly at around 15 minutes but decreased after 40 minutes. Suspended moxibustion with tail temperature increase significantly strengthened the efficacy of suspended moxibustion in stroke rats, which was associated with suppression of tumor necrosis factor-α and interleukin-1β mRNA. However, continuing suspended moxibustion could not increase its efficacy when the tail temperature began to decrease.

MATERIALS AND METHODS

Design
A randomized, controlled, animal study.

Time and setting
This experiment was performed at the Laboratory Animal Center, Jiangxi University of Traditional Chinese Medicine, China from April to May 2011.

Materials
Animals
A total of 120 adult, male, Sprague-Dawley rats, 8 weeks

old, weighing 220–250 g, of clean grade were purchased from the Shanghai Laboratory Animal Resources Center (license No. SCXK (Hu) 2003-0002), Shanghai, China. The rats were maintained in a cage at room temperature 22 ± 2°C, with controlled humidity 60 ± 5% and 12-hour day/night cycle, with a maximum of five rats per cage. All experimental studies were performed in accordance with the *National Institutes of Health Guide for the Care and Use of Laboratory Animals*.

Instrument
Moxa stick, weighing 6 g, 12 cm in length, 0.6 cm in diameter, was prepared by the Affiliated Hospital of Jiangxi University of Traditional Chinese Medicine, China.

Methods
Preparation of experimental stroke model in rats
Rats were anesthetized with an intraperitoneal injection of sodium pentobarbital (3%) at a dose of 30 mg/kg. Core body temperature was monitored using a rectal probe (Shenchao Transducer Co., Ltd, Shenzhen, Guangdong Province, China) and maintained at 37 ± 0.5°C by a heating lamp and a heating pad. Middle cerebral artery occlusion was performed using the intraluminal filament method as described previously[8]. After 2 hours of occlusion, the fishing line advanced to the origin of the middle cerebral artery was unclamped to allow reperfusion. Adequacy of vascular occlusion and reperfusion was assessed by Laser Doppler Monitoring (PeriFlux 5000, Perimed AB, Stockholm, Sweden) of cerebral cortical perfusion. Regional cerebral blood flow in the middle cerebral artery territory was reduced to < 20% of baseline after advancing the fishing line to the origin of the middle cerebral artery, and reconstituted to > 60% of baseline after removal of the fishing line. Rats dying within 24 hours after surgery, or displaying a neurological score of 0 or subarachnoid hemorrhage (as macroscopically assessed), were excluded from the final analysis.

Suspended moxibustion treatment
Stimulation of suspended moxibustion was performed 6 hours after reperfusion on the first day. A special cage in which the rat could maintain a comfortable position and the motion was restricted was used while testing. The cage was convenient for performing suspended moxibustion. Room temperature was maintained at 25 ± 2°C for the entire experimental process. The acupoint *Dazhui* (at C_7–T_1), which is very important for brain function[5], was heated by suspended moxibustion using a moxa (used specifically for animals) at approximately

Chen RX, et al. / Neural Regeneration Research. 2013;8(12):1132-1138.

3 cm (held by hand) over the hairless skin once a day for 3 days (in the first part of the experiments) or 7 days (in the second part of the experiments).

Tail temperature measurement

The midpoint tail temperature of rats was recorded once every 2 minutes precisely by an electro-digital thermometer (Shanghai Medical Instrument Factory, Shanghai, China) during suspended moxibustion treatment. The testing environment was maintained quiet, and room temperature was maintained at $25 \pm 2°C$. Rats were placed in a cage for 30 minutes before the experiment was started.

Assessment of neurological function

In the second part of experiments, neurological assessment, using a modified neurological severity scale (as described previously[9]), was performed at 0, 1, 3 and 7 days after transient middle cerebral artery occlusion by an investigator who was blinded to the experimental groups. In brief, scores on this scale were derived by evaluating animals for hemiparesis, sensory deficits, beam balance tests, absent reflexes, and abnormal movement. Neurological deficit scores were graded on a scale of 0 to 18 (normal score, 0; maximal deficit score, 18). One point was awarded for the inability to perform a task or the lack of a reflex.

Real time PCR analysis for tumor necrosis factor-α and interleukin-1β mRNA expression in rat cortex

Rats were sacrificed by cervical dislocation. Infarcted cortex was separated from the brain. Total RNA from cortex was reverse-transcribed into cDNA using oligo (dT) 18 primers and Avian Myeloblastosis reverse transcriptase (Gibco, Carlsbad, CA, USA). Real-time PCR was performed in the presence of a fluorescent dye (Evagreen, BIOTIUM, Hayward, CA, USA). The primer sequences used in this study were as described previously[10]:

Primer	Sequence	Product size (bp)
Tumor necrosis factor-α	Forward: 5'- CCC AGA CCC TCA CAC TCA GAT-3' Reverse: 5'- TTG TCC CTT GAA GAG AAC CTG-3'	215
Interleukin-1β	Forward: 5'- CAC CTT CTT TTC CTT CAT CTT TG-3' Reverse: 5'- GTC GTT GCT TGT CTC TCC TTG TA-3'	241
GAPDH	Forward: 5'- TGC CAA GTA TGA TGA CAT CAA GAA G-3' Reverse: 5'- AGC CCA GGA TGC CCT TTA GT-3'	80

The PCR protocol consisted of 5-minute enzyme activation at 95°C, followed by 45 cycles of 20-second denaturation at 95°C, 30-second annealing at 55°C and 23-second extension and fluorescence measurement at 72°C. Relative absorbance of mRNA was calculated after normalization to GAPDH ribosomal RNA and determined using crossing point analysis of log/linear plots of fluorescence/cycle number. The experiments were performed at least three times. ABI 7500 PCR system (ABI Carlsbad, CA, USA) was used.

Statistical analysis

Data were presented as mean $\pm$ SD and analyzed using one-way analyses of variance with *post hoc* Newman-Keuls multiple range tests for multiple groups. SPSS 13.0 (SPSS, Chicago, IL, USA) was used for analysis. A value of $P < 0.05$ was considered statistically significant.

Funding: This study was supported by the Major State Basic Research Development Program of China, No. 2009CB522902; the National Natural Science Foundation of China, No. 81160453; and the Traditional Chinese Medicine Research Fund of Health Department of Jiangxi Province, No. 2011A008.

Author contributions: Rixin Chen and Mingren Chen designed and carried out the study, and supervised the project. Zhimai Lv and Dangdang Huang established the models. Zhimai Lv, Dangdang Huang and Fan Yi performed the moxibustion, temperature measurement, neurological assessment and real-time PCR. Rixin Chen and Zhimai Lv collected and analyzed the data, discussed the interpretation of the results, and wrote the manuscript. All authors read and approved the final manuscript.

Conflicts of interest: None declared.

Ethical approval: All experimental procedures involving the use of animals were approved by the Animal Use and Care Committee for Jiangxi University of Traditional Chinese Medicine.

Author statements: The manuscript is original, has not been submitted to or is not under consideration by another publication, has not been previously published in any language or any form, including electronic, and contains no disclosure of confidential information or authorship/patent application/funding source disputations.

REFERENCES

[1]   Lee MS, Shin BC, Kim JI, et al. Moxibustion for stroke rehabilitation: systematic review. Stroke. 2010;41(4): 817-820.

[2]   Chen RX, Chen MR, Kang MF. Practical Reading of Heat-sensitization Moxibustion. Beijing: People's Medical Publishing Press. 2009.

Chen RX, et al. / Neural Regeneration Research. 2013;8(12):1132-1138.

[3] Chen R, Chen M, Xiong J, et al. Comparison of heat-sensitive moxibustion versus fluticasone/salmeterol (seretide) combination in the treatment of chronic persistent asthma: design of a multicenter randomized controlled trial. Trials. 2010;11:121.

[4] Chen RX, Lv ZM, Chen MR, et al. Stroke treatment in rats with tail temperature increase by 40-min moxibustion. Neurosci Lett. 2011;503(2):131-135.

[5] Luo YF. Subject of Acupoint. 5th ed. Shanghai: Shanghai Science and Technology Press. 2000.

[6] Wang Q, Tang XN, Yenari MA. The inflammatory response in stroke. J Neuroimmunol. 2007;184(1-2):53-68.

[7] Huang J, Upadhyay UM, Tamargo RJ. Inflammation in stroke and focal cerebral ischemia. Surg Neurol. 2006; 66(3):232-245.

[8] Longa EZ, Weinstein PR, Carlson S, et al. Reversible middle cerebral artery occlusion without craniectomy in rats. Stroke. 1989;20(1):84-91.

[9] Chen J, Sanberg PR, Li Y, et al. Intravenous administration of human umbilical cord blood reduces behavioral deficits after stroke in rats. Stroke. 2001;32(11): 2682-2688.

[10] van Neerven S, Mey J, Joosten EA, et al. Systemic but not local administration of retinoic acid reduces early transcript levels of pro-inflammatory cytokines after experimental spinal cord injury. Neurosci Lett. 2010; 485(1):21-25.

(Reviewed by Apricò K, Frenchman B, Tian N, Zhou MQ)
(Edited by Yu J, Su LL, Li CH, Wang L)

Hindawi Publishing Corporation
Evidence-Based Complementary and Alternative Medicine
Volume 2013, Article ID 140581, 4 pages
http://dx.doi.org/10.1155/2013/140581

Research Article

The Characterization of Deqi during Moxibustion in Stroke Rats

Zhimai Lv,[1] Zhongyong Liu,[2] Dandan Huang,[3] Rixin Chen,[2] and Dingyi Xie[2]

[1] *The First Affiliated Hospital of Gannan Medical University, Ganzhou, Jiangxi Province 341000, China*
[2] *Affiliated Hospital of Jiangxi University of TCM, Nanchang, Jiangxi Province 330006, China*
[3] *Gannan Medical University, Ganzhou, Jiangxi Province 341000, China*

Correspondence should be addressed to Rixin Chen; jxchenrixin@163.com

Received 8 May 2013; Revised 2 August 2013; Accepted 7 August 2013

Academic Editor: Fan-rong Liang

The efficacy of acupuncture and moxibustion is closely related to Deqi phenomenons, which are some subjective feelings. However, no one has reported the objective characterization of Deqi. Our preliminary research has found a phenomenon of tail temperature increasing (TTI) obviously in some stroke rats by suspended moxibustion at the acupoint dà zhuī (DU 14), which is similar to one characterization of Deqi during moxibustion that moxibustion heat is transferred from the original moxibustion acupoint to the other areas of the body. We wonder whether TTI is the objective indicator of Deqi characterization in animals. The present study showed that the stroke rat's recovery was also associated with TTI phenomenon. This suggests that TTI phenomenon is one objective characterization of the Deqi in stroke rats. Application of the TTI phenomenon contributes to explore the physiological mechanism of Deqi.

1. Introduction

It is considered that the clinical efficacy of acupuncture and moxibustion is closely related to Deqi phenomenon in traditional Chinese medicine. The characterizations of the Deqi during acupuncture treatment have been elaborated in acupuncture textbooks, which are some subjective feelings, such as soreness and heaviness [1]. Meanwhile, the characterizations of the Deqi during moxibustion treatment have also been clarified in clinical heat-sensitive moxibustion practice over the past decade [2], including the following: (a) moxibustion heat penetrates deep into the tissues or internal organs of the body; (b) moxibustion heat is transferred from the original moxibustion acupoint to the other areas of the body; (c) moxibustion heat could elicit other sensations, including pressure, soreness, heaviness, and dull pain, at the surface of the skin or deep tissues. However, the above characterizations are also some subjective feelings. The objective characterization of Deqi during moxibustion has not been reported yet. Our preliminary research has found a phenomenon of tail temperature increasing (TTI) obviously in some stroke rats by suspended moxibustion (SM) at the acupoint dà zhuī (DU 14), which is similar to the characterization (b) of Deqi during moxibustion in

humans [3]. We hereby propose the hypothesis that TTI is the objective indicator of Deqi characterization in stroke rats during moxibustion. The present study was designed to verify this hypothesis.

2. Methods

2.1. Animal Preparation. A total of 75 adult male Sprague-Dawley rats (220 to 250 g) were used in the experiment. The rats were maintained in a cage at room temperature $23 \pm 2°C$, with controlled humidity $60 \pm 5\%$ and 12-hour day/night cycle, with a maximum of five rats per cage. Firstly, 30 rats were divided randomly into 2 groups: (1) Sham operation with SM for 60 min group (sham, $n = 10$) and (2) ischemia with SM for 60 min group (M, $n = 20$). They were all treated for 3 days. According to the tail temperature change, the M group was further divided into two subgroups, including a nonincreasing subgroup ($\leq 1°C$ an average of 3 days, non-TTI group) and an increasing subgroup ($>1°C$ an average of 3 days, TTI group). Then, four points around the rat's torso were heated in five TTI rats. Secondly, another 45 rats with transient middle cerebral artery occlusion (tMCAO) operation were divided randomly into 2 groups: (1) ischemic control group (C, $n = 15$) (2) ischemia with SM for 60 min group (M60, $n = 30$). Rats in M60 group were treated with SM for 7 days. Like the first part of the experiment, the M60 group was also further divided into two subgroups, respectively, including the M60-non-TTI subgroup and the M60-TTI subgroup. All experimental procedures involving the use of animals were conducted in accordance with NIH Guidelines and approved by the Animal Use and Care Committee for Jiangxi University of TCM.

2.2. Preparation of Experimental Stroke Model in Rats. The rats were anesthetized with an intraperitoneal injection of sodium pentobarbital (3%) at a dose of 30 mg/kg. Core body temperature was monitored using a rectal probe and maintained at $37 \pm 0.5°C$ by a heating lamp and a heating pad. The middle cerebral artery occlusion was achieved by the Intraluminal Filament method as previously described [4]. After 2 h of occlusion, the fishing line advanced to the origin of the middle cerebral artery was withdrawn to allow for reperfusion. Sham-operated rats were manipulated in the same way, but the MCA was not occluded. Adequacy of vascular occlusion and reperfusion was assessed by Laser Doppler Monitoring (PeriFlux 5000, Perimed AB, Stockholm, Sweden) of cerebral cortical perfusion. Regional cerebral blood flow in the middle cerebral artery territory was reduced to <20% of baseline, after advancing the fishing line to the origin of the MCA, and reconstituted to >60% of baseline after removal of the fishing line. Rats dying within 24 hours after surgery or displaying a neurological score of 0 were excluded from the final analysis.

2.3. Suspended Moxibustion. A special cage in which the rat can maintain a comfortable position and the rat's motion is restricted was used while testing. The cage was convenient to the operation of SM. Room temperature was maintained at $25 \pm 2°C$ for the entire experimental process. In the first part of the experiment, DU 14, which is considered very important for brain functions [5], was heated by SM using a moxa (exclusively used on animals, length 12 cm, diameter 0.6 cm, made by the Affiliated Hospital of Jiangxi University of TCM, China). Then, five rats, selected randomly from the TTI group, received SM operation at four points. The first point was DU 14. The second point was located at the one that was 2 centimeters right beside the acupoint of DU 14. Both of them were heated at approximately 3 cm high over the hairless skin. The third point was located at the extension line of the longitudinal axis of the rat. The fourth point was located at perpendicular of the tail's midpoint. The third and fourth points both had the same distance far from rat's tail midpoint, which was identical to the distance between the acupoint of DU 14 and rat's tail midpoint. In the second part of the experiment, the heating point was also the acupoint of DU 14.

2.4. Tail Temperature Measurement. The rats' midpoint tail temperature was recorded once every 2 minutes precisely by an electrodigital thermometer (Shanghai Medical Instrument Factory, Shanghai, China) in process of SM treatment. The testing environment was kept quiet, and the room temperature was maintained at $25 \pm 2°C$. The rats were placed in a cage for 30 min before the experiment started.

2.5. Neurological Assessment. Neurological assessment was performed at 0, 1, 3, and 7 days after transient middle cerebral artery occlusion by a researcher who was unaware of the experimental groups, using a modified neurological severity score, which were graded on a scale of 0 to 18 (normal score, 0; maximal deficit score, 18), as previously described [6].

2.6. Statistical Analysis. Data was analyzed using one-way analysis of variance (ANOVA) with post hoc Newman-Keuls multiple-range test for multiple groups. The pearson correlation coefficient was also calculated between the neurological deficits score and change of tail temperature. SPSS 10.0 was used for analysis. $P < 0.05$ was considered statistically significant. All values were expressed as the mean $\pm$ SD.

3. Results

3.1. Quantitative Analysis of Experimental Animals. In the first part of the experiment, 2 of the 20 ischemic rats (1 death and 1 displaying 0 score) met at least one of the exclusion criteria. 9 ischemic rats exhibited TTI, and 9 subjects showed non-TTI. In the second part, 2 of the 15 rats in C group (2 death) and 3 of the 30 rats in M60 group (2 death and 1 displaying 0 score) met at least one of the exclusion criteria. There were 13 subjects in M60-non-TTI subgroup and 14 subjects in M60-TTI subgroup. Thus, 28 rats of the first part and 40 rats of the second part were included in the final analysis.

3.2. Tail Temperature Change following Suspended Moxibustion. In the first part of the experiment, tail temperature began to quickly increase immediately after suspended moxibustion. At about 5–10 min, the temperature reached a relatively stable level but less than 1°C on average. 9 tMCAO rats, as well as the sham rats, maintained this level (non-TTI) throughout the treatment session. However, the other 9 tMCAO rats exhibited TTI (more than 2°C on average). Furthermore, the tail temperature in the rats with TTI increased to a peak value at around 15 min, and the peak temperature was maintained until 40 min, at which a decline began to appear. At about 50 min, the tail temperature decreased to a level similar to that of the non-TTI or sham rats. The results were similar during the 3 consecutive days (Figure 1). Five stroke rats were randomly selected from TTI group and received SM operation for 60 min at four points, respectively. The tail temperature exhibited TTI by heating the first point. However, heating the other three points did not elicit TTI (Figure 2).

3.3. Neurological Deficits Score. To investigate the efficacy of SM for 60 min with TTI, we examined the neurological deficit score of tMCAO rats in the second part of the experiment. The results revealed that the M60-TTI group significantly reduced neurological deficit score at 3 days after reperfusion, compared with the C group ($P < 0.05$). This group further ameliorated the neurological deficit score at 7 days after reperfusion, compared with the C and M60-non-TTI ($P < 0.05$) groups. The M60-non-TTI group reduced neurological

Evidence-Based Complementary and Alternative Medicine

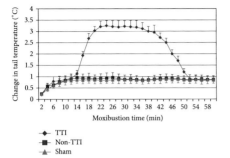

FIGURE 1: Change in tail temperature induced by SM in the first part of the experiment. Because the change of tail temperature was similar among the three consecutive testing days, data of the first day were presented as a representative. Data were expressed as mean ± SD.

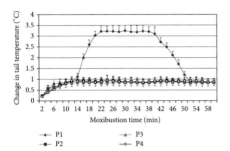

FIGURE 2: Change in tail temperature induced by SM at four points, respectively, around TTI rat's torso. Data were expressed as mean ± SD. P1: first point; P2: second point; P3: third point; P4: fourth point.

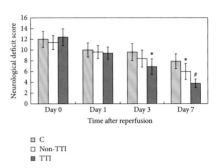

FIGURE 3: SM on neurological deficit score in the tMCAO rats. Data were presented as mean ± SD. $^{*}P < 0.05$ versus C group; $^{#}P < 0.05$ versus C and M60-non-TTI groups using one-way analyses of variance.

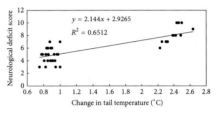

FIGURE 4: The change of tail temperature increase correlated with the neurological deficits score. $r = 0.807$, $P < 0.01$.

deficits score markedly at 7 days compared to the C group ($P < 0.05$) (Figure 3).

3.4. Behavior Correlation with Tail Temperature Increase. In order to explore the relationship between the reduction of neurological deficits score and the change of tail temperature increase induced by SM, we calculated the intersubject Pearson correlation coefficient between both mentioned above. We found that the reduction of neurological deficits score was positively correlated with the change of tail temperature increase induced by SM ($R = 0.807$, $P < 0.01$) (Figure 4).

4. Discussion

Deqi is a composite of unique sensations that is produced during acupuncture or moxibustion stimulation. We have paid attention to the clinical characterizations of Deqi during moxibustion for 20 years and summarized its characterizations as previously described. Furthermore, we have confirmed the efficacy of SM with Deqi is superior to that without

Deqi in clinic [2, 7–9]. Further investigation of the biological mechanism of Deqi during moxibustion depends on establishing the objective assessment of Deqi characterization, especially in animal study. However, few investigators have reported the objective characterization of Deqi in animals. In our previous study, we have accidentally found a TTI phenomenon in some stroke rats by SM at the DU 14 [10]. Based on the TTI phenomenon similar to one of Deqi characterizations during SM in clinic, we wonder whether TTI is the objective indicator of Deqi characterization in animals.

In this study, we have observed the change rule of TTI induced by SM at the DU 14 of tMCAO rats. The tail temperature in the rats with TTI increased beyond other subjects at about 15 min, and the peak temperature was maintained until 40 min, at which the decline began to appear. At about 50 min, the tail temperature decreased to a level similar to that of the non-TTI or sham rats. The results also suggested that TTI did not appear in sham-operated rats. This indicates that TTI is relevant to the model of stroke. It is consistent with the fact in clinic that Deqi phenomenon during SM is highly relevant to the morbid condition of human body [2, 11].

The tail is far from the heating acupoint. How is the TTI induced? In order to exclude the impacts of the conductive (the second point) and radiant (the third and fourth points)

heat on TTI generation, we set three other heating points except DU 14 as comparisons. The results showed that heating on three other heating points, respectively, exhibited no TTI. This proclaimed that conductive heat and radiant heat were not the reasons of inducing TTI phenomenon. However, in traditional Chinese channel theory, DU 14 and the tail are both on the DU channel (Governor Vessel) [5]. Stimulating the DU14 with SM could provide heat for the tail through the channel. The results of neurological deficit score further revealed that the tMCAO rats with TTI during SM recovered better than those without. This confirmed that the efficacy of SM was closely related to TTI phenomenon. It is also consistent with the fact in clinic that clinical efficacy of moxibustion is closely related to Deqi phenomenon. From this perspective, TTI could be considered as a characterization of Deqi in tMCAO rats during SM.

Why did not the other 13 tMCAO rats exhibit TTI? It is similar to the observation in clinic that acupoints that can be stimulated to cause Deqi phenomenon may have different locations in subjects who are afflicted with the same disease [2]. In the present study, the point (DU 14) for SM treatment was fixed. Therefore, some of them exhibited TTI, while others did not. Acupoints other than DU 14 were stimulated in the 13 tMCAO rats in order to produce TTI. As the occurrence rate of TTI is 40–60% in our previous study [3], the number of moxibustion-treated groups we designed is twice of the other groups (such as sham or C group) so that the number of non-TTI or TTI rats selected from the total tMCAO rats is almost the same as the sham or C group.

In conclusion, this study reported a TTI phenomenon in tMCAO rats with SM and proved this phenomenon was associated with the tMCAO rat's recovery. There was enough reason to believe that TTI phenomenon was one of the Deqi characterizations in tMCAO rat. Application of the TTI phenomenon contributes to explore the physiological mechanism of Deqi.

Abbreviations

SM: Suspended moxibustion
TTI: Tail temperature increase
tMCAO: Transient middle cerebral artery occlusion.

Conflict of Interests

The authors declare that they have no conflict of interests.

Authors' Contribution

R. X. Chen designed and carried out the study and supervised the project. Z. M. Lv and Z. Y. Liu established the models. Z. M. Lv, D. D. Huang, and Z. Y. Liu performed the moxibustion and temperature measurement. D. Y. Xie performed the neurological assessment. R. X. Chen and Z. M. Lv collected and analyzed the data, discussed the interpretation of the results, and wrote the paper. All authors read and approved the final paper. Zhimai Lv and Zhongyong Liu contributed equally to this work.

Acknowledgments

This study was supported by the Major State Basic Research Development Program of China, no. 2009CB522902; the National Natural Science Foundation of China, no. 81160453; and the Traditional Chinese Medicine Research Fund of Health Department of Jiangxi Province, no. 2012A049.

References

[1] X. M. Shi, *Acupuncture*, China press of traditional Chinese medicine, Beijing, China, 5th edition, 2007.

[2] R. X. Chen, M. R. Chen, and M. F. Kang, *Practical Reading of Heat-Sensitization Moxibustion*, People's Medical Publishing Press, Beijing, China, 1st edition, 2009.

[3] R.-X. Chen, Z.-M. Lv, M.-R. Chen, F. Yi, X. An, and D.-Y. Xie, "Stroke treatment in rats with tail temperature increase by 40-min moxibustion," *Neuroscience Letters*, vol. 503, no. 2, pp. 131–135, 2011.

[4] E. Z. Longa, P. R. Weinstein, S. Carlson, and R. Cummins, "Reversible middle cerebral artery occlusion without craniectomy in rats," *Stroke*, vol. 20, no. 1, pp. 84–91, 1989.

[5] Y. F. Luo, *Subject of Acupoint*, Shanghai Science and Technology Press, Shanghai, China, 5th edition, 2000.

[6] J. Chen, P. R. Sanberg, Y. Li et al., "Intravenous administration of human umbilical cord blood reduces behavioral deficits after stroke in rats," *Stroke*, vol. 32, no. 11, pp. 2682–2688, 2001.

[7] M. R. Chen, R. X. Chen, J. Xiong et al., "Evaluation of different moxibustion doses for lumbar disc herniation: multicentre randomised controlled trial of heat-sensitive moxibustion therapy," *Acupuncture in Medicine*, vol. 30, no. 4, pp. 266–272, 2012.

[8] R. X. Chen, J. Xiong, Z. H. Chi et al., "Heat-sensitive moxibustion for lumbar disc herniation: a meta-analysis of randomized controlled trials," *Journal of Traditional Chinese Medicine*, vol. 32, no. 3, pp. 322–328, 2012.

[9] R. X. Chen, M. R. Chen, J. Xiong et al., "Is there difference between the effects of two-dose stimulation for knee osteoarthritis in the treatment of heat-sensitive moxibustion?" *Evidence-Based Complementary and Alternative Medicine*, vol. 2012, Article ID 696498, 7 pages, 2012.

[10] R. Chen, Z. Lv, M. Chen, X. An, D. Xie, and J. Yi, "Neuronal apoptosis and inflammatory reaction in rat models of focal cerebral ischemia following 40-minute suspended moxibustion," *Neural Regeneration Research*, vol. 6, no. 15, pp. 1180–1184, 2011.

[11] R. Chen, M. Chen, J. Xiong, F. Yi, Z. Chi, and B. Zhang, "Comparison of heat-sensitive moxibustion versus fluticasone/salmeterol (seretide) combination in the treatment of chronic persistent asthma: design of a multicenter randomized controlled trial," *Trials*, vol. 11, article 121, 2010.

Hindawi Publishing Corporation
Evidence-Based Complementary and Alternative Medicine
Volume 2014, Article ID 154941, 7 pages
http://dx.doi.org/10.1155/2014/154941

Hindawi

Research Article

A 3-Arm, Randomized, Controlled Trial of Heat-Sensitive Moxibustion Therapy to Determine Superior Effect among Patients with Lumbar Disc Herniation

Rixin Chen,[1] Mingren Chen,[1] Tongsheng Su,[2] Meiqi Zhou,[3] Jianhua Sun,[4] Jun Xiong,[1] Zhenhai Chi,[1] Dingyi Xie,[1] and Bo Zhang[1]

[1] *The Affiliated Hospital with Jiangxi University of TCM, No. 445 Bayi Avenue, Nanchang 330006, China*
[2] *Shanxi TCM Hospital, Xian 710003, China*
[3] *The First Affiliated University with Anhui University of TCM, Hefei 230031, China*
[4] *Jiangsu TCM Hospital, Nanjing 210029, China*

Correspondence should be addressed to Rixin Chen; chenrixin321@163.com

Received 15 April 2014; Revised 16 June 2014; Accepted 7 July 2014; Published 24 July 2014

Academic Editor: Xueyong Shen

Systematic reviews of moxibustion for LDH have identified ponderable evidence, especially for heat-sensitive moxibustion (HSM). Therefore, we designed and carried out the large sample trial to evaluate it. 456 patients were recruited from 4 centers in China and were randomly divided into three groups by the ratio of $1:1:1$ to HSM (152) group, conventional moxibustion (152) group, and conventional drug plus acupuncture (152) group. Compared with usual care, there was a statistically significant reduction in mean M-JOA score at 2 weeks and 6 months for HSM (3.8 ± 2.6 versus 8.5 ± 2.9; 3.7 ± 2.2 versus 10.1 ± 2.9) and conventional moxibustion (7.9 ± 3.0 versus 8.5 ± 2.9; 8.9 ± 3.1 versus 10.1 ± 2.9). Compared with conventional moxibustion group, HSM group showed greater improvement in all the outcomes. The mean dose of moxibustion was 41.13 ± 5.26 (range 21–60) minutes in the HSM group. We found that HSM was more effective in treating patients with LDH, compared with conventional moxibustion and conventional drug plus acupuncture. This finding indicated that the application of moxibustion on the heat-sensitive points is a good moxibustion technique in treating disease.

1. Background

Therapies to strengthen the motor function and relieve low back pain are the most commonly recommended treatment for lumbar disc herniation (LDH), such as acupuncture and moxibustion [1]. They have the advantage better than other therapies (especially surgery) that they have no physical side-effects or adverse reactions [2, 3]. Moxibustion is a traditional oriental therapy that treats diseases through thermal stimulation of burning herbs, primarily *Artemisia vulgaris*, at specific acupuncture and moxibustion point on the skin [4]. Traditional Chinese medicine (TCM) considers LDH to be the result of an unbalanced state among interfunctioning organs or a block vital energy (called Qi) condition with characteristic blood symptoms [5]. A large number of clinical studies have shown positive results of moxibustion remedies on LDH

[6]. And moxibustion therapy has been important treatment in China. In particular, moxibustion treatment is effective for functional limitation and pain symptom because it provides warm energy, expels Qi-blood stagnation, and enhances local blood circulation [7]. Experimental studies showed moxibustion had anti-inflammatory or immunomodulatory effects against chronic inflammatory conditions in humans [8].

For moxibustion therapy, many factors influenced the therapeutic effect. However, the first thing to think about is the selection of location for manipulating moxa [9]. Conventional moxibustion applied moxibustion on fix acupuncture points based on pattern differentiation. Different patients received treatments on the same acupuncture points. However, heat-sensitive moxibustion (HSM) selected location that received moxibustion differently [10]. Heat-sensitive moxibustion administered moxibustion on heat-sensitive acupuncture points, which are extremely sensitive to the heat stimulation of burning moxa [11]. By using such acupuncture points, it is easier for channel Qi to transmit to and to allow a strong response to be produced by weak stimulation. Patients felt heat-sensitive sensation on these acupuncture points [12].

According to acupuncture point sensitized theory, there are two kinds of state in acupuncture points in human body: stimulated state and resting state. When people get sick, the acupoints on the body surface area are activated and sensitized. Our research found that the heat-sensitive phenomenon to acupuncture point or an area is a new type of reaction in a pathological state. The sensitive areas are susceptible to heat stimulation and called "heat-sensitive acupuncture points." A feature of these areas is that these areas are specific or closely relevant to acupuncture points and produce the same clinical effect as "a small stimulation induces a large response." This heat-sensitive acupuncture point is not only the pathological phenomenon reflection of the diseases but also an effective stimulating location with acupuncture and moxibustion. These heat-sensitized locations are not fixed, but may, during the progression of disease, dynamically change within a certain range centered on acupuncture points [13]. Our empirical evidence engaged us in formulating the following hypothesis: moxibustion at the heat-sensitive acupuncture points showed better efficacy than that at fixed acupuncture points.

However TCM theory in China agreed that the best place to apply moxibustion was on heat-sensitive acupuncture points, because using them led to better stimulation and transmission of channel Qi. When Qi arrives at one part of the body, it can treat the diseases nearby. In the part of *Miraculous pivot, the chapter of nine needles and twelve sources* said: "The key point of acupuncture is the arrival of Qi, it ensures therapeutic effect." However, there is little high-quality clinical evidence of its effectiveness. Therefore, we designed and carried out the large sample trial to evaluate it.

The results of a recent meta-analysis of six randomized controlled trials (RCTs) on moxibustion for LDH manifested that heat-sensitive therapy presented a favorable effect on LDH symptom scores compared with that of the drug [RR = 1.91, 95% CI (1.01, 3.60)] [14]. However, because of the number of eligible RCTs and the high risk of bias in the assessment of the available RCTs, the evidence supporting this conclusion is limited. Therefore, this well-designed and big sample RCT was needed to establish the efficacy of heat sensitive moxibustion for LDH.

2. Methods

2.1. Objective.
The aim of this study is to assess the effectiveness of heat-sensitive moxibustion for treating LDH compared with conventional drug plus acupuncture as well as conventional moxibustion.

2.2. Sample Size.
An effect size on the M-JOA was sought when comparing the heat-sensitive with conventional moxibustion. In our previous pilot study, the effective rate in heat-sensitive moxibustion group is 65% and 45% in the other

groups. An allocation ratio of $1:1:1$ was chosen in order to increase power to detect statistically significant differences between the three groups. With 90% power and a two-sided significance level of 5%, the required group sizes were 126. Allowing for 20% attrition, the total sample size required was 456 (i.e., groups of 152, 152, 152, resp.):

$$n = \frac{p_1 \times (1 - p_1) + p_2 \times (1 - p_2)}{(p_2 - p_1)^2} \times f(\alpha, \beta). \quad (1)$$

2.3. Design.
We performed a multicenter (four centers in China), randomized, assessor blinded, and positive controlled trial. Our trial was carried out in four hospitals in China, including the Affiliated Hospital of Jiangxi University of Traditional Chinese Medicine (TCM) in Nanchang, the first Affiliated Hospital of Anhui University of TCM in Hefei, Jiangsu TCM Hospital in Nanjing, and Shanxi TCM Hospital in Xian. Patients were recruited through hospital-based recruitment and newspaper advertisements. After a baseline phase of one week, we used a central randomization system (random list generated with computer telephone integration by the statistician from China Academy of Chinese Medical Sciences) to randomize patients [15]. All study participants provided written, informed consent, and the study conformed to common guidelines for clinical trials (Declaration of Helsinki, ICH-GCP, including certification by external audit). The evaluation of participants and the analysis of the results were performed by professionals blinded to the group allocation.

2.4. Participants

2.4.1. Recruitment.
Patients were recruited in China from December 30, 2011, to January 30, 2013. Informed consent was obtained from each subject, and the Ethics Committee of Affiliated Hospital of Jiangxi Institute of Traditional Chinese Medicine, China, approved the study protocol, authorization number: 2008(11).

2.4.2. Inclusion Criteria.
Inclusion criteria were a diagnosis of LDH according to the guiding principle of clinical research on new drugs (GPCRND) [16], at least 10 scores in M-JOA in the baseline period, age 18–65 years, pain occurring in lower back and radiating to the lower limb, completed baseline LDH diary, and written informed consent. Meanwhile, heat-sensitive acupuncture points were found in the triangle region formed with bilateral Dachangshu (BL25) and Yaoshu (Du2) of patients (Dachangshu-Yaoshu-contralateral Dachangshu intraregion).

2.4.3. Exclusion Criteria.
Main exclusion criteria were patients with serious life-threatening disease, such as disease of the heart and brain, blood, vessels, liver, kidney, and hematopoietic system, pregnant or lactating female, and psychotic patients. We also excluded patients with a single nerve palsy, or cauda equina nerve palsy, manifested as muscle paralysis or having rectum or bladder problems; complicated with lumbar spinal canal stenosis and space-occupying lesions or for

Evidence-Based Complementary and Alternative Medicine

3

other reasons; complicated with lumbar spine tumors, infections, tuberculosis; complicated with moxibustion syncope and unwilling to be treated with moxibustion; patients do not sign informed consent.

2.5. Study Interventions.

We developed the study interventions in a consensus process with China acupuncture experts and societies. Physicians trained and experienced (at least five years) in acupuncture delivered the interventions. All treatment regimens were standardized between four centers practitioners via video, hands-on training, and internet workshops. In the moxibustion groups, 22 mm (diameter) × 120 mm (length) moxa-sticks (Jiangxi Traditional Chinese Medicine Hospital, China) were used. The patient was usually in the comfortable supine position for treatment, with 24°C to 30°C temperature in the room.

2.5.1. Heat-Sensitive Moxibustion Group.

For the heat-sensitive moxibustion group, moxibustion treatment was defined as burning a moxa-stick with the patient lying on his or her back. The moxa-sticks were lit by the therapist and held over the region among two Dachangshu (BL25) and Yaoshu (Du 2) of patients. The moxa-stick suspended at an approximate distance of 3 cm was used to search for acupuncture points showing the heatsensitisation phenomenon. The following patients sensation suggested the special heat-sensitization acupuncture points: heat penetration, patients reporting heat penetrating from the skin into subcutaneous tissues; heat expansion, heat expanding away from the stimulation site to surrounding cutaneous and subcutaneous tissues; heat transmission, patients perceiving a stream of heat conducting in certain directions or perceiving heat in some body regions or into the joint cavity; nonthermal sensations, instead of thermal sensations, some patients perceiving aching, heaviness, pain, numbness, pressure, or cold in local or distant locations of stimulation. When such an acupuncture point was found, the therapists marked the point. We tried our best to seek all the special acupuncture points in each patient by the repeated manipulation.

The therapists began to treat patients from the most heat-sensitive intensity acupoint. Treatment sessions ended when patients felt the acupoint heat-sensitization phenomenon had disappeared. Generally speaking, one point was selected each time. One point was treated 30~60 minutes. Patients received the treatment for two times daily in the first four days and for one time daily in remaining ten days. The whole treatment contained 18 sessions over 14 days.

2.5.2. Conventional Moxibustion Group.

A licensed doctor performed fixed acupuncture point moxibustion. Common practices were similar to the first group. The different manipulation was that the therapists carry out warming moxibustion in traditional acupuncture point, selecting Dachangshu (BL25), Weizhong (BL40), and A-shi Xue. One point is treated 15 minutes a time. The whole process of moxibustion took about 45 minutes for each session. Patients usually felt local warmth without burning pain and might experience mild hyperemia in the local region. The sensation of acupuncture point heat-sensitization phenomenon was not pursued and not avoided in the treatment. Patients received the treatment for two times daily in the first four days and for one time daily in the remaining ten days. The whole treatment contained 18 sessions over 14 days.

2.5.3. Conventional Drug Plus Acupuncture Group.

For conventional drug, patients received the 20% mannitol (250 mL, intravenously) and Voltaren tablets (75 mg, 2 times a day) in the first 3 days. Voltaren tablets were continued to be used in the subsequent 11 days. At the same time, acupuncture needles were used and acupuncture points selected from Bladder Meridian of Foot-Taiyang and Gallbladder Meridian of Foot-Shaoyang. Acupoints included Dachangshu (BL25), Yaojiaji (EX-B2), Huantiao (GB30), Weizhong (BL40), Yanglingquan (GB34), Xuanzhong (GB39), and Qiuxu (GB40). We selected bilateral acupoints located in waist and ipsilateral acupoints located in lower limbs. Needles remained in acupuncture point for 30 minutes. Patients received the acupuncture needle treatment one time/day in two weeks for a total of 14 sessions over 14 days.

2.6. Outcome Measures.

Our primary outcome measure was the M-JOA. The JOA has proposed a series of criteria to define patient response in the context of clinical trials of LDH. M-JOA scale is a modified edition of JOA Back Pain Evaluation Questionnaire. According to these criteria, a patient with LDH is assessed for pain, the ability to conduct daily life and work, functional impairment, and particular clinical examinations. M-JOA scores range from 0 to 24, with LDH considered mild (0–9), moderate (10–20), or severe (21 and above). The M-JOA was used as a preference-based measure of health outcome. All patients were assessed before randomization (baseline phase), 2 weeks after randomization, and 6 months after the last treatment. This trial also recorded adverse effects reported by patients during treatment.

We ensured assessor blinding in this trial. Patients were informed not to tell outcome assessors the treatment they received. The outcome assessor was not involved in treatment administration.

2.7. Statistical Methods.

Data were analysed on an intention-to-treat (ITT) basis including all randomised patients with at least one measurable outcome report. The statistician conducting the analyses remained blinded to treatment groups. All analyses were conducted using SPSS 11.5. The groups were compared on 2 weeks, with t-tests used to assess changes between baseline and 2 weeks within each arm. ANOVA was used to compare these changes among the three treatment arms of the trial. Where a significance difference was found among the three groups, pair-wise tests were used to determine specifically which groups differed significantly. Student-Newman-Keuls was used for pairwise comparison. All adverse reactions manifested were listed with detailed explanations. A significance level of 5% was used in all analyses.

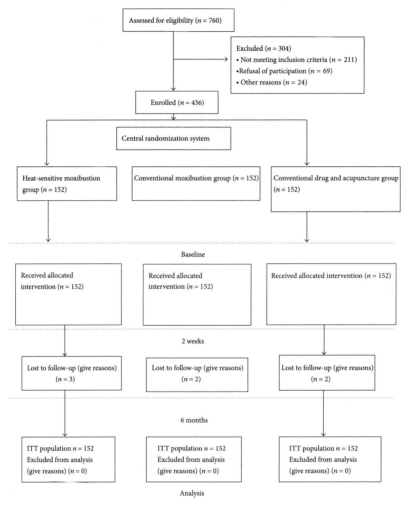

FIGURE 1: A flowchart of the study process.

3. Results

3.1. Population and Baseline. Participants were recruited from outpatients and inpatients in the four study centers. Patient flow in the trial was presented in Figure 1. After screening 760 patients, 456 were randomly assigned to treatment. 304 could not be included in the study, mainly because they did not meet all eligibility criteria. After six months, 7 patients missed. Reasons for missing follow-up data were not contactable. Participants had a mean age of 46.3 years, and 52.4% were female. Table 1 presented the history of LDH of the subjects. The mean M-JOA score was 17.6. Baseline patient characteristics were balanced between trial arms. There was no difference in attrition rate among the groups at 6-month follow-up ($P > 0.05$, Fisher exact test).

TABLE 1: Baseline characteristics of participants.

Items	Heat-sensitive moxibustion group	Conventional moxibustion group	Conventional drug plus acupuncture group
Age, mean (SD), years	45.5 (10.6)	47.3 (11.2)	46.6 (10.5)
Age, min~max, years	18~59	20~58	18~59
Age, >60 y, n (%)	9 (5.92)	10 (6.6)	9 (5.92)
Sex n (%)			
Female	78 (51.3)	80 (52.6)	81 (53.3)
Male	74 (48.7)	72 (47.4)	71 (46.7)
Duration of pain n (%)			
<1 m	32 (21.1)	30 (19.7)	30 (19.7)
2~6 m	40 (26.3)	42 (27.6)	43 (28.2)
7~12 m	40 (26.3)	33 (21.7)	31 (20.3)
1~5 y	33 (21.7)	38 (25.1)	40 (26.3)
>5 y	7 (4.6)	9 (5.9)	8 (5.2)
BMI, mean (SD), kg/m$'$	22.2 (3.3)	22.4 (3.1)	21.1 (4.0)
BMI, min~max, kg/m$'$	14.3~30.1	16.2~29.2	13.1~28.9
M-JOA score n (%)			
Severe	115 (75.6)	113 (73.4)	119 (78.3)
Moderate	37 (24.4)	39 (25.6)	33 (21.7)
M-JOA score, mean (SD)	18.6 (3.8)	17.5 (3.3)	17.2 (4.4)

BMI, Body Mass Index; M-JOA, Improvement Japanese Orthopedic Association (M-JOA) Lumbago Score Scale; SD, standard deviation; LDH, lumbar disc herniation.

3.1.1. Total M-JOA Score. There was a significant reduction in mean M-JOA score from baseline in all three groups ($P < 0.01$). ANOVA test showed significant difference in the three groups at both time points. Mixed-effects model analysis (q-test) showed that subjects in the heat-sensitive moxibustion group had significantly greater reduction in M-JOA scores than those in conventional moxibustion group or conventional drug plus acupuncture group at 2 weeks and 6 months; however, there was no significant difference between conventional moxibustion and conventional drug plus acupuncture at both time points (Table 2).

3.2. Moxibustion Time in the Heat-Sensitive Moxibustion Group. Different from the conventional moxibustion group, moxibustion dose was individual in the heat-sensitive moxibustion group. According to the record of individual moxibustion time, the dose differed in terms of patients' conditions and moxibustion sensation, which had been measured about 21~60 minutes in the treatment of LDH. The range of mean moxibustion dose was about 41.13 ± 5.26 minutes in the conventional moxibustion group. We used a linear correlation to measure the strength of a relationship between change in M-JOA score and stimulation duration in the conventional moxibustion group. The Pearson coefficient $r = 0.0006$, showing a poor correlation between the two values.

3.3. Safety. No adverse events were reported in the 456 participants.

4. Discussions

The heat-sensitive moxibustion intervention tested in this study was significantly more effective than conventional moxibustion treatment and significantly more effective than the conventional drug plus acupuncture intervention in patients with LDH. No serious cases of adverse reactions related to treatment were reported. This study had a clear and practical research question with an appropriate trial design, namely, a pragmatic randomized controlled trial, which modelled closely what would happen if patient refers to moxibustion. Compared with available studies of moxibustion for LDH, which included a maximum amount of 120 patients [17–19], our study has a much larger sample size. Other advantages included adherence to current guidelines for acupuncture trials, strictly concealed central randomization, blinded evaluation of statistics and measurement, interventions based on expert consensus provided by qualified and experienced medical acupuncturists, and high follow-up rates. Trial physicians could not be blinded. It was not possible to blind the conventional drug plus acupuncture patients. Therefore, the large and significant difference between HSM and conventional moxibustion and between HSM and conventional drug plus acupuncture could be due to performance bias and detection bias. The results of this study proved the superiority of heat-sensitive moxibustion in patients suffering from LDH. That is, selecting the heat-sensitive acupuncture point obtained therapeutic effect far better than moxibustion at acupuncture point of routine resting states. These heat-sensitive acupuncture points are not fixed, but may, during the progression of disease, dynamically change within

TABLE 2: Comparison of M-JOA scores.

Variable	Week 2			Month 6		
	Mean (SD)		95% CI	Mean (SD)		95% CI
Group A	3.8 (2.6)		3.4~4.2	3.7 (2.2)		3.3~4.1
Group B	7.9 (3.0)		7.4~8.4	8.9 (3.1)		8.4~9.4
Group C	8.5 (2.9)		8.0~9.0	10.1 (2.9)		9.5~10.6
Comparison between the three groups						
F value		3.8			5.2	
P value		0.016			0.008	
Group A versus Group B						
q value		4.1			5.9	
P value		0.022			0.013	
Group A versus Group C						
q value		5.1			6.7	
P value		0.017			0.002	
Group C versus Group B						
q value		2.0			3.2	
P value		0.146			0.041	

Comparison between the three groups by ANOVA test. Pairwise comparison for the two groups by Student-Newman-Keuls (q-test). All data are intended to treat. Each group $n = 152$. SD: standard deviation; M-JOA: Improvement Japanese Orthopedic Association (M-JOA) Lumbago Score Scale; SD: standard deviation; LDH: lumbar disc herniation; Group A: Heat-sensitive moxibustion group; Group B: Conventional moxibustion group; Group C: Conventional drug plus acupuncture group.

a certain range centered on acupuncture points. Several types of heat-sensitization responses might appear alone or in combination. Patients become thermally sensitized to moxibustion stimulation at certain locations on the body, indicated by sensations of strong warmth or heat penetrating into the body (heat penetration), warmth spreading around the stimulation site (heat expansion), warmth conducting in certain directions and reaching some body regions or even internal organs remote from stimulation sites (heat transmission), or other nonthermal sensations [20]. These responses gradually disappear with disease recovery.

In summary, we have provided high-quality evidence that heat-sensitive moxibustion showed significant reduction in symptoms of LDH in the short and long term compared with other two treatments (conventional moxibustion, conventional acupuncture plus medicine). The importance of the therapeutic relationship providing heat-sensitive acupuncture point should not be underestimated in the moxibustion therapy. Therefore, the success of this project is more than providing the efficacy of heat-sensitive moxibustion as a treatment modality in patients with LDH. The findings will be helpful to provide better therapeutic options to enhance the efficacy of moxibustion and to perfect acupuncture point heat-sensitive theory.

Conflict of Interests

The authors declare that they have no conflict of interests.

Authors' Contribution

Mingren Chen and Rixi Chen obtained fund of the research project. Jun Xiong wrote the final paper. Rixin Chen, Tongsheng Su, Jianhua Sun, Meiqi Zhou, Zhenhai Chi, Dingyi Xie, and Bo Zhang contributed to the trial implement. All authors read and approved the final paper. Rixin Chen and Mingren Chen contributed equally to this work.

Acknowledgments

This study was supported by the Major State Basic Research Development Program of China (Grant no. 2009CB522902), the National Natural Science Foundation of China (Grant no. 81160453), the National Natural Science Foundation of China (Grant no. 81202854), Jiangxi Key R&D Project, and traditional Chinese medicine scientific research plan of Jiangxi Province Health Department (Grant no. 2012A113).

References

[1] L. C. Paramore, "Use of alternative therapies: estimates from the 1994 Robert Wood Johnson Foundation National Access to Care Survey," *Journal of Pain and Symptom Management*, vol. 13, no. 2, pp. 83–89, 1997.

[2] A. K. Hopton, S. Curnoe, M. Kanaan, and H. MacPherson, "Acupuncture in practice: mapping the providers, the patients and the settings in a national cross-sectional survey," *BMJ Open*, vol. 2, no. 1, Article ID e000456, 2012.

[3] K. J. Thomas, J. P. Nicholl, and P. Coleman, "Use and expenditure on complementary medicine in England: a population based survey," *Complementary Therapies in Medicine*, vol. 9, no. 1, pp. 2–11, 2001.

[4] World Health Organization, *WHO International Standard Terminologies on Traditional Medicine in the Western Pacific Region*, World Health Organization, Western Pacific Region, Maynila, Philippines, 2007.

[5] L. Fanrong, *Acupuncture (Zhen Jiu Xue)*, China Traditional Chinese Medicine Publishing, Beijing, China, 2005.

[6] X. H. Wang, "Advances in lumbar disc herniation treatment research," *Chinese Journal of Health Industry*, vol. 10, no. 8, pp. 38–39, 2012 (Chinese).

[7] Z. H. Cho, S. C. Hwang, E. K. Wong et al., "Neural substrates, experimental evidences and functional hypothesis of acupuncture mechanisms," *Acta Neurologica Scandinavica*, vol. 113, no. 6, pp. 370–377, 2006.

[8] W. Chen, A. Yang, M. Dai, and Q. Fu, "Observation on therapeutic effect of electroacupuncture under continuous traction for treatment of lumbar disc herniation," *Zhongguo Zhen Jiu*, vol. 29, no. 12, pp. 967–969, 2009 (Chinese).

[9] C. RiXin and K. Mingfei, *Acupuncture Point Heat-Sensitive Moxibustion and New Therapy*, People's Medical Publishing House, Beijing, China, 2006.

[10] C. RiXin, C. Mingren, and K. Mingfei, *An Practical Book of Heat-Sensitive Moxibustion*, Press by People's Medical Publishing House, Beijing, China, 1st edition, 2009.

[11] R. Chen and M. Kang, "Clinical application of acupoint heat-sensitization," *Zhongguo zhen jiu*, vol. 27, no. 5, pp. 199–202, 2007 (Chinese).

[12] R. Chen and M. Kang, "Key point of moxibustion, arrival of qi produces curative effect," *Zhongguo Zhen Jiu*, vol. 28, no. 1, pp. 44–46, 2008.

[13] X. Dingyi, L. Zhongyong, and H. Xiaoqin, "Heat sensitization in suspended moxibustion: features and clinical relevance," *Acupuncture in Medicine*, vol. 31, no. 4, pp. 422–424, 2013.

[14] R. Chen, J. Xiong, Z. Chi, and B. Zhang, "Heat-sensitive moxibustion for lumbar disc herniation: a meta-analysis of randomized controlled trials," *Journal of Traditional Chinese Medicine*, vol. 32, no. 3, pp. 322–328, 2012 (Chinese).

[15] B. Liu, T. Wen, C. Yao et al., "The central randomization system in multi-center clinical trials," *Chinese Journal of New Drugs and Clinical Remedies*, vol. 12, no. 3, pp. 931–935, 2006 (Chinese).

[16] "JOA Back Pain Evaluation Questionnaire," Japanese Orthopedic Association, http://www.joa.or.jp/english/english_frame .html.

[17] F. Y. Tang, C. J. Huang, R. X. Chen, M. Xu, B. X. Liu, and Z. Liang, "Observation on therapeutic effect of moxibustion on temperature-sensitive points for lumbar disc herniation," *Chinese Acupuncture & Moxibustion*, vol. 29, no. 5, pp. 382–384, 2009 (Chinese).

[18] C. Zhang, H. Xiao, and R. Chen, "Observation on curative effect of moxibustion on heat-sensitive points on pressure sores," *China Journal of Traditional Chinese Medicine and Pharmacy*, vol. 25, no. 6, pp. 478–488, 2010 (Chinese).

[19] M. F. Kang, R. X. Chen, and Y. Fu, "Observation on curative effect of moxibustion on heat-sensitive points on knee osteoarthritis," *Jiangxi Journal of Traditional Chinese Medicine and Pharmacy*, vol. 18, no. 2, pp. 27–28, 2006 (Chinese).

[20] C. Rixin, C. Mingren, and K. Mingfei, *Heat-sensitive Moxibustion Therapy*, People's Medical Publishing House, Beijing, China, 1st edition, 2012.

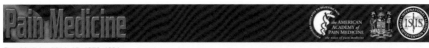

Pain Medicine 2014; 15: 1272–1281
Wiley Periodicals, Inc.

GENERAL SECTION

Original Research Articles

Characterizing Heat-Sensitization Responses in Suspended Moxibustion with High-Density EEG

Feifei Liao, MSc,* Chan Zhang, MPhil,*
Zhijie Bian, PhD,† Dingyi Xie, MD,‡
Mingfei Kang, MD,‡ Xiaoli Li, PhD,†§
You Wan, PhD,*¶ Rixin Chen, MD,‡ and Ming Yi, PhD*

*Neuroscience Research Institute and ¶Key
Laboratory for Neuroscience, Ministry of
Education/National Health and Family Planning
Commission, Peking University, Beijing; †Institute of
Electrical Engineering, Yanshan University,
Qinhuangdao; ‡Affiliated Hospital of Jiangxi University
of TCM, Nanchang; §National Key Laboratory of
Cognitive Neuroscience and Learning, Beijing Normal
University, Beijing, China

Reprint requests to: Ming Yi, PhD, Neuroscience
Research Institute, Peking University, 38 Xueyuan
Road, Beijing 100191, China. Tel: +86 (0)10 8280 552;
Fax: +86 (0)10 8280 1151; E-mail:
mingyi@bjmu.edu.cn. Rixin Chen, MD, The Affiliated
Hospital of Jiangxi University of TCM, No. 445 Bayi
Avenue, Nanchang, Jiangxi Province, 330006, PR
China. Tel: +86 (0) 791 8859 6387; Fax: +86 (0) 791
8859 6387; E-mail: chenrixin321@163.com.

Abstract

Objective. We have reported "heat-sensitization" responses during suspended moxibustion, whose occurrence is associated with significantly better therapeutic effects. The present study aimed to characterize the electrophysiological features of this interesting phenomenon with high-density electroencephalography (EEG).

Methods. We performed EEG recording in a group of patients with chronic low back pain before, during, and after moxibustion treatment at DU3.

Results. 12 out of 25 subjects experienced strong heat-sensitization during moxibustion, which was accompanied by increased power spectral densities (PSDs) at the theta, alpha, and beta frequency bands. The scalp topographies of averaged power indicated that the theta and beta PSD changes were most obvious in fronto–central regions, whereas those of the alpha band were more global. In addition, nonsensitized and sensitized groups showed distinct activity patterns, with heat-sensitization inducing increased phase coherence at the theta and beta ranges.

Conclusions. These data were the first objective evidence of heat-sensitization responses during suspended moxibustion, which were characterized by widespread oscillatory changes in scalp EEG.

Key Words. Moxibustion; Heat-sensitization; Chronic Low Back Pain; Electroencephalography; Acupuncture

Introduction

Acupuncture and moxibustion have been used to treat a variety of diseases in China for over 2,000 years. Unlike acupuncture which uses mechanical stimulation, moxibustion is primarily a type of thermal stimulation with burning dried plant materials (*Artimisia moxa*). It can be applied either with a small amount of burning *moxa* directly on the skin (direct moxibustion) or with heat generated from burning *moxa* 3–5 cm away from the skin surface (suspended or indirect moxibustion, supplementary Figure S1). Moxibustion exerts antinociceptive, anti-inflammatory, and immunomodulatory effects in humans, and gains increasing popularity from both clinicians and researchers worldwide [1–7].

We previously reported a "heat-sensitization" phenomenon during suspended moxibustion [1]. That is, patients often become sensitized to moxibustion stimulation at certain locations on the body. They experience strong warmth or heat spreading around the stimulating site or penetrating into the body, which quite frequently is accompanied by pleasant feelings. These locations are not always acupoints anatomically, but may change within a certain range centered by specific acupoints during the progression of disease. Each disease has a specific set of such sensitized acupoints, and such phenomenon is not

1272

Table 1 Clinical characteristics of recruited CLBP patients

	Nonsensitized Group	Sensitized Group	P
Number of patients	13	12	>0.05
Gender: M/F	8/5	6/6	>0.05
Age: mean in years (SE)	42.7 (3.4)	47.3 (4.0)	>0.05
Duration of pain: mean in months (SE)	45.9 (17.4)	44.2 (11.0)	>0.05

CLBP = chronic low back pain.

commonly seen in healthy volunteers. For example, patients with chronic low back pain (CLBP) frequently showed heat-sensitization around Yaoyangguan (DU3) areas [2–4]. Recent randomized controlled trials revealed that patients with heat-sensitization responses during moxibustion had significantly better clinical outcomes than those without [1–3,5], and that performing moxibustion on these functionally sensitized locations yields better therapeutic effects than the anatomically defined but nonsensitized acupoints [3]. These studies suggest a potential link between the sensitization responses induced by moxibustion and its modulatory effects on pain and inflammation. However, there are no objective evidences for the presence of these responses, nor information about their biological mechanisms.

The noninvasive feature of electroencephalography (EEG) allows its application in conscious human subjects. Oscillatory and coherent activities recorded from scalp EEG reflect intra- and inter-regional interactions in the brain and their characteristic changes have been identified in a number of physiological and pathological conditions [8–10]. The strong perceptual and emotional responses during heat-sensitization in moxibustion almost definitely implicate cortical activities. In the present study, we performed high-density EEG recording in a group of patients with CLBP before, during, and after moxibustion treatment and studied EEG changes associated with the heat-sensitization responses.

Methods

Subjects and Ethics Statement

Twenty-five right-handed Chinese patients suffering from CLBP were recruited to receive moxibustion treatment in the Affiliated Hospital of Jiangxi University of TCM (Table 1). The diagnosis of CLBP was in accordance with previous guidelines [11]. These patients aged between 18 and 60 years and none had a history of major medical illness, head trauma, neuropsychiatric disorders, evidence of root damages, or other diseases that would affect brain activities. A previous study had shown that quantitative EEG of such patients was comparable with healthy volunteers [12]. The experimental procedures were approved by the Local Ethical Committee on Human Studies based in Jiangxi University of TCM and in accordance with the ethical standards laid down in the 1964 Declaration of Helsinki and its later amendments. All patients were given written informed consent before the experiment.

Moxibustion and Grouping

The patients took a comfortable prone position in a quiet and dimly lit room. An experienced clinician performed suspended moxibustion with two *moxa* sticks over Yaoyangguan (DU3), which locates between the fourth and fifth lumbar vertebra. The *moxa* sticks were fixed 3–5 cm above the skin surface to get a skin surface temperature of 41°C (supplementary Figure S1). The treatment lasted 30 minutes. Patients who experienced strong warmth or heat penetrating into the body, spreading around the stimulating site, or conducting along the spine [1] fell into the heat-sensitized group (N = 12), whereas those experiencing only mild local warmth entered the nonsensitized group (N = 13) (Figure 1).

EEG Recording and Preprocessing

Spontaneous resting EEG was recorded via a 128 channel EGI (Electrical Geodesics, Inc.) system. Patients were requested to keep relaxed but alert with eyes closed. The central electrode Cz served as the reference during

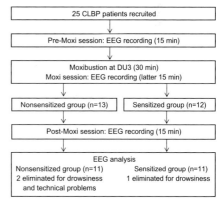

Figure 1 Experimental flowchart.

Liao et al.

recording which was re-referenced to the averaged ear lobe off-line. The sample frequency was 1,000 Hz with a notch filter at 50 Hz. The electrode impedances were under 50 kΩ. Three sessions(15 minutes each) of resting EEG were recorded for each patient: one before moxibustion (pre-Moxi session), one during the last 15 minutes of moxibustion (Moxi session), and one immediately after moxibustion (post-Moxi session).

EEG data were resampled at 250 Hz with a band pass filtered off-line in the frequency range of 1–100 Hz for removing linear trends. The middle 5 minutes of each session was chosen for further analysis. Conspicuous artifacts were eliminated by visual inspection on time series and data exceeding ±80 μV in any channel were rejected by manual, remaining data: 252.67 ± 42.69 seconds per subject in a range of 144.92–299.63 seconds. Due to equipment problems, data from two of the original 128 channels were off-line replaced by the average data from the neighboring channels. In addition, 38 out-line channels were excluded because of their vulnerability against muscle activities or eye movements, leaving a total of 90 channels for further off-line analysis (supplementary Figure S2).

Power Spectral Densities (PSDs)

Data were analyzed off-line in Matlab interface (The Mathworks, Natick, MA) using Matlab and EEGLAB (http://www.sccn.Ucsd.edu/eeglab/index.html). Spectra power analysis used the EEGLAB spectopo method (with a window length of 512 points, fast Fourier transform (fft) length of 1,024 points, non-overlap) to estimate and plot PSDs of EEGs per frequency. To compare spectral parameters, all P values are two sided from nonparametric Wilcoxon tests. To summarize the data, we first averaged the log-transformed spectra of the 90 scalp electrodes for each subject (spectra from all electrodes had similar shapes and scales). The EEG data were further divided into five different bands: delta (δ, 1–4 Hz), theta (θ, 4–8 Hz), alpha 1 (α1, 8–10 Hz), alpha 2 (α2, 10–13 Hz) and beta (β, 13–30 Hz), and the PSDs of each band were estimated again using Welch's averaged modified periodogram method (MATLAB function: window length: 256, fft length: 256, overlap 50%).

Phase Coherence Analysis

To calculate the correlation coefficient among signals from regions of interest, magnitude squared coherence (MSCxy) in the theta, alpha, and beta frequency bands was measured. The coherence (value lies between 0 and 1) was a function of the averaged PSD (Pxx and Pyy) and the averaged cross PSD (Pxy) of x and y signals. Mathematically, MSCxy is equal to Pxy normalized by Pxx and Pyy, namely, MSCxy = |Pxy|2/(Pxx × Pyy). MSCxy equals 0 means that the two signals have no linear relationship at a given frequency. However, when two signals are completely phase-locked and have a constant amplitude ratio, MSCxy = 1, which means the two signals are in a good phase synchronization. Here we chose 18 out of 90 chan-

nels according to the standard 10–20 system, including Fp1/Fp2, Fz/F3/F4/F7/F8, C3/C4, T3/T4, Pz/P3/P4, T5/T6, O1/O2 (Cz, as the reference in recording session, was excluded here). The coherence spectra of frequency bands for all pairs of the 18 electrodes were calculated with a window length of 2 seconds, fft length of 1 second, and 50% overlap. The correlation coefficients of phase coherence of each electrode pair were compared with paired t-tests.

Results

Heat-Sensitization Responses During Moxibustion

With 30 minutes moxibustion at DU3, 12 out of 25 CLBP patients experienced moderate to strong heat-sensitization, whereas 13 reported only local warmth. They fell into the sensitized and nonsensitized groups, respectively. The general information of these patients did not differ between groups (Table 1).

Increased PSDs at Theta, Alpha1 and Beta Bands During Heat-Sensitization

To determine the EEG correlates of heat-sensitization during moxibustion, PSDs of the pre-Moxi, Moxi, and post-Moxi sessions were analyzed. In the nonsensitized group where patients experienced only local warmth, no differences of averaged PSDs were found at any frequency bands between the three sessions ($P > 0.05$, Wilcoxon tests, Figure 2A and C). In contrast, heat-sensitization responses in the sensitized group during moxibustion were accompanied by significant increases of PSDs in the theta, alpha1, and beta bands ($P < 0.05$, Wilcoxon tests, Figure 2B and D). The PSD increase in the beta range persisted to the post-moxibustion phase. Direct comparisons of PSDs of 90 electrodes at each frequency points from 1.2 to 30 Hz also indicated significantly more changes in the sensitized group (Figure 3A–D, and supplementary Figure S2).

The scalp topographies of average PSDs indicated that changes in the theta and beta bands were strongest in frontal–central regions, whereas those in the alpha1 band were more global (Figure 3E).

Increased Phase Coherence at Theta and Beta Bands During Heat-Sensitization

We next examined the phase coherence for theta, alpha, and beta frequency bands between pre-Moxi and Moxi sessions and between pre-Moxi and post-Moxi sessions. For all frequency bands, relatively few changes were detected in the nonsensitized group, whereas many electrode pairs showed significantly increased phase coherence between the pre-Moxi and Moxi sessions in the sensitized group. For the theta band (Figure 4), coherence between electrodes at the central–frontal regions significantly increased during heat sensitization, which was in sharp contrast to that of the nonsensitized patients. But these changes were not present in the post-Moxi phase.

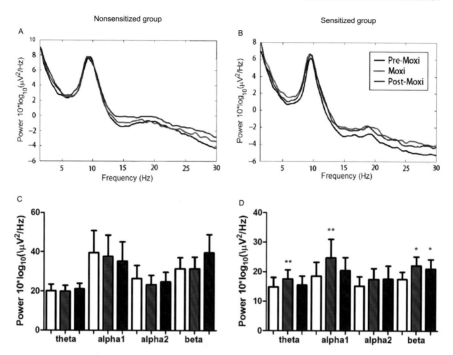

Figure 2 Average PSDs of 90 channels before (pre-Moxi session, black), during (Moxi session, red) and after (post-Moxi session, blue) moxibustion. No changes were detected at any frequency bands in the nonsensitized group (A and C). In the sensitized group (B and D), PSDs of theta, lower alpha, and beta bands significantly increased during moxibustion. Changes in the beta band persisted after moxibustion. *$P < 0.05$, **$P < 0.01$, two-sided Wilcoxon tests.

No obvious changes in the alpha band were present during moxibustion, regardless of the occurrence or absence of heat-sensitization (Figure 5). Phase coherence changes at the beta band were more global during heat-sensitization, and persisted even after the end of moxibustion (Figure 6). The clear difference between the nonsensitized and sensitized groups indicated distinct brain activity patterns between the two states, and implied potential inter-regional cross-talks during the heat-sensitization of moxibustion.

Discussion

The present study was designed to characterize moxibustion-induced heat-sensitization responses with EEG. Rhythmical activities of different frequency ranges recorded from EEG have their specific behavioral or cognitive correlates. For example, beta oscillations considered as an index of cortical arousal and beta synchronization between temporal and parietal cortexes appear during multimodal semantic processing, whereas long range frontal–parietal interactions during cognition induce theta and alpha oscillations [8–10]. Here we showed significant increases of the PSDs of theta, alpha, and beta bands in the central–frontal–parietal areas during heat-sensitization. Moreover, heat-sensitization was accompanied with increased phase coherence, indicating strong interactions between these regions. These changes were not observed in patients without heat-sensitization responses.

As far as we knew, the present study was the first EEG study of moxibustion. An interesting finding was that significant EEG changes were not observed in all subjects, but only in a proportion of patients with heat-sensitization responses. These changes provided objective indications of the subjective perceptions. One clear factor affecting

1275

Liao et al.

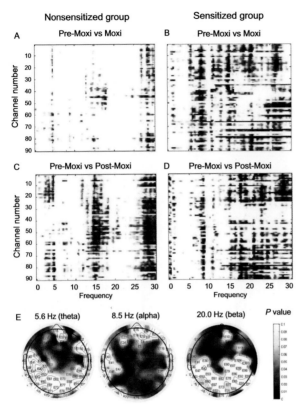

Nonsensitized group   Sensitized group

A   Pre-Moxi vs Moxi   B   Pre-Moxi vs Moxi

C   Pre-Moxi vs Post-Moxi   D   Pre-Moxi vs Post-Moxi

E   5.6 Hz (theta)   8.5 Hz (alpha)   20.0 Hz (beta)   P value

Figure 3 Statistical comparison of PSDs at each frequency points. Shown were the P values from Wilcoxon tests between pre-Moxi and Moxi sessions of nonsensitized (A) and sensitized (B) groups, and those between pre-Moxi and post-Moxi sessions of nonsensitized (C) and sensitized (D) groups. (E) The scalp topographies of PSD differences between pre-Moxi and Moxi sessions at 5.6 Hz (theta, left), 8.5 Hz (alpha, middle), and 20.0 Hz (beta, right) of the sensitized group. Changes at the theta and beta ranges were most obvious in the frontal–central regions, whereas changes at the alpha1 range were more global. No changes were detected in the nonsensitized group.

the occurrence of heat-sensitization is the state of the subject. Heat-sensitization could be induced in no more than 30% of healthy volunteers, but 50–70% under morbid states [1]. In the present study, heat-sensitization at DU3 appeared in 12 out of 25 CLBP patients. However, it is needed to note that failure to induce heat-sensitization at DU3 did not exclude the presence of such responses in other regions of the body. So the grouping in the present study only served for EEG characterization of heat-sensitization but could not reflect the presence or absence of such responses in each patient *per se*. It is still unclear why this phenomenon occurs in some patients but not others. Clinical data from the present study did not support gender, age, and pain duration as crucial factors, consistent with results from our previous studies [2–6].

It is interesting to compare current findings from moxibustion with those on acupuncture, which had been more intensively studied for years. Previous neuroimaging studies have shown that deqi sensation of acupuncture is associated with the deactivation of a limbic–paralimbic–neocortical network and activation of somatosensory brain regions [13]. Data from EEG recording during acupuncture were not consistent across studies due to different experimental designs and stimulating protocols, but all revealed widespread electrophysiological changes [14–20]. Sakai et al. [14] showed that acupuncture nonspecifically increased power of all spectral bands except the gamma band. Zhang et al. [15] and Tanaka et al. [16] reported similar results and further showed that these electrophysiological changes were correlated with analgesic effects. These results were comparable with our data from moxibustion, indicating some overlapping mechanisms under both situations, for example, widespread cortical and subcortical interactions. But they bear significant differences as well. The deqi response in acupuncture includes a variety of sensations such as aching, pressure, soreness, heaviness, fullness, warmth, cooling,

1276

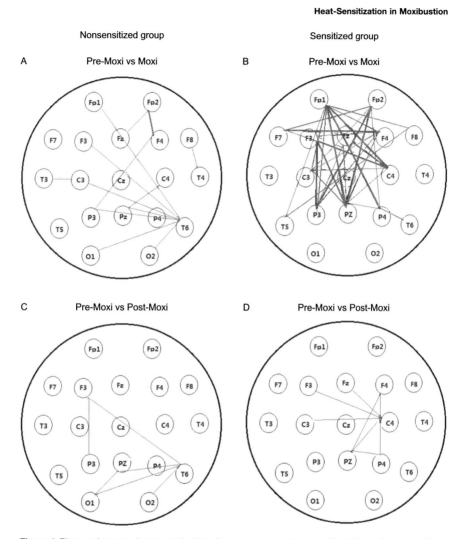

Heat-Sensitization in Moxibustion

Figure 4 Phase coherence changes at the theta frequency range of nonsensitized (A and C) and sensitized (B and D) groups. Significant changes were observed in the sensitized group between pre-Moxi and Moxi sessions (B). Blue lines indicated coherence decrease and red indicated increase. Line thickness indicated the level of statistical significance (thin lines: $P < 0.05$; thick lines: $P < 0.01$; paired t tests).

1277

Liao et al.

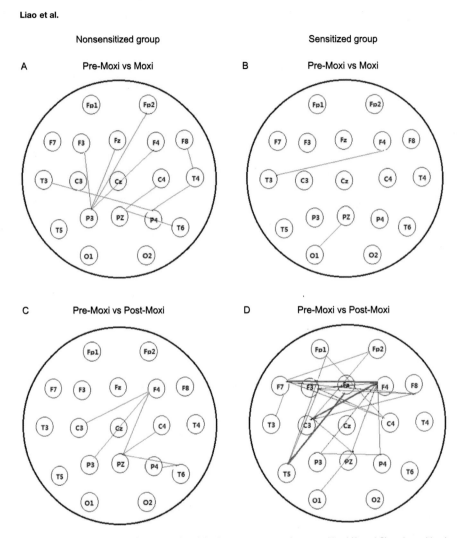

Figure 5 Phase coherence changes at the alpha frequency range of nonsensitized (A and C) and sensitized (B and D) groups. Blue lines indicated coherence decrease and red indicated increase. Line thickness indicated the level of statistical significance (thin lines: $P < 0.05$; thick lines: $P < 0.01$; paired t tests).

numbness, tingling, and dull pain [13], and is not disease specific. In contrast, the heat-sensitization in moxibustion is not commonly observed in healthy subjects and is mainly composed of strong warmth or heat spreading around the stimulating site or penetrating into the body [1]. The clear difference in induction (mechanical vs thermal stimulation) and sensory modalities implies distinct nature between them.

1278

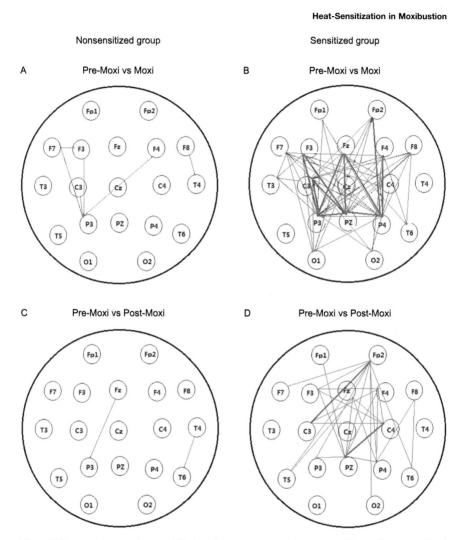

Figure 6 Phase coherence changes at the beta frequency range of nonsensitized (A and C) and sensitized (B and D) groups. Significant changes were observed in the sensitized group between pre-Moxi and Moxi sessions (B) and between pre-Moxi and post-Moxi sessions (D). Blue lines indicated coherence decrease and red indicated increase. Line thickness indicated the level of statistical significance (thin lines: $P < 0.05$; thick lines: $P < 0.01$; paired t tests).

Liao et al.

What are the mechanisms of heat-sensitization? Most of the sensitized points sit around the pathological regions, but they can be detected at distant locations as well. So local, spinal, and supra-spinal mechanisms may all contribute. Furthermore, the dynamically changed sites of sensitization with disease progression do not support a pure structural explanation. Functional mechanisms such as peripheral or central sensitization may be involved. A number of pain conditions, such as myofascial pain syndrome, are characterized by the presence of "trigger points," points tender to applied stimuli. These trigger points share many similarities with heat-sensitized sites, suggesting some common pathophysiological basis [21]. It is known that moxibustion promotes the local release of neuropeptides such as substance P and calcitonin gene-related peptide [22,23]. Heat shock proteins are also induced in the local areas [24]. In the central nervous system, moxibustion modulates dopaminergic and serotonergic metabolism in reward-related regions [25,26]. This is consistent with our clinical observation that heat-sensitization during moxibustion is frequently accompanied with pleasant feelings [1].

A crucial clinically relevant question is the behavioral correlates of heat-sensitization and/or the corresponding EEG changes. Previous clinical trials indicated that the presence of heat-sensitization during moxibustion treatment is correlated with better therapeutic effects, not only in low back pain [2–4] but also in other diseases such as knee osteoarthritis [5,6] and persistent asthma [7]. Although increasing evidence confirms the therapeutic effects of moxibustion, very few studies have addressed the underlying mechanisms. This was not the aim of the present study, but it was rational to hypothesize that the significant EEG changes accompanying heat-sensitization reflected pain and inflammatory modulation. Pain itself significantly affects central neuroplasticity and EEG [12,15,20,27,28], and as discussed earlier, analgesic manipulations such as acupuncture induce widespread EEG changes. The increases of the PSDs of theta, alpha, and beta bands in patients with heat-sensitization were most obvious in the frontal–central regions. These areas include a number of pain-related cortices, including pre-frontal cortex and anterior cingulate cortex (ACC). ACC has been shown crucial for at least some types of acupuncture [29]. Considering the presence of pleasant feelings during heat-sensitization, cognitive and affective modulation would be one rational mechanism of moxibustion analgesia.

In conclusion, our pilot EEG data provided the first objective evidence of heat-sensitization responses during suspended moxibustion, which were accompanied with widespread oscillatory changes in scalp EEG. Further investigation is required to elucidate its behavioral correlates and the underlying mechanisms.

Acknowledgments

This work was supported by the Major State Basic Research Development Program of People's Republic of China (2009CB522902) and the National Natural Science Foundation of China (81160453) to Rixin Chen, and the National Natural Science Foundation of China (31200835) to Ming Yi. The funders had no role in study design, data collection and analysis, decision to publish, or preparation of the manuscript.

References

1 Xie D, Liu Z, Hou X, et al. Heat-sensitization in suspended moxibustion: Features and clinical relevance. Acupunct Med 2013;31(4):422–4.

2 Chen R, Chen M, Xiong J, et al. Influence of the deqi sensation by suspended moxibustion stimulation in lumbar disc herniation: Study for a multicenter prospective two arms cohort study. Evid Based Complement Alternat Med 2013;2013:718593.

3 Chen R, Xiong J, Chi Z, Zhang B. Heat-sensitive moxibustion for lumbar disc herniation: A meta-analysis of randomized controlled trials. J Tradit Chin Med 2012;32:322–8.

4 Chen M, Chen R, Xiong J, et al. Evaluation of different moxibustion doses for lumbar disc herniation: Multicentre randomised controlled trial of heat-sensitive moxibustion therapy. Acupunct Med 2012;30:266–72.

5 Chen R, Chen M, Xiong J, et al. Comparative effectiveness of the deqi sensation and non-deqi by moxibustion stimulation: A multicenter prospective cohort study in the treatment of knee osteoarthritis. Evid Based Complement Alternat Med 2013;2013: 906947.

6 Chen R, Chen M, Xiong J, et al. Is there difference between the effects of two-dose stimulation for knee osteoarthritis in the treatment of heat-sensitive moxibustion? Evid Based Complement Alternat Med 2012;2012:696498.

7 Chen R, Chen M, Xiong J, et al. Curative effect of heat-sensitive moxibustion on chronic persistent asthma: A multicenter randomized controlled trial. J Tradit Chin Med 2013;33(5):584–91.

8 Klimesch W. EEG alpha and theta oscillations reflect cognitive and memory performance: A review and analysis. Brain Res Rev 1999;29:169–95.

9 von Stein A, Sarnthein J. Different frequencies for different scales of cortical integration: From local gamma to long range alpha/theta synchronization. Int J Psychophysiol 2000;38:301–13.

10 Fries P. A mechanism for cognitive dynamics: Neuronal communication through neuronal coherence. Trends Cogn Sci 2005;9:474–80.

11 Deyo RA, Weinstein JN. Low back pain. New Engl J Med 2001;344:363–70.

1280

12 Schmidt S, Naranjo JR, Brenneisen C, et al. Pain ratings, psychological functioning and quantitative EEG in a controlled study of chronic back pain patients. PLoS ONE 2012;7:e31138.

13 Hui KK, Marina O, Liu J, et al. Acupuncture, the limbic system, and the anticorrelated networks of the brain. Auton Neurosci 2010;157:81–90.

14 Sakai S, Hori E, Umeno K, et al. Specific acupuncture sensation correlates with EEGs and autonomic changes in human subjects. Auton Neurosci 2007;133:158–69.

15 Zhang W, Luo F, Qi Y, et al. Modulation of pain signal processing by electric acupoint stimulation: An electroencephalogram study. Beijing Da Xue Xue Bao 2003;35:236–40.

16 Tanaka Y, Koyama Y, Jodo E, et al. Effects of acupuncture to the sacral segment on the bladder activity and electroencephalogram. Psychiatry Clin Neurosci 2002;56:249–50.

17 Chen AC, Liu FJ, Wang L, Arendt-Nielsen L. Mode and site of acupuncture modulation in the human brain: 3D (124-ch) EEG power spectrum mapping and source imaging. Neuroimage 2006;29:1080–91.

18 Hori E, Takamoto K, Urakawa S, et al. Effects of acupuncture on the brain hemodynamics. Auton Neurosci 2010;157:74–80.

19 Streitberger K, Steppan J, Maier C, et al. Effects of verum acupuncture compared to placebo acupuncture on quantitative EEG and heart rate variability in healthy volunteers. J Altern Complement Med 2008;14:505–13.

20 Wang J, Li D, Li X, et al. Phase-amplitude coupling between θ and γ oscillations during nociception in rat electroencephalography. Neurosci Lett 2011;499: 84–7.

21 Melzack R, Stillwell DM, Fox EJ. Trigger points and acupuncture points for pain: Correlations and implications. Pain 1977;3:3–23.

22 Kashiba H, Nishigori A, Ueda Y. Expression of galanin in rat primary sensory afferents after moxibustion to the skin. Am J Chin Med 1992;20:103–14.

23 Nakanishi H. Moxibustion modulates SP and c-fos-immunoreactivity of mouse spinal neurons by peripheral noxious stimuli. Acta Med Kinki Univ 2000;25:7–20.

24 Kobayashi K. Induction of heat-shock protein (hsp) by moxibustion. Am J Chin Med 1995;23:327–30.

25 Fukuda F, Shinbara H, Yoshimoto K, et al. Effect of moxibustion on dopaminergic and serotonergic systems of rat nucleus accumbens. Neurochem Res 2005;30:1607–13.

26 Yano T, Kato B, Fukuda F, et al. Alterations in the function of cerebral dopaminergic and serotonergic systems following electroacupuncture and moxibustion applications: Possible correlates with their antistress and psychosomatic actions. Neurochem Res 2004;29:283–93.

27 Stern J, Jeanmonod D, Sarnthein J. Persistent EEG overactivation in the cortical pain matrix of neurogenic pain patients. Neuroimage 2006;31:721–31.

28 Yi M, Zhang H. Nociceptive memory in the brain: Cortical mechanisms of chronic pain. J Neurosci 2011;31:13343–5.

29 Yi M, Zhang H, Lao L, et al. Anterior cingulate cortex is crucial for contra- but not ipsi-lateral electro-acupuncture in the formalin-induced inflammatory pain model of rats. Mol Pain 2011;7:61.

Supporting information

Additional Supporting Information may be found in the online version of this article at the publisher's Website:

Figure S1 Suspended moxibustion was performed with burning *moxa* sticks suspended above the body. The exact distance was adjusted to reach a skin surface temperature of around 41°C.

Figure S2 Scalp localization of 90 out of 128 EEG channels included in data analysis.

1281

Original paper

Heat-sensitive moxibustion in patients with osteoarthritis of the knee: a three-armed multicentre randomised active control trial

Rixin Chen,[1] Mingren Chen,[1] Tongsheng Su,[2] Meiqi Zhou,[3] Jianhua Sun,[4] Jun Xiong,[1] Zhenhai Chi,[1] Dingyi Xie,[1] Bo Zhang[1]

For numbered affiliations see end of article.

Correspondence to Professor Rixin Chen, The Affiliated Hospital with Jiangxi University of TCM, No 445 Bayi Avenue, Nanchang City 330006, People's Republic of China; chenrixin321@163.com

RC and MC contributed equally.

Accepted 25 April 2015

ABSTRACT

Background In China, heat-sensitive moxibustion (HSM) is used for knee osteoarthritis (KOA) to reduce pain and improve physical activity. However, there is little high-quality evidence of its effectiveness.

Objective To evaluate the effectiveness of HSM in the treatment of KOA compared with usual care.

Methods We performed a multicentre, randomised controlled trial. In total, 432 patients with KOA were randomly assigned to one of three groups (HSM, conventional moxibustion, or conventional injection with sodium hyaluronate). The primary end point was the guiding principle of clinical research on new drugs in the treatment of KOA (GPCRND-KOA). Measurements were obtained at baseline and after 1 and 6 months (month 7) of study.

Result For GPCRND-KOA, there were significant differences among the three groups after treatment at months 1 and 7. Pairwise comparisons showed that HSM was more effective than the conventional drug. There was no difference in any measures between conventional moxibustion and the conventional drug. Compared with conventional moxibustion, HSM resulted in greater improvement in all outcomes.

Conclusions This trial provided some evidence of the superiority of HSM in patients with KOA, suggesting that the observed differences might be due to superiority effects of a heat-sensitive point, although the effect of expectation cannot be ruled out.

Trial registration number The trial was registered at Controlled Clinical Trials: ChiCTR-TRC-09000600.

BACKGROUND

Knee osteoarthritis (KOA) is a common and disabling health problem in the elderly and significantly affects the lives of many.[1 2] Management of KOA is primarily aimed at pain relief and functional recovery.[3] Although pharmacological treatments are widely used, they are associated with adverse events, such as gastrointestinal irritation and bleeding, perforating ulcers and renal and hepatic toxicity.[4] Therefore, patients are recommended to follow non-pharmacological treatments in China, including complementary and alternative medicines, such as acupuncture and moxibustion.

Moxibustion has been studied sufficiently to demonstrate that it does have benefits for KOA.[5 6] One recent systematic review evaluated moxibustion for osteoarthritis and included six randomised controlled trials (RCTs) for KOA; meta-analysis showed favourable effects of moxibustion on the response rate.[7] An experimental study found that indirect moxibustion could relieve pain in an experimental rat model of KOA and suggested the existence of sustained inhibitory modulation by endogenous opioids.[8]

Heat-sensitive moxibustion (HSM) is a form of treatment for pain and dysfunction associated with musculoskeletal conditions in China that involves administering suspended moxibustion at heat-sensitive acupuncture points.[9 10] It has been used for various diseases, such as KOA, lumbar disc herniation and fibromyalgia syndrome. It originated from the observation that suspended moxibustion at certain body locations elicited heat sensitisation.[11–13] Patients appear to become thermally sensitised to moxibustion stimulation at certain locations, as indicated by sensations of strong warmth or heat penetrating into the body (heat penetration), warmth spreading

To cite: Chen R, Chen M, Su T, et al. Acupunct Med Published Online First: [please include Day Month Year] doi:10.1136/acupmed-2014-010740

1

around the stimulation site (heat expansion), or warmth conducted in certain directions and reaching some body regions or even internal organs remote from the stimulation sites (heat transmission).[13] These heat-sensitised locations are not fixed, but may, during the progression of disease, change within a certain range, centred on acupuncture points. However, conventional moxibustion is applied at fixed acupuncture points. From our empirical evidence we formulated the following hypothesis: moxibustion at heat-sensitive acupuncture points has better efficacy than that at fixed acupuncture points.[12 13]

Some small sample studies have evaluated the effect of HSM. For example, Kang *et al*[14] treated 40 patients with KOA by suspended moxibustion. The HSM group showed a higher recovery rate than the conventional moxibustion group (n=80) (80.95% vs 21.05%, respectively).[14] Xie *et al*[15] observed that HSM treatment reduced joint pain and improved functional disability, compared with the conventional moxibustion (n=120). However, these studies do not provide conclusive evidence of the effect of HSM, as the RCTs were limited by methodological defects, including small sample size, variability of control group, poor clinical practice and missing information. We therefore carried out a rigorous multicentre RCT with a large sample size, with the aim of assessing the effectiveness of HSM for treating KOA compared with conventional moxibustion or conventional drug.

METHODS
Design
We performed a multicentre (four centres in China), randomised, active controlled trial. Our trial was carried out in four hospitals, including the Affiliated Hospital of Jiangxi University of Traditional Chinese Medicine (TCM) in Nanchang, the first Affiliated Hospital of Anhui University of TCM in Hefei, Jiangsu TCM Hospital in Nanjing and Shanxi TCM Hospital in Xian. Patients were gathered through hospital-based recruitment and newspaper advertisements. Eligible participants were randomly allocated into one of three groups (the HSM group, the conventional moxibustion group, or the conventional drug treatment group) with a 1:1:1 allocation ratio by the central randomisation system (figure 1). This system was provided by the China Academy of Chinese Medical Sciences, using computer telephone integration technology to integrate computer, internet and telecom. The random number list was assigned by interactive voice response and interactive web response.[16] The evaluation of participants and the analysis of results were performed by professionals blinded to the group allocation.

Sample size
We calculated the sample size according to our previous pilot study. A two-sided 5% significance level and 95% power were considered to detect an effective rate difference (70% for HSM and 50% in the other groups). It was calculated that about 120 participants in each group were required. Assuming a dropout rate of 20%, the sample size would be 144 for each group (total n=432).

Participants
Recruitment
Patients were recruited in China between 30 December 2011 and 30 January 2013. Written consent was obtained from each participant before the start of this trial. We obtained oral and written consent from each participant before collecting information at the first visit.

Inclusion criteria
We included participants who met the following criteria: diagnosed with idiopathic KOA according to the guiding principle of clinical research on new drugs (GPCRND-KOA),[17] with a score of more than five points; moderate to severe swelling KOA; aged 38–70 years and of either sex. Additionally, according to the KOA diagnosis standard, knee joints appeared swollen; a floating patella test was negative; patients accepted the treatment protocol in this trial; and acupuncture point heat-sensitisation phenomenon was present in the region bounded by SP9 (*Yinlingquan*), GB34 (*Yanglingquan*), ST34 (*Liangqiu*) and SP10 (*Xuehai*).

The patients were instructed not to take any regular drugs before and during the treatment periods and were provided with the usual care instructions and rescue medication for KOA.

Exclusion criteria
Participants were excluded if they were experiencing or had a history of the following: serious life-threatening disease, such as heart disease or disease of brain blood vessels, liver, kidney and haematopoietic system, or if they were psychotic; diabetes, diabetic polyneuropathy and polyneuropathic disturbances; were pregnant or in the lactation period. The following conditions also led to exclusion: acute knee joint trauma or ulceration of local skin; complications of serious genu varus/valgus and flexion contraction.

Study interventions
The treatments, which included moxibustion treatments, were provided by specialised acupuncturists who had at least 5 years' training and 5 years' experience using a standardised protocol. All treatment regimens and outcome assessment methods were standardised between the four centres and basic information about this study and the monitoring process was disseminated through workshops before the start of the study. All the patients were asked not to use any additional treatments such as physiotherapy or regular pain-killing drugs.

Chen R, *et al. Acupunct Med* 2015;**0**:1–8. doi:10.1136/acupmed-2014-010740

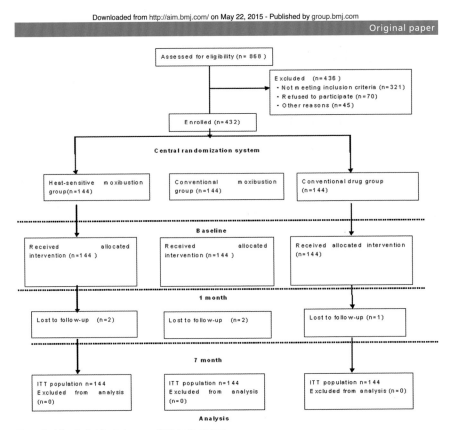

Figure 1   A flowchart of the study process. ITT, intention to treat.

In the two moxibustion groups, a moxa stick (diameter 22 mm, length 120 mm) was applied (produced by Jiangxi provincial TCM Hospital, China). The patients usually lay down in a comfortable supine position for treatment, with 24–30°C temperature in the room. Patients were asked to wear loose trousers, to allow the knees to be exposed.

HSM group

For the HSM group, the moxa sticks were lit by the therapist and held over the rectangle bounded by SP9, GB34, ST34 and SP10 to identify any heat sensitisation phenomenon present. The smouldering moxibustion stick was suspended about 3 cm over the skin to search for the acupuncture point heat-sensitisation phenomenon (box 1). When an acupuncture point showed at least one sensation listed in box 1, the therapists marked the point as a heat-sensitive point. We attempted to identify all sensitive points in each patient by repeated testing.

The therapists then began treatment, starting with the most heat-sensitive point. Treatment sessions ended when patients felt that the acupuncture point

---

Box 1   Heat-sensitisation phenomenon at acupuncture points

Heat penetration
Heat penetrating from the skin into subcutaneous tissues.
Heat expansion
Heat expanding away from the stimulation site to surrounding cutaneous and subcutaneous tissues.
Heat transmission
Perceiving a stream of heat conducted in certain directions, or perceiving heat in some body regions or in the joint cavity.
Non-thermal sensations
Instead of thermal sensations, some patients perceiving aching, heaviness, pain, numbness, pressure, or cold in local or distant locations of stimulation.

Chen R, *et al. Acupunct Med* 2015;**0**:1–8. doi:10.1136/acupmed-2014-010740

3

heat-sensitisation phenomenon had disappeared, usually after 30–60 min. Patients received the treatment twice a day in the first week (5 days a week) and once a day from the second week to sixth week (a total of 35 sessions over 30 days).

Conventional moxibustion group

A licensed doctor performed moxibustion at three acupuncture points around the affected knee—EX-LE5 (*Xiyan*, two points) and EX-LE2 (*Heding*)—for a total of 35 sessions for 30 days throughout the trial. Most procedures were similar to those used in the first group, except that each point was treated for 15 min at a time, according to current practice.[18] The total time comprised 45 min for every treatment. In the treatment, patients usually felt local warmth without burning pain and might experience mild hyperaemia in the local region. The sensation of acupuncture point heat-sensitisation phenomenon was not pursued and not avoided in the treatment.

Conventional drug group

According to pragmatic design, the control group did not use a placebo procedure, but received sodium hyaluronate intra-articular injection as the conventional drug. Many studies have confirmed the efficacy and safety of intra-articular hyaluronan for KOA.[19] The injection was given every 6 days (2 mL) for a total of five times.

Outcome measures

The primary outcome with respect to the effectiveness on KOA was the mean change in the global scale score of the GPCRND-KOA scale from baseline to month 1 and month 7. The GPCRND-KOA scale is one of the most widely used instruments in China and composed of six items to assess disability related to osteoarthritis.[17] It is recommended by the Ministry of Health of the People's Republic of China. The scale assesses pain, the relation between activity and pain and functional impairment (table 1). This scoring system has been validated.[17] The severity of KOA was divided into three levels: mild <5; moderate 5–9; severe >9. The maximum possible score on GPCRND-KOA is 18.

For swelling of the knee, knee circumference was selected as a secondary outcome. The parameter was measured in centimetres across the middle of a patella, with an ordinary tape measure.[20]

The outcomes were measured at baseline, 1 month and 7 months in all participants. All outcomes were collected by a patient self-report questionnaire and mailed back to the investigators. Age, gender, weight, duration and nature (unilateral/bilateral) of knee symptoms and previous treatment for knee joint problems were obtained by the questionnaire at baseline for descriptive purposes.

We defined adverse events as unfavourable or unintended signs and symptoms or disease presenting after

Table 1 List of items in the guiding principle of clinical research on new drugs in the treatment of knee osteoarthritis (GPCRND-KOA)

Item	Grade/classification	Score
Pain or discomfort in night when lying in bed	No	0
	Pain in activity or some position	1
	Pain in non-activity	2
Morning stiffness or pain worse when getting out of bed	No	0
	<30 min	1
	≥30 min	2
Pain or discomfort in walking	No	0
	After walking in some distance	1
	Pain at beginning of walk or worse	2
Arise from seat	Independent	0
	Need assistance	1
Maximum walking distance (accompanied by pain)	Unrestricted	0
	Restricted	
	>1 km	1
	300 m–1 km	2
	<300 m	3
Daily activities	Climbing standard stairs	
	Independent	0
	Difficulty	1
	Unable	2
	Descending standard stairs	
	Independent	0
	Difficulty	1
	Unable	2
	Squat or bend knees	
	Independent	0
	Difficulty	1
	Unable	2
	Walk over rough terrain	
	Independent	0
	Difficulty	1
	Unable	2

treatment, even if not necessarily related to the moxibustion intervention.

Statistical methods

All statistical analyses were performed using SAS V.9.1.3 (SAS Institute, Cary, North Carolina, USA). A significance level of 5% was used in all analyses. For baseline characteristics, continuous data were represented by the mean, SD, minimum value and maximum value, whereas categorical data were represented by a frequency table. Results were presented as mean or proportion with SD and/or 95% CI.

4

To compare the results among the groups, an analysis of variance test was used when the data were normally distributed; the Kruskal–Wallis test was used otherwise. The χ^2 test was used for categorical data. If any imbalances in baseline characteristics between groups were found, we conducted an analysis of covariance using these imbalanced variables as covariates and allocated group as the fixed factor. If a significant difference was identified among the three groups, then multiple comparisons were conducted to determine which groups were different. A Student–Newman–Keuls test was used for pairwise comparison. Reasons for dropout or missing data were explored descriptively. Multiple imputation was used to ensure that dropouts did not affect the conclusions.

All adverse reactions reported were listed with detailed explanations. The frequencies of abnormal reactions correlated and not correlated with the treatment were recorded. A Fisher exact test was performed to determine whether there were any differences among the groups with respect to the incidence of abnormal reactions as reported by the subjects.

Participant protections and ethics

The protocol was established according to general ethical guidelines including the Declaration of Helsinki and China Good Clinical Practice and was approved by the ethics committee of the Affiliated Hospital of Jiangxi Institute of TCM: registration number 2008(9).

RESULTS

Population and baseline

After screening 868 patients, 432 were randomly assigned to treatment (figure 1). After 7 months, five patients had dropped out and were not contactable. Participants had a mean age of 54 years and 62.0% were male. Table 2 presents the baseline characteristics of the patients with KOA. Participants had been diagnosed with KOA for an average of 4.6 years. More than half (54.6%) were taking a pharmaceutical agent, about one tenth were using physiotherapy and 12% were using various acupuncture and moxibustion treatments. The mean GPCRND-KOA score was 11.4; 78.8% of the sample scored ≥11, suggesting a history of pharmacotherapy failure. The baseline parameters did not differ significantly among the groups (table 1). There was no difference in attrition rate among the groups at 6 months' follow-up (month 7, p>0.05, Fisher exact test).

Outcome measures

Total GPCRND-KOA score

Table 3 presents a comparison of GPCRND-KOA scores. The total score for each group decreased significantly during the 1-month trial and the 6-month follow-up visit (p<0.01). An analysis of covariance showed a significant difference in the three groups at both time points. Mixed-effects model analysis (q test) showed that subjects in the HSM group had significantly greater reduction in GPCRND-KOA scores

Table 2 Baseline characteristics of participants

Characteristics	Heat-sensitive moxibustion group (n=144)	Conventional moxibustion group (n=144)	Conventional drug group (n=144)
Age (years), mean (SD)	55 (5.1)	53 (5.2)	56 (5.0)
Age (years), min–max	41–70	40–70	42–66
Age >60 years, n (%)	19 (3.2)	20 (13.8)	18 (12.5)
Sex, n (%)			
Female	56 (38.9)	53 (36.8)	57 (39.6)
Male	88 (61.1)	91 (63.2)	87 (60.4)
Duration of knee pain, n (%)			
<5 Years	78 (54.2)	75 (52.1)	73 (50.7)
5–10 Years	39 (27.1)	46 (31.9)	40 (35.1)
>10 Years	27 (18.8)	23 (15.0)	31 (21.5)
BMI (kg/m^2), mean (SD)	22.1 (2.1)	23.2 (2.2)	23.1 (2.3)
BMI (kg/m^2), min–max	15.4–30.2	16.2–31.1	13.4–33.1
GPCRND-KOA grade, n (%)			
Severe	85 (59.0)	88 (61.1)	82 (56.9)
Moderate	59 (40.1)	56 (38.9)	62 (43.1)
Knee circumference (cm), mean (SD)	41.2 (3.2)	42.2 (3.2)	41.3 (2.7)
GPCRND-KOA score, mean (SD)	11.2 (3.3)	11.3 (3.2)	12.1 (2.9)
Previous treatment (past half year), n (%)			
Pharmaceutical intervention	76 (52.8)	81 (56.3)	79 (54.9)
Physiotherapy	12 (8.3)	16 (11.1)	13 (9.0)
Previous acupuncture treatment	18 (12.5)	16 (11.1)	16 (11.1)

BMI, body mass index; GPCRND-KOA, guiding principle of clinical research on new drugs in the treatment of knee osteoarthritis score .

Chen R, et al. Acupunct Med 2015;0:1–8. doi:10.1136/acupmed-2014-010740

5

Table 3 Comparison of GPCRND-KOA scores*

Variable	Month 1		Month 7	
	Mean (SD)	95% CI	Mean (SD)	95% CI
Heat-sensitive moxibustion group (n=144)	2.8 (1.8)	2.6 to 3.0	3.6 (1.6)	3.3 to 3.9
Conventional moxibustion group (n=144)	4.9 (2.8)	4.4 to 5.3	6.4 (1.5)	6.2 to 6.6
Conventional drug group (n=144)	5.6 (2.1)	5.4 to 5.9	7.0 (1.9)	6.6 to 7.3
Comparison of the three groups				
F Value	3.6		4.2	
p Value	0.031		0.020	
Heat-sensitive moxibustion group versus conventional moxibustion group				
q Value	3.8		5.9	
p Value	0.035		0.023	
Heat-sensitive moxibustion group versus conventional drug group				
q Value	6.2		8.2	
p Value	0.011		0.0096	
Conventional moxibustion group versus conventional drug group				
q value	2.1		2.7	
p Value	0.130		0.091	

*Comparison of the three groups by analysis of covariance. Pairwise comparison for the two groups by Student–Newman–Keuls (q test). All data are based on an intention to treat.
GPCRND-KOA, guiding principle of clinical research on new drugs in the treatment of knee osteoarthritis score.

than those in conventional moxibustion group or conventional drug group at 1 and 7 months; however, there were no significant differences between the conventional moxibustion and conventional drug groups at either time point.

Knee circumference
In comparison with baseline, significant reductions in each group were seen at months 1 and 7 ($p<0.05$). Significant differences between the three groups are shown in table 4. A comparison of the scores between the HSM and conventional moxibustion groups was significant at both time points. Significant differences between the HSM group and the conventional drug group were also evident; however, there was no significant difference between the conventional moxibustion and conventional drug groups at both time points.

Moxibustion in the HSM group
The mean number of heat-sensitive points located in the group was 2.1 ± 0.52. The range of moxibustion

Table 4 Comparison of knee circumference*

Variable	Month 1		Month 7	
	Mean (SD)	95% CI	Mean (SD)	95% CI
Heat-sensitive moxibustion group (n=144)	36.8 (2.7)	36.3 to 37.2	35.7 (1.8)	35.4 to 35.9
Conventional moxibustion group (n=144)	38.3 (2.6)	37.8 to 38.7	37.4 (1.6)	37.1 to 37.7
Conventional drug group (n=144)	38.6 (2.2)	38.2 to 38.9	37.2 (1.4)	36.9 to 37.4
Comparison of the three groups				
F Value	3.1		3.3	
p Value	0.042		0.039	
Heat-sensitive moxibustion group versus conventional moxibustion group				
q Value	3.4		3.8	
p Value	0.035		0.028	
Heat-sensitive moxibustion group versus conventional drug group				
q Value	3.6		3.7	
p Value	0.031		0.029	
Conventional moxibustion group versus conventional drug group				
q Value	1.8		2.1	
p Value	0.141		0.187	

*Comparison of the three groups by analysis of covariance. Pairwise comparison for the two groups by Student–Newman–Keuls (q test). All data are based on an intention to treat.

Chen R, *et al. Acupunct Med* 2015;**0**:1–8. doi:10.1136/acupmed-2014-010740

time was 27–63 min, with mean of 46±5.2 min, in the HSM group. We used linear correlation to measure the strength of a relationship between change in GPCRND-KOA score and stimulation duration in the HSM group. The Pearson coefficient was r=0.0011, showing no significant correlation between the two values.

Safety
No adverse events were reported in the 432 participants.

DISCUSSION
This multicentre RCT, comparing HSM, conventional moxibustion and conventional drug treatment, showed a statistically significantly greater improvement in GPCRND-KOA score and knee circumference in the HSM group at both 1 and 7 months. We found no relevant differences between the conventional moxibustion and conventional drug treatment groups. Therefore, HSM treatment in this study had the most significant impact on KOA symptoms and functional disorder.

This trial used random sequence generation and allocation concealment using the central randomisation system, to overcome limitations of previous trials.[7 21–25] Concealment is the most critical factor of the allocation process and a high risk of bias is generated by unconcealed allocation. Therefore, to the best of our knowledge, our study is the largest reported RCT comparing effectiveness of HSM and conventional moxibustion groups in the treatment of patients with KOA. The statistical analysis was carried out in a blind fashion.

One limitation of this study is the possibility of a high risk of bias from lack of blinding because we used usual care as a control instead of a sham procedure. In view of the special nature of KOA, an active control had to be used to help the patient's condition. Also, owing to the nature of the intervention, it was not possible to blind acupuncturists to treatment. A sham device is difficult to use because of the high prevalence of moxibustion use in China. Additionally, it is more appropriate to use a pragmatic design to answer our research question, which is whether HSM treatment is effective in treating KOA in real practice.

The evidence from our previous research indicated that three essential elements influence the therapeutic effect of moxibustion: location, dose and sensation.[26] HSM differs from conventional moxibustion in all three aspects. First, HSM treats diseases at heat-sensitive acupuncture points. The sensitised locations are not always anatomical acupuncture points, but may change within a certain range centred on fixed acupuncture points during the progression of disease. Each disease has a specific set of such sensitised acupuncture points. However, conventional moxibustion, which applies stimulation at fixed acupuncture points, has some therapeutic effects. A number of clinical trials have shown that selecting the heat-sensitive acupuncture points might produce a better therapeutic effect than moxibustion at fixed acupuncture points.[27 28] Second, patients feel local warmth and experience mild hyperaemia in the local region in conventional moxibustion. For HSM, this phenomenon resembles *de qi*, which appears after moxibustion, rather than local heat sensation and surface glow of the skin; *de qi* is essential to achieve the prospective therapeutic effects.[18] Third, our team's experimental evidence with HSM suggests that the most appropriate dose at each acupuncture point is the dose that causes the heat-sensitisation phenomenon to disappear. This dose varies depending on the person and disease. We called this the 'individualised sensitivity elimination dose'.[29] Meanwhile, conventional moxibustion uses a standardised dose, such as 15 min at each acupuncture point. Some studies have suggested that the effectiveness of the individualised sensitivity elimination dose is better than that of the standardised dose.[30] Our findings support the suggestion that HSM for about 46 min is better than conventional moxibustion for KOA. We note that HSM had an additional psychological impact, making the patients feel they were receiving more individualised attention, which might have influenced the improvement of KOA symptoms.

This study provides some evidence of the superiority of HSM over conventional moxibustion in patients with KOA. Further studies are needed to provide independent support for the intervention and to explore underlying mechanisms of moxibustion in patients with KOA, including the influence of expectation.

Summary points

▶ In heat-sensitive moxibustion, treatment is given only at locations that show increased sensitivity to the heat.
▶ We found that heat-sensitive moxibustion was more effective for knee osteoarthritis pain and disability than conventional moxibustion or hyaluronic acid injection, though patient expectation might have influenced this result.

Author affiliations
[1]The Affiliated Hospital with Jiangxi University of TCM, Nanchang, People's Republic of China
[2]Shanxi TCM Hospital, Xian, People's Republic of China
[3]The first Affiliated Hospital with Anhui University of TCM, Hefei, People's Republic of China
[4]Jiangsu TCM Hospital, Nanjing, People's Republic of China

Chen R, et al. Acupunct Med 2015;0:1–8. doi:10.1136/acupmed-2014-010740

7

Original paper

Acknowledgements This study was supported by the major state basic research development programme of the People's Republic of China (grant number 2015CB554503), the National Natural Science Foundation of China (grant number 81160453), the National Natural Science Foundation of China (grant number 81202854) and the Jiangxi key R&D project.

Contributors MC and RC obtained funding for the research project. JX wrote the final manuscript. RC, TS, JS, MZ, ZC, DX and BZ contributed to implementation of the trial. All authors read and approved the final manuscript.

Competing interests None declared.

Ethics approval The ethics committee of the Affiliated Hospital of Jiangxi Institute of Traditional Chinese Medicine approved this trial (code 2008(9)).

Provenance and peer review Not commissioned; externally peer reviewed.

REFERENCES

1　National Collaborating Centre for Chronic Condition. *Osteoarthritis: national clinical guideline for care and management in adults*. London: Royal College of Physicians, 2008.

2　Peat G, McCarney R, Croft P. Knee pain and osteoarthritis in older adults: a review of community burden and current use of primary health care. *Ann Rheum Dis* 2001;60:91–7.

3　Zhang W, Moskowitz RW, Nuki G, *et al*. OARSI recommendations for the management of hip and knee osteoarthritis. Part II: OARSI evidence-based, expert consensus guidelines. *Osteoarthritis Cartilage* 2008;16:137–62.

4　Towheed TE, Maxwell L, Judd MG, *et al*. Acetaminophen for osteoarthritis. *Cochrane Database Syst Rev* 2006;(1):CD004257.

5　Choi TY, Kim TH, Kang JW, *et al*. Moxibustion for rheumatic conditions: a systematic review and meta-analysis. *Clin Rheumatol* 2011;30:937–45.

6　Manheimer E, Cheng K, Linde K, *et al*. Acupuncture for peripheral joint osteoarthritis. *Cochrane Database Syst Rev* 2010;(1):CD001977.

7　Choi TY, Choi J, Kim KH, *et al*. Moxibustion for the treatment of osteoarthritis: a systematic review and meta-analysis. *Rheumatol Int* 2012;32:2969–78.

8　Uryu N, Okada K, Kawakita K. Analgesic effects of indirect moxibustion on an experimental rat model of osteoarthritis in the knee. *Acupunct Med* 2007;25:175–83.

9　Chen R, Kang M. *Acupuncture point heat-sensitive moxibustion and new therapy*. 1st edn. Beijing, China: Press by People's Medical Publishing House, 2006 [Chinese].

10　Chen R, Chen M, Kang M. *A practical book of heat-sensitive moxibustion*. 1st edn. Beijing, China: Press by People's Medical Publishing House, 2009 [Chinese].

11　Chen M, Kang M. Clinical application of acupoint heat-sensitization. *Zhongguo Zhen* 2007;27:199–202 [Chinese].

12　Chen R, Kang M. Key point of moxibustion, arrival of qi produces curative effect. *Zhongguo Zhen Jiu* 2008;28:44–6 [Chinese].

13　Xie D, Liu Z, Hou X, *et al*. Heat sensitization in suspended moxibustion: features and clinical relevance. *Acupunct Med* 2013;31:422–4.

14　Kang M, Chen R, Fu Y. Observation on curative effect of moxibustion on heat-sensitive points on knee osteoarthritis. *Jiangxi J Tradit Chin Med Pharm* 2006;18:27–8 [Chinese].

15　Xie HW, Chen RX, Xu FM, *et al*. Comparative study of heat-sensitive moxibustion in the treatment of knee osteoarthritis. *Zhongguo Zhen Jiu* 2012;32:229–32 [Chinese].

16　Liu B, Wen T, Yao C, *et al*. The central randomization system in multi-center clinical trials. *Chin J New Drugs Clin Rem* 2006;12:931–5 [Chinese].

17　Zhen XY. *The guideline of the latest Chinese herbs to clinical research*. 1st edn. Beijing: Medicine Science and Technology Press of China, 2002 [Chinese].

18　Park JE, Ryu YH, Liu Y, *et al*. A literature review of de qi in clinical studies. *Acupunct Med* 2013;31:132–42.

19　Hamburger MI, Lakhanpal S, Mooar PA, *et al*. Intra-articular hyaluronans: a review of product-specific safety profiles. *Semin Arthritis Rheum* 2003;32:296–309.

20　Nicholas JJ, Taylor FH, Buckingham RB, *et al*. Measurement of circumference of the knee with ordinary tape measure. *Ann Rheum Dis* 1976;35:282–4.

21　Zhang QJ, Cao L, Li Z, *et al* Clinical efficacy and safety obvervation of moxibustion and celecoxib in the treatment of knee osteoarthritis. *Chin J Traumatol* 2011;19:13–15 [Chinese].

22　Liu X, Wang P, Zhang C, *et al*. Clinical efficacy observation of moxibustion in the treatment of knee osteoarthritis. *Chin J Bone Joint Damage* 2009;24:1115–16 [Chinese].

23　Chen H. Clinical observation of foam moxibustion in the treatment of knee osteoarthritis. *Zhejiang TCM J* 2013;48:522–3 [Chinese].

24　Xu M. Clinical efficacy observation of moxibustion plus injection of medication in the treatment of knee osteoarthritis. *Shanghai J Acu-mox* 2011;30:318–9 [Chinese].

25　Wang B, Han JS. 30 cases observation of moxibustion plus TCM fomenting therapy in the treatment of knee osteoarthritis. *Chin Tradit Chin Med Sci Technol* 2012;19:175–6 [Chinese].

26　Chen R, Chen M, Kang M. *Heat-sensitive moxibustion therapy*. 1st edn. Beijing, China: Press by People's Medical Publishing House, 2012 [Chinese].

27　Tang FY, Huang CJ, Chen R, *et al*. Observation on therapeutic effect of moxibustion on temperature-sensitive points for lumbar disc herniation. *Zhongguo Zhen Jiu* 2009;29:382–4 [Chinese].

28　Zhang C, Xiao H, Chen R. Observation on curative effect of moxibustion on heat-sensitive points on pressure sores. *China J Tradit Chin Med Pharm* 2010;25:478–88 [Chinese].

29　Chen M, Chen R, Xiong J, *et al*. Evaluation of different moxibustion doses for lumbar disc herniation: multicentre randomized controlled trial of heat-sensitive moxibustion therapy. *Acupunct Med* 2012;30:266–72.

30　Chen R, Chen M, Xiong J, *et al*. Is there difference between the effects of two-dose stimulation for knee osteoarthritis in the treatment of heat-sensitive moxibustion? *Evid Based Complement Altern Med* 2012;12:1–7.

Chen R, *et al. Acupunct Med* 2015;**0**:1–8. doi:10.1136/acupmed-2014-010740

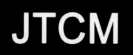

Journal of Traditional Chinese Medicine

Online Submissions:http://www.journaltcm.com
info@journaltcm.com

J Tradit Chin Med 2013 October 15; 33(5): 584-591
ISSN 0255-2922

CLINICAL STUDY

Curative effect of heat-sensitive moxibustion on chronic persistent asthma: a multicenter randomized controlled trial

Rixin Chen, Mingren Chen, Jun Xiong, Zhenhai Chi, Bo Zhang, Ning Tian, Zhenhua Xu, Tangfa Zhang, Wanyao Li, Wei Zhang, Xiaofeng Rong, Zhen Wang, Gang Sun, Baohe Ge, Guoxiong Yu, Nanchang Song

Rixin Chen, Mingren Chen, Jun Xiong, Zhenhai Chi, Bo Zhang, Department of Acupuncture and Rehabilitation, Hospital Affiliated to Jiangxi University of Traditional Chinese Medicine, Nanchang 330006, China
Ning Tian, Department of Rehabilitation, Guangdong Hospital of Combination of Traditional Chinese Medicine with Western Medicine, Foshan 528000, China
Zhenhua Xu, Department of Pneumology, Guangdong Hospital of Traditional Chinese Medicine, Guangzhou 519015, China
Tangfa Zhang, Department of Acupuncture, First Hospital of Wuhan, Wuhan 430032, China
Wanyao Li, Institute of Acupuncture and Massage, Guangzhou University of Traditional Chinese Medicine, Guangzhou 510405, China
Wei Zhang, Department of Pneumology, First Hospital Affiliated to Nanchang University, Nanchang 330006, China
Xiaofeng Rong, Department of Rehabilitation, First Hospital Affiliated to Chongqing Medical University, Chongqing 400016, China
Zhen Wang, Department of Acupuncture, First Hospital Affiliated to Zhejiang University of Traditional Chinese Medicine, Hangzhou 310018, China
Gang Sun, Department of Acupuncture, Suzhou Hospital of TCM, Suzhou 215003, China
Baohe Ge, Department of Acupuncture, Hospital Affiliated to Shandong University of Traditional Chinese Medicine, Jinan 250011, China
Guoxiong Yu, Department of Acupuncture, Guangdong Disabled Soldier Hospital, Guangzhou 510260, China
Nanchang Song, Department of Acupuncture, Nanchang Hospital of combination of Traditional Chinese Medicine with Western Medicine, Nanchang 330003, China
Supported by the Major State Basic Research and Development Program of People's Republic of China (No. 2009CB522902); National Key Technology R&D Program (No. 2006BAI12B04-2); National Natural Science Foundation of China (No. 81160453); National Natural Science Foundation of China (No. 81202854); Jiangxi Key R&D Project
Correspondence to: Prof. Rixin Chen, Department of Acupuncture and Rehabilitation, Hospital Affiliated to Jiangxi University of TCM, Nanchang 330006, China
Telephone: +86-91-86363653; +86-13870995605
Accepted: January 10, 2013

Abstract

OBJECTIVE: To compare the curative effects of heat-sensitive moxibustion with conventional drugs on chronic persistent asthma and seek a valuable therapy to replace Western Medicine.

METHODS: The participants in this multi-center, randomized, and controlled study were randomly divided into two groups: group A ($n=144$), treated with heat-sensitive moxibustion (50 sessions) and group B ($n=144$), treated with Seretide (salmeterol 50 μg/fluticasone 250 μg, twice a day). The scores of asthma control test (ACT), forced expiratory volume in 1 second (FEV1), peak expiratory flow (PEF), and attack frequency were measured after 15, 30, 60, and 90 days of treatment. Patients followed up 3 and 6 months after treatment.

RESULTS: There was a significant difference ($P=0.0002$) in the ACT score and lung function between the two groups after 3 months of treatment and ($P=0.000\ 03$) during the follow-up visits. In addition, heat-sensitive moxibustion reduced attack frequency in the period from inclusion to the 6-month follow-up visit.

CONCLUSION: This study shows that heat-sensitive moxibustion may have a comparable curative effect to Seretide (salmeterol/fluticasone) on asthma.

352

Key words: Moxibustion; Asthma; Randomized controlled trial; Heat sensitive; Seretide

INTRODUCTION

Bronchial asthma is a significant burden on healthcare and the social economy.[1-5] In 2010, there were 300 million asthma patients worldwide.[6] At present, no single therapy can effectively cure it. Therefore, asthma treatment aims to control the disease and improve the quality of life.[7,8]

Western Medicine can cause discomfort and influence daily life.[9] Therefore, acupuncture or moxibustion has been gradually accepted as a complementary or alternative treatment in China and Western countries for preventing asthma attacks and relieving symptoms.[10-12]

Heat-sensitive moxibustion is a new therapy in which a burning moxa-roll is placed over a heat-sensitive acupoint.[13] Studies have shown that it can treat diseases such as myofascial pain syndrome,[14] lumbar disc herniation,[15] pressure sores,[16] knee osteoarthritis,[17] primary dysmenorrhea,[18] neck pain,[19] and allergic rhinitis.[20]

We have found that moxibustion over heat-sensitive acupoints on the back of asthma patients[21,22] can improve their clinical asthma symptoms.[23,24] Two trials suggesting that heat-sensitive moxibustion can treat asthma[23,24] were not randomized and controlled trials with large sample sizes.

Therefore, we designed this rigorous trial to provide evidence to confirm the curative effect of heat-sensitive moxibustion on chronic persistent asthma. Heat-sensitive moxibustion could be a valuable asthma-controlling therapy to replace Western Medicine. The designed plan of this study was published in Trials in October 2010.[25]

DATA AND METHODS

Estimation of sample size

We estimated the sample size according to the requirements of a non-inferiority clinical trial. Non-inferiority critical value δ was determined with a small sample pilot study. ACT score after 3 months of treatment was used as the terminal index. The difference in means between the two groups was 0.45. Considering clinical relevance and statistical judgment, $\delta=0.15$ (30% of Δ). We calculated that 120 patients ($\alpha=0.05$, $\beta=0.2$) were needed. Allowing for a 20% loss, 144 participants were required in each group, with 288 participants in total.

Randomization

Central randomization used in this trial was performed by the China Academy of Chinese Medical Sciences (Beijing, China). Patients meeting the inclusion criteri-

on were randomly and equally divided into two groups. Before randomization, the patients gradually stopped medication and were routinely nursed for asthma.

Ethics

The ethics committee of the Hospital Affiliated to Jiangxi Institute of Traditional Chinese Medicine approved this trial with the code 2008 (13).

Inclusion criterion

Patients meeting the asthma-diagnosing standard according to the guideline of asthma treatment and prevention in China (GATPC)[24] were grouped into three categories: acute exacerbation, chronic persistence, and clinical remission. GATPC severity includes intermittent, mild, moderate, and severe grades. Our trial only chose patients with chronic moderate persistent asthma. All patients aged 18-65 years provided written informed consent. Moreover, heat-sensitivity appeared within the rectangular area consisting of the two outer lines of the dorsal Bladder Meridian of Foot-Taiyang and two horizontal lines of Fei Shu (BL 13) and Geshu (BL 17), 6 inches from the intercostals space between the first rib and second rib of the anterior aspect of the chest. Patients were asked to take no medicine during the treatment and acknowledge acceptance of treatment and related inquiries 24 h before and after treatment.

Exclusion criterion

Patients with one of the following conditions were excluded: (a) other diseases that also cause breathlessness or dyspnea, such as bronchiectasis, cor pulmonale, pulmonary fibrosis, tuberculosis, pulmonary abscess, and chronic obstructive pulmonary disease; (b) pregnancy or lactation; (c) hormone-dependent patients, or patients using adrenal cortical hormone within 4 weeks of recruitment; (d) life-threatening complications, such as cerebrocardiovascular diseases, diseases of liver, kidney, and hematopoietic system; and (e) psychotic patients.

Baseline data

Two hundred and thirty of 518 patients in our trial from September 2008 to December 2010 were excluded from the study (Figure 1). According to the definition of intention-to-treat (ITT), the ITT population comprised 288 patients in the twelve hospitals. The groups were comparable in baseline characteristics (Table 1), including the objective parameters of age, sex, duration of asthma, and ACT scores. There were no statistically significant differences between the two groups ($P>0.05$).

Data collection

Assessors, who did not participate in the treatment and were blind to the allocation results, performed the outcome assessment. The statistician conducting the

353

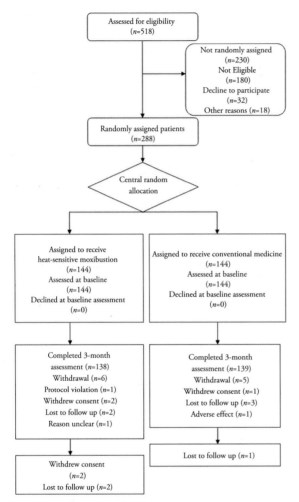

Figure 1 Diagram for procedure of the trial

analyses remained blind to treatment group. Data were made public once they were summarized and analyzed.

Treatment

The treatment plan in this study was developed over a 3-month period. Patients were randomly divided into a heat-sensitive moxibustion group (treatment group) and a control group. In the treatment group, all acupoints were stimulated with the burning of moxa-sticks, 22 mm in diameter and 160 mm in length, (produced by Jiangxi Hospital of Traditional Chinese Medicine, China). Patients lay in a comfortable position with the moxibustion site fully exposed in a room at 24℃-30℃.

Heat-sensitive moxibustion

An ignited moxa-stick was held over the rectangular area consisting of two outer lines of the dorsal Bladder Meridian of Foot-Taiyang and two horizontal lines of Feishu (BL 13) and Geshu (BL 17), 6 inches from the intercostal space between the first rib and second rib of the anterior aspect of the chest. The burning moxa-stick was held about 3 cm from the skin to look for heat-sensitive acupoints. When patients felt the heat penetrating to deep tissue or spreading to the surrounding area or transmitting in a direction, the therapists marked the point as having a heat-sensitive phenomenon. Therapists attempted to find all heat-sensitive acupoints in each patient.

Having found all heat-sensitive acupoints possible, therapists treated patients at the acupoint most sensitive to heat until the patient nearly felt the disappearance of the heat-sensitivity. The heat-sensitivity tended to decrease but could be still identified even at the end of treatment. After treatment, the therapist recorded the duration of moxibustion. During the first month, patients were treated once a day in the first 8 days and 12 times in the following 22 days. The treatment was given 15 times a month in the remaining two months.

Control group (Seretide)
Seretide Accuhaler (GlaxoSmithKline Plc, UK), containing fluticasone propionate and salmeterol xinafoate, is recommended by Global Initiative for Asthma (GINA) as a regular treatment of asthma.[26] In our trial, patients were treated with Seretide (salmeterol 50 μg/ fluticasone 250 μg) twice a day for 90 days.

Index of observation
ACT score, a primary index of observation, was measured before treatment and after 15, 30, 60, and 90 days of treatment. ACT, recommended by GINA in 2002,[7] is a validated and patient-completed

measurement of asthma control comprising five questions on limitation of activity, difficulty in breathing, symptoms at night, use of drugs and frequency of attack over the previous four weeks. The questions are scored from 1 (worst) to 5 (best), and the ACT score is the sum of the responses, giving the maximum score of 25. The ACT in Chinese, provided by China Asthma Alliance in 2006,[26] was tested by Chinese researchers previously. Some studies suggested that the score system was useful for identifying patients in China.[27,28]

Secondary indexes of observation were forced expiratory volume in 1 second (FEV1), peak expiratory flow (PEF), and frequency of attack. All patients filled in asthma diaries during 3 weeks before randomization and every visit after randomization. In the diaries they documented the time of attack from beginning to end, the intensity, the frequency, and the associated symptoms during each asthma attack. Patients documented whether or not they took medicine during treatment periods. If they did, they were required to document its name and dosage, the time of administration, the time of the relief of the symptoms and the side-effects

Table 1 Baseline characteristics of patients with chronic moderate persistent asthma

Item		Experimental group	Control group
Age [mean (*SD*), years]		43.8 (13.00)	43.6 (12.2)
Age	Age (min-max, years)	18-65	20-65
	Age>50 years [*n* (%)]	51 (35.42)	50 (34.72)
Sex [*n* (%)]	Male	58 (40.28)	62 (43.06)
	Female	86 (59.72)	82 (56.94)
Patient source [*n* (%)]	Specialized outpatient center	108 (37.50)	110 (38.19)
	Primary care	40 (13.89)	30 (10.42)
History of asthma [*n* (%)]	<5 year	63 (43.75)	69 (47.92)
	5-10 year	40 (27.78)	45 (31.25)
	>10 year	41 (28.47)	30 (20.83)
Body mass index [mean (*SD*) (kg/m²)]		23.07 (2.31)	21.53 (2.13)
ACT [mean (*SD*)]		15.10 (4.05)	15.70 (3.78)
Baseline FEV₁ [mean (*SD*) (L)]		74.90 (16.70)	75.10 (18.50)
Baseline PEF [mean (*SD*) (m/s)]		72.81 (22.25)	73.83 (24.33)
Attack frequency [mean (*SD*) (/w)]		4.53 (1.02)	4.36 (1.13)
Prior ICS use [*n* (%)]	Beclomethasone	33 (22.92)	29 (20.14)
	Budesonide	30 (20.83)	27 (18.75)
	Ciclesonide	6 (4.17)	4 (2.78)
	Fluticasone	27 (18.75)	53 (36.81)
	Mometasone	8 (5.56)	6 (4.17)
ICS + LABA [*n* (%)]	Budesonide/formoterol	30 (20.83)	20 (13.89)
	Fluticasone/salmeterol	10 (6.94)	5 (3.47)

Notes: experimental group was treated with heat-sensitive moxibustion; control group was treated with fluticasone/salmeterol (Seretide). ACT: asthma control test; FEV1: forced expiratory volume in 1 second; PEF: peak expiratory flow; IICS: inhaled corticosteroid, LABA: long-acting β2-agonist.

of the medicine. Adverse reactions were recorded during the 3-month treatment and 6-month follow-up visit.

Quality monitoring

Monitoring the quality of moxibustion is mainly based on quality control program (QCP) including the design of case report form (CRF) and the training of qualified investigators, researchers and data-managers.[29] According to good clinical practice (GCP), a standard QCP was established to monitor the quality of our trial. Monitors directly appointed by the project leader completed the quality control program, guaranteed data accuracy, and prevented or detected plan violations. Clinical centers and clinicians, the randomization system of the centers, and the treatment processes were monitored. In addition, the case report forms were reviewed for completeness and internal consistency, the eligibility and validity of the patients in the study were verified, and data were monitored for compliance and accuracy.

Compliance analysis

In the control group, data were collected with an electronic timed inhaler (Nebulizer Chronolog), which can automatically count and record each actual inhaled dosage. The testees were given an initialized Nebulizer Chronolog and a diary card used to record their daily symptoms. The card included instructions on how to use the inhaler. After 3 months of treatment, the Nebulizer Chronolog and diary cards were returned. Days of good compliance were defined as days a patient took a fixed dosage of drug at the appropriate time.

Patients' compliance to receiving heat-sensitive moxibustion was assessed with three oral questions: "Does the patient receive moxibustion treatment in hospital regularly?" "Has the patient ever had any history of not using moxibustion treatment?" "Does the patient still receive last prescribed moxibustion?" The higher the score, the better the compliance.

Statistical analysis

The intention-to-treat (ITT) population is defined as the randomized patients. The data analysis of baseline characteristics is based on the ITT population as well as the primary and secondary indexes. In the ITT population, none of the patients were excluded and the patients were analyzed according to the randomization scheme. The basic ITT principle was that patients in the trials should be analyzed, regardless of whether they receive or adhere to treatment.

Data were analyzed with SAS 9.0 statistical software (Cary, NC, USA). The first step of analysis was to compare baseline characteristics between the two groups. The second step was to check whether the treatment group was inferior or not to the control group in treating asthma.

For data in a normal distribution (normality, homogeneity of variances), repeated analyses were used in assessments. Mann-Whitney U, *t*-test, and Wilcoxon test

were used for comparison of variables. Two-sided test was applied to all available data, and P value <0.05 was considered statistically significant. Missing data were replaced according to the principle of the last observation.

RESULTS

ACT score

There was an obvious difference ($P<0.001$) in ACT score at each time-point as compared to baseline. Comparisons of data at six time-points between groups were multiple testing. We used the Bonferroni adjustment *t*-test.[30] The differences in ACT score between the two groups at each time-point are shown in Table 2, indicating significant differences in the ACT score after 3 months of treatment ($P=0.0002$) and highly significant difference during the 6-month follow-up visit ($P=0.000\ 03$). Figure 2 shows that the mean ACT score of both groups increased sharply after half a month of treatment and continually increased up to the end of 6-month follow-up visit. In the control group, the ACT score remained stable during 3- and 6-month follow-up visit, and patients continued to take the drug with gradually reduced dosage during follow-up visit.

Lung function

Tables 3 and Table 4 show the secondary indexes of FEV1, PEF, and attack frequency derived from ITT analyses. FEV1 and PEF in both groups after 3 months of treatment were much higher than those before treatment (Table 3). The improvement of lung function in the heat-sensitive moxibustion group was better than that in the control group ($P=0.035$ for FEV1, $P=0.011$ for PEF). Moreover, there were noticeable differences between the two groups during the 6-month follow-up visit ($P=0.042$ for FEV1, $P=0.0012$ for PEF). The frequency of asthma attack after 3 months of treatment in the heat-sensitive moxibustion group was much lower than that in the control group ($P=0.000\ 17$). There was still an obvious difference between the two groups during 6-month follow-up visit ($P=0.047$).

In the control group, the majority of patients were able to correctly use the inhaler. The days of inhaling inadequate dosage accounted for 9% and the days of inhaling excessive dosage accounted for 2%. In the heat-sensitive moxibustion group, 90% of patients were regularly treated in hospitals, and only 1.5% of patients were irregularly treated.

Adverse reactionsAmong the 9 patients (5.1%) with mild adverse reactions during treatment were 5 cases of headache and 4 cases of palpitation. However, after the treatment, all the symptoms disappeared. No patient reported any severe adverse reactions.

DISCUSSION

This trial used subjective and objective indexes to as-

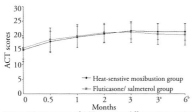

Figure 2 Comparison of ACT scores at different time-points ACT: asthma control test. ᵃ: 3-month follow-up visit; ᵇ: 6-month follow-up visit.

sess curative effect on asthma using standard treatment or heat-sensitive moxibustion. ACT score was markedly enhanced in both groups, there was an obvious difference in ACT score and lung function between the two groups, and asthma attack frequency was noticeably lower in the heat-sensitive moxibustion group. This indicates that heat-sensitive moxibustion is not inferior to Seretide in curative effect on bronchial asthma.

In contrast to acupuncture, heat-sensitive moxibustion indirectly stimulates acupoints. Adverse reactions, such as infection, minor hemorrhage and pain in the moxibustion region, and uncomfortable reactions, such as dizziness, nausea or vomiting, aggravation of complaint, malaise, fever and numbness, were not observed in the heat-sensitive moxibustion group. Meanwhile, several patients in the control group had adverse reactions. The most common adverse reactions to Seretide are upper respiratory tract infection, mouth infection, nausea, headache, muscle and bone pain, and bronchitis.[31,32] The superiority of heat-sensitive moxibustion is manifested in its safety. Large-scale surveys have provided evidence that moxibustion is a relatively safe treatment.[33]

To our knowledge, this is the first randomized controlled trial with large sample to compare the curative effect of heat-sensitive moxibustion and Western Medicine on asthma. Published studies have methodological deficiencies, including deficient randomization descrip-

Table 2 Comparison of ACT scores at different time-points between groups

Variable	Experimental group		Control group		t test ᵃ	P value	Mean difference, MD (95% CI)
	Mean	SD	Mean	SD			
Observed ACT score							
Before treatment	15.10	4.05	15.70	3.78	1.30	0.19	− 0.60 (− 1.50, 0.30)
After half a month of treatment	17.86	3.69	18.54	4.13	− 1.18	0.14	− 0.68 (− 1.58, 0.22)
After 1 month of treatment	19.54	3.68	19.81	3.99	− 0.31	0.56	− 0.27 (− 1.17, 0.63)
After 2 months of treatment	20.65	3.22	20.98	3.27	− 0.52	0.39	− 0.33 (− 1.08, 0.42)
After 3 months of treatment	21.60	2.77	21.20	3.61	3.15	0.0002	0.40 (− 1.34, 1.14)
3-month follow-up visit	21.35	2.75	20.47	3.58	2.68	0.0009	0.88 (0.14, 1.62)
6-month follow-up visit	21.29	2.88	20.35	3.72	4.42	0.000 03	0.94 (0.17, 1.71)

Notes: experimental group was treated with heat-sensitive moxibustion; control group was treated with fluticasone/salmeterol (Seretide). ACT: asthma control test. Bonferroni adjustment *t*-test was used for group differences. The adjusting of *P*-values was 0.008.

Table 3 Comparison of FEV1 and PEF between groups at each time point

Lung function	Experimental group		Control group		t test ᵃ	P value	Mean difference, MD (95% CI)
	Mean	SD	Mean	SD			
Observed FEV1 (L)							
Before treatment	74.90	16.70	75.10	18.50	0.37	0.92	− 0.20 (− 4.27, 3.87)
After 3 months of treatment	87.29	17.44	83.39	22.29	1.86	0.035	3.90 (− 0.72, 8.52)
6-month follow-up visit	83.34	22.29	80.52	20.93	1.69	0.042	2.82 (− 2.33, 7.97)
Observed PEF (m/s)							
Before treatment	72.81	22.25	73.83	24.33	0.10	0.71	− 1.02 (− 6.40, 4.36)
After 3 months of treatment	86.16	21.27	81.64	26.27	2.07	0.011	4.52 (− 1.00, 10.04)
6-month follow-up visit	84.89	23.01	80.01	25.75	2.19	0.0012	4.88 (− 0.76, 10.52)

Notes: experimental group was treated with heat-sensitive moxibustion; control group was treated with fluticasone/salmeterol (Seretide). FEV1: forced expiratory volume in 1 second; PEF: peak expiratory flow.

Chen RX *et al.* / Clinical Study

Table 4 Comparison of attack frequency between two groups							
Variable	Experimental group		Control group		*t* test[a]	*P* value	Mean difference, MD (95% *CI*)
	Mean	*SD*	Mean	*SD*			
Observed attack frequency (w)							
Before treatment	4.53	1.02	4.36	1.13	0.21	0.18	0.17 (− 0.08, 0.42)
After 3 months of treatment	0.81	0.29	1.28	0.25	3.56	0.000 17	− 0.47 (− 0.53, − 0.41)
6-month follow-up visit	0.59	0.25	1.12	0.33	1.74	0.047	− 0.53 (− 0.60, − 0.46)

Notes: experimental group was treated with heat-sensitive moxibustion; control group was treated with fluticasone/salmeterol (Seretide).

tions, no concealment of therapeutic plan, data heterogeneity between groups, and different periods of follow-up visits. Unlike previous studies on moxibustion, our study required participating therapists to have corresponding medical education and TCM clinical practice before performing treatment according to a series of strict standards. In addition, our study used central randomization to ensure adequate concealment of group assignment. Both evaluation and statistical analysis were carried out blindly. High quality follow-up visits were an important guarantee for the quality of our trial.

However, it was impossible for doctors to conduct a blind manipulative intervention method in this study. Zhao *et al*[34] has developed a moxa cone fixed to a special base to carry out sham or real moxibustion. Sham moxibustion is identical to real moxibustion in the shape, burning process, and residue of moxa cone but distinct in only the production of heat and smoke and isolation from skin. Of course, such a method is suitable for direct moxibustion. It is necessary for experienced therapists to carry out heat-sensitive moxibustion, an indirect moxibustion. Furthermore, it is very easy for bronchial asthma patients to distinguish heat-sensitive moxibustion from Seretide. However, it is possible for patients to carry out a blind method. Acupoints unrelated to asthma treatment can be selected for sham moxibustion in the control group. Meanwhile, a placebo could be taken in real moxibustion group. We intended to try the blind method in future trials.

In our trial, we selected acupoints in the back, which are used to treat bronchial asthma and other lung diseases according to TCM theory. For example, Fei Shu (BL 13) on the Bladder Meridian of Foot-Taiyang, is used to treat bronchitis, asthma, pleurisy, and night sweating and can regulate lung *Qi*, improve lung function, and build Stomach *Qi*. Some experimental studies have indicated that the mechanism of moxibustion may be related to adjusting the release of inflammatory substances in the lung, improving respiratory tract spasms, and inhibiting respiratory tract inflammation.[33-35] A study of 32 patients with both asthma and rheumatoid arthritis showed the effects of acupuncture and moxibustion on immunoglobulin.[36,37] A study in 1995 of 94 patients with bronchial asthma showed

that acupuncture and moxibustion can affect the nervous and immune systems, cause metabolic changes, and effectively reduce the sensitivity and reactivity of bronchioles. In other words, acupuncture and moxibustion can reduce the reactivity of bronchioles to asthma-inducing factors.[37,38] Although studies from China have investigated the mechanisms of moxibustion on the nervous system,[39] further study is still necessary.

Because adverse reactions caused by long-term use of asthma drugs can influence their continuous use, other treatment courses are necessary. This study has demonstrated that the curative effect of heat-sensitive moxibustion is not inferior to that of Seretide on asthma. Therefore, our study has clinical significance for providing a potential non-drug therapy to control asthma.

REFERENCES

1   **Anderson HR**, Gupta R, Strachan DP, Limb ES. 50 years of asthma: UK trends from 1955 to 2004. Thorax 2007; 9 (62): 85-90.

2   **Brogger J**, Bakke P, Eide GE, Johansen B, Andersen A, Gulsvik A. Long-term changes in adult asthma prevalence. Eur Respir J 2003; 3(21): 468-472.

3   **Ekerljung L**, Ronmark E, Larsson K, et al. No further increase of incidence of asthma: incidence, remission and relapse of adult asthma in Sweden. Respir Med 2008; 12 (102): 1730-1736.

4   **Pallasaho P**, Lundback B, Meren M, et al. Prevalence and risk factors for asthma and chronic bronchitis in the capitals. Respir Med 2002; 5(96): 759-769.

5   **Lotvall J**, Ekerljung L, Ronmark EP, et al. West sweden asthma study: prevalence trends over the last 18 years argue no recent increase in asthma. Respir Res 2009; 10 (10): 94.

6   Global initiative for asthma (GINA). Global strategy for asthma management and prevention: NHLBI/WHO work shop Report. Bethesda: National Institutes of Health, National Heart, Lung and Blood Institute. Available from URL: http://www.ginasthma.org/pdf/GINA_Report_2010.pdf.

7   Global Initiative for Asthma (GINA). Global strategy for asthma man- agement and prevention: NHLBI/WHO work shop Report. Bethesda: National Institutes of Health, National Heart, Lung and Blood Institute, 2002: 2-3659.

8   British thoracic society (BTS) and scottish intercollegiate

guidelines network. British guideline on the management of asthma. Thorax 2003; SupplI(58): 11-19.

9 **Lundback B**, Ronmark E, Lindberg A, et al. Control of mild to moderate asthma over 1-year with the combination of salmeterol and fluticasone propionate. Respir Med 2006; 1(100): 2-10.

10 **McCarney RW**, Brinkhaus B, Lasserson TJ, Linde K. Acupuncture for chronic asthma. Cochrane database of systematic reviews 2003; (3): CD000008.

11 **Jobst K**. A critical analysis of acupuncture in pulmonary disease: efficacy and safety of the acupuncture needle. J Altern Complement Med 1995; 1(1): 57-84.

12 **Davis PA**, Chang C, Hackmann RM, Stern JS, Gershwin ME. Acupuncture in the treatment of asthma: a critical review. Allergol et Immunopathol 1998; 6(26): 263-271.

13 **Chen RX**, Kang MF. Acupoint heat-sensitive moxibustion a new therapy. Beijing: People's Medical Publishing House, 2006: 48-49.

14 **Chen RX**, Kang MF, He WL, Chen SY, Zhang B. Moxibustion on heat-sensitive acupoints for treatment of myofascial pain syndrome: a multi-central randomized controlled trial. Zhong Guo Zhen Jiu 2008; 28(6): 395-398.

15 **Tang FY**, Huang CJ, Chen RX, Xu M, Liu BX, Liang Z. Observation on therapeutic effect of moxibustion on temperature-sensitive points for lumbar disc herniation. Zhong Guo Zhen Jiu 2009; 29(7): 382-384.

16 **Zhang C**, Xiao H, Chen RX. Observation on curative effect of moxibustion on heat-sensitive points on pressure sores. Zhong Hua Zhong Yi Yao Za Zhi 2010; 25(5): 478-488.

17 **Kang MF**, Chen RX, Fu Y. Observation on curative effect of moxibustion on heat-sensitive points on knee osteoarthritis. Jiangxi Zhong Yi Yao 2006; 18(3): 27-28.

18 **Zhang B**, Chen RX, Chen MR, Kang MF. The distribution and clinical observation of heat-sensitive points on asthma. Jiangxi Zhong Yi Yao 2011; 22(6): 45.

19 **Tang FY**, Huang CJ, Xu M. Observation on curative effect of moxibustion on heat-sensitive points on cervical spondylotic radiculopathy (neck pain). Zhong Guo Lin Chang Yi Xue Za Zhi 2010; 17(6): 120.

20 **Yang SR**, Chen H, Xie Q. Observation on curative effect of moxibustion on heat-sensitive points on allergic rhinitis. Zhong Guo Zhen Jiu 2008; 28(2): 81.

21 **Chen RX**, Kang MF. Key point of moxibustion, arrival of *Qi* produces curative effect. Zhong Guo Zhen Jiu 2008; 28 (1): 44-46.

22 **Chen RX**, Chen MR, Kang MF. Heat-sensitive moxibustion therapy practical clinical book. Beijing: People's Medical Publishing House, 2009: 56-59.

23 **Liang C**, Huang GF, Yang K, Zhang TF. Short-and long-term effects of Heat-sensitive Moxibustion therapy on lung ventilation function of patients with chronic asthma. Zhong Guo Kang Fu Yi Xue Za Zhi 2010; 25(4): 19-23.

24 **Liang C**, Yang K, Zhang TF. Comparative observation on therapeutic effect of chronic persistent bronchial asthma treated with heat-sensitive moxibustion and medication. Zhong Guo Zhen Jiu 2010; 29(11): 1-4.

25 **Chen RX**, Chen MR, Xiong J, Yi F, Chi ZH, Zhang B. Comparison of heat-sensitive moxibustion versus fluticasone/salmeterol (seretide) combination in the treatment of chronic persistent asthma: design of a multicenter randomized controlled trial. Trials 2010; 11(2): 121.

26 Asthma group of Chinese society of respiratory diseases: the guideline of asthma treatment and prevention. Clin J Tuberc Respir Dis 1997; 7(20): 261-267.

27 **Zhou WY**. An exploratory research of asthma control test (ACT) in China. Zhong Hua Xiao Chuan Za Zhi 2009; 5 (9): 21-25.

28 **Lei Y**, Wen JZ. Asthma patients serum high sensitive C-reaction protein and asthma control test scores: a correlational study. Chengdu Yi Xue Za Zhi 2012; 24(2): 77-79.

29 **Zhang J**, Dai G, Shang H, Cao H, Ren M, Xiang Y. Data audit in large scale clinical trial of Traditional Chinese Medicine. Zhong Guo Xun Zheng Yi Xue Za Zhi 2007; 7 (3): 230-232.

30 **Bland M**, Altman DG. Multiple significance tests. the Bonferroni method. BMJ 1995; 6973(310): 170.

31 **Edward J**. Lamb, eHow Contributor. What Are the Side Effects of Seretide? Cited 2012-10-01; 1(1): 12 screens. Available from URL: http://www.ehow.com/about_ 5194814_side-effects-seretide_.html.

32 **Guittier MJ**, Klein TJ, Dong HG, Andreoli N, Irion O, Boulvain M. Side-effects of moxibustion for cephalic version of breech presentation. The Journal of Alternative and Complementary Medicine 2008; 10(14): 1231-1233.

33 **Ernst G**, Strzyz H, Hagmeister H. Incidence of adverse effects during acupuncture therapy a multicentre survey. Complement Ther Med 2003; 2(11): 93-97.

34 **Zhao B**, Wang X, Lin Z, Liu R, Lao L. A novel sham moxibustion device: a randomized, placebo-controlled trial. Complement Ther Med 2006; 1(14): 53-60.

35 **Zhao C**, Zhang W, Zhu HH. Progress and comment on mechanism of moxibustion treating asthma. Zhong Guo Xian Dai Zhong Xi Yi Jie He Za Zhi 2004; 27(3): 213-215.

36 **Wu YC**, Shi Y. Clinical progress on moxibustion treatment of asthma. Zhen Jiu Tui Na Za Zhi 2004; 2(3): 54-57.

37 **Li Q**, Dong J. Review on the study of the mechanism of acupuncture and moxibustion in the treatment of asthma. Zhong Guo Zhong Xi Yi Jie He Za Zhi 2000; 20(5): 391-396.

38 **Guan Z**, Zhang J. Effects of acupuncture and moxibustion on immunoglobulin in patients with asthma and rheumatoid arthritis. Zhong Yi Za Zhi 1995; 15(2): 102-105.

39 **Miller AL**. The etiologies, pathophysiology, and alternative/complementary treatment of asthma. Altern Med Rev 2001; 1(6): 20-47.

Hindawi Publishing Corporation
Evidence-Based Complementary and Alternative Medicine
Volume 2013, Article ID 906947, 7 pages
http://dx.doi.org/10.1155/2013/906947

Hindawi

Research Article

Comparative Effectiveness of the Deqi Sensation and Non-Deqi by Moxibustion Stimulation: A Multicenter Prospective Cohort Study in the Treatment of Knee Osteoarthritis

Rixin Chen,[1] Mingren Chen,[1] Jun Xiong,[1] Tongsheng Su,[2] Meiqi Zhou,[3] Jianhua Sun,[4] Zhenhai Chi,[1] Bo Zhang,[1] and Dingyi Xie[1]

[1] The Affiliated Hospital with Jiangxi University of TCM, Nanchang 330006, China
[2] Shanxi TCM Hospital, Xian 710003, China
[3] The First Affiliated Hospital with Anhui University of TCM, Hefei 230031, China
[4] Jiangsu TCM Hospital, Nanjing 210029, China

Correspondence should be addressed to Rixin Chen; chenrixin321@163.com

Received 10 May 2013; Revised 21 July 2013; Accepted 23 July 2013

Academic Editor: Lin-Peng Wang

Substantial evidence has supported that moxibustion stimulates a unique phenomenon of Deqi, heat-sensitive moxibustion sensation. This study consisted of a multicenter, prospective cohort study with two parallel arms (A: heat-sensitive moxibustion sensation group; B: nonheat-sensitive moxibustion sensation group). All forms of moxibustion were applied unilaterally on the right leg with a triangle shape of three acupuncture points simultaneously (bilateral Xi Yan (EX-LE5) and He Ding (EX-LE2)). After one month the primary outcome parameter GPCRND-KOA showed significant differences between groups: trial group 5.23 ± 2.65 (adjusted mean $\pm$ SE) 95% CI [4.44~6.01] versus control group 7.43 ± 2.80 [6.59~8.26], $P = 0.0001$. Significant differences were manifested in total M-JOA score during the follow-up period ($P = 0.0006$). Mean knee circumference indicated significant difference between the groups ($P = 0.03$; $P = 0.007$). Overall, this evidence suggested that the effectiveness of the Deqi sensation group might be more superior than the non-Deqi sensation one in the treatment of KOA. This study was aimed at providing scientific evidence on the Deqi sensation of moxibustion and at showing that heat-sensitive moxibustion sensation is essential to achieve the preferable treatment effects of KOA.

1. Background

Acupuncture stimulates the Deqi, a sensory response which literally means "the arrival of meridian Qi" according to traditional Chinese medicine (TCM) [1, 2]. The classical TCM textbook of *Huangdi Neijing* states that the Deqi must be felt by the therapist, and it is also necessary for therapist to concentrate in order to ensure the Deqi [3]. The essence of acupuncture therapy was expressed in *Nine Needle* and *Twelve Sources* (from *Huangdi Neijing*), "the arrival of meridian Qi ensures the therapeutic effects." This chapter describes the importance of activating meridian Qi and prompting it to transmit to the affected body part. Therefore, a lot of researchers confirmed that the Deqi is the key experience related to clinical efficacy of acupuncture [4, 5].

For acupuncture needle, multiple unique sensations experienced by the patient around the applied part of needle manipulation are often described as suan (aching or soreness), ma (numbness or tingling), zhang (fullness/distention or pressure), and zhong (heaviness) [6]. The Deqi stimulated by needle is believed to be closely related to clinical effects [7]. And there is also evidence to support that the increasing clinical effects were associated with the Deqi by needle stimulation [8–10].

Unlike acupuncture needle, which involves thrusting or twisting of needles and induces various Deqi phenomena, moxibustion implements heat stimulation of various temperature levels from mild skin warming to acupuncture points. Suspended moxibustion is the most common therapy in China. It involves burning of moxa on the acupuncture points at a distance. The Deqi by moxibustion stimulation is different from the one simulated by acupuncture needle as well. Substantial evidence has supported that moxibustion stimulates a unique of Deqi, that is, heat-sensitive moxibustion sensation [11]. A lot of observations and researches were adopted to confirm this phenomenon in the 1990s [12].

For humans, acupuncture points include two states: stimulated state and resting state. For healthy people, acupuncture points are in a resting state, and moxibustion only stimulates local superficial heat sensation. When people get sick, the acupuncture points on the surface of body are activated and sensitized. Several Deqi sensations are induced and called heat-sensitive moxibustion sensation. The first of all, penetrating heat, is the feeling from the applied part of the skin sinking into the underlying tissues or organs. In the second, expanding heat is the feeling of heat spreading out from the spot receiving moxibustion. The third, transmitting heat, refers to the sensation of heat moving from spot receiving moxibustion along a certain route. These sensations indicate that meridian Qi has been stimulated, and transmission has occurred [13]. However, there is lack of experimental data to indicate how heat-sensitive moxibustion sensation (the Deqi by moxibustion stimulation) compares with conventional local superficial heat sensation (non-Deqi by moxibustion stimulation).

Moreover, several articles and research reports have reported the effectiveness and safety of moxibustion for the treatment of knee osteoarthritis (KOA) [14–17]. Moxibustion has anti-inflammatory or immunomodulatory effects to fight against chronic inflammatory conditions in humans. For KOA, especially, is it necessary for moxibustion to produce the phenomenon of obtaining Qi in order to improve the curative effect? Therefore, it would be valuable to know whether there is difference between the moxibustion sensations in the treatment of KOA. The rigorous multicenter prospective cohort study trial was planned in order to determine the relationship of the Deqi by moxibustion stimulation and therapeutic effect.

2. Methods

2.1. Objective. The aim of this study is to compare the effectiveness of heat-sensitive moxibustion sensation and nonheat-sensitive moxibustion sensation in the treatment of patients with moderate-to-severe swelling KOA in China.

2.2. Sample Size. The sample size for testing the difference between the effective rates was calculated by the SPSS 13.0 programme. The outcome was the guiding principle of clinical research on new drugs in the treatment of KOA (GPCRND-KOA) [18]. According to previous pilot study, the effective rate in heat-sensitive moxibustion sensation group is 80% and 50% in the other group. If we apply a two-sided 5% significance level, 90% power the calculated required sample size is approximately 36 participants in each group. Allowing

for a 20% loss to followup, a total of 45 participants were required in two groups:

$$n = \left\{ \frac{Z_{1-a}\sqrt{2pq} + Z_{1-\beta}\sqrt{p_1(1-p_1) + p_2(1-p_2)}}{p_1 - p_2} \right\}^2, \quad (1)$$

$$p = \frac{(p_1 + p_2)}{2}, \qquad q = 1 - p.$$

2.3. Design. A multicenter (four centers in China), prospective cohort study was conducted by the Affiliated Hospital of Jiangxi University of Traditional Chinese Medicine (TCM) in Nanchang, the first Affiliated Hospital of Anhui University of TCM in Hefei, Jiangsu TCM Hospital in Nanjing, and Shanxi TCM Hospital in Xian. The patients were recruited at either outpatient service or inpatient department and had already made their own choice of moxibustion therapy. Thus, the groups were divided by the appearance of acupuncture point's Deqi sensation stimulated by suspended moxibustion. In trial group, patients felt the Deqi sensation when the acupuncture point was stimulated by moxibustion heat. In the control group, patients felt local superficial heat sensation (non-Deqi sensation) when the acupuncture point was stimulated by moxibustion heat.

2.4. Participants

2.4.1. Recruitment. Patients were recruited in China for this nonrandomized prospective multicenter open comparative cohort study from July 30, 2010 to July 30, 2011. The ethics committees of the Affiliated Hospital with Jiangxi University of TCM approved the study and the consent procedure. Oral and written informed consent was obtained after verbal information about the study was provided by the physician. The signed consent form was sent to the central study center, and a copy was kept at the physician's office.

2.4.2. Inclusion Criteria. Participants meeting the following criteria were included: patients met the diagnostic criteria for GPCRND-KOA; the GPCRND-KOA scale for KOA count should be more than 5 points, moderate-to-severe swelling KOA; the age of patients was from at least 38 years to no more than 70 years, and regardless of genders. According to the following KOA diagnosis standard, the following criteria were included simultaneously: knee joints appeared swelling; floating patella test was negative; patients accepted the treatment protocol in this trial; patients had stopped receiving previous treatment before recruitment for two weeks.

2.4.3. Exclusion Criteria. Participants with one or more than one of the following criteria should be excluded: participants suffered from serious life-threatening disease, such as the heart disease or disease of brain and blood vessels, liver, kidney, and hematopoietic system, as well as psychotic patients; patients with diabetes, diabetic polyneuropathy, and polyneuropathic disturbances; the pregnant patients or patients in lactation period. The following conditions were also excluded items: acute knee joint trauma or ulceration in its local skin, complicated with serious genu varus/valgus and flexion contraction.

2.5. Study Interventions. The moxibustion therapies were implemented by qualified specialists of acupuncture in TCM with at least five years of clinical experience in this study. All treatment regimens were standardized between four centers practitioners by means of video, hands-on training, and internet. Both groups of patients were requested to receive no other treatments such as physical therapies, pain-killing medicines, or acupuncture treatment from other places.

In the two groups, 22-millimeter (diameter) × 120-millimetre (length) moxa sticks (produced by Jiangxi provincial TCM Hospital, China) were applied. The patients usually laid in the comfortable supine position for treatment, with 24°C~30°C temperature in the room. Loose trousers are suggested to wear, in order to make knee joints to be exposed.

2.5.1. The Heat-Sensitive Moxibustion Sensation Group. The moxa sticks were ignited by the therapist, and three acupuncture points (bilateral Xi Yan (EX-LE5) and He Ding (EX-LE2)) with triangle shape should be implemented simultaneously by suspended moxibustion. The warm suspended moxibustion was applied 3 centimetres away from the surface of the skin to search for the heat-sensitive moxibustion sensation. In this group, these acupuncture points were brought mild warmth without burning by moxa sticks and manipulated until the patient reported the characteristic of heat sensitization sensation; it is commonly called Deqi. Patients felt comfortable in the moxibustion manipulation.

The following patients' sensation suggested the Deqi: penetrating heat sensation due to moxa heat, defining as the heat sensation conducting from the moxa local skin surface into deep tissue or even into the joint cavity; expanding heat sensation due to moxa heat, defining as the heat sensation spreading the surrounding little by little around the moxa point; transmitting heat sensation due to moxa heat, defining as the heat sensation transferring along some pathway or direction, even to the ankle or hip conduction. In the course of manipulation, the therapist continued for 15 minutes in per treatment session. Patients received the treatment two times/day in 1st week (one time/day from 2nd week) for a total of 35 sessions over 30 days.

2.5.2. The Nonheat-Sensitive Moxibustion Sensation Group. Common practices were similar to the first group. Only one difference was that patients in this group felt local superficial heat sensation. No Deqi sensations were stimulated in this group.

2.6. Outcome Measures. Ministry of Health of the People's Republic of China (MHPRC) has proposed the GPCRND-KOA [18]. The GPCRND-KOA scale was used widely and authoritatively recommended by China Clinic Trial. In the scale, a patient with KOA was assessed, including pain, the relation between activity and pain, function impairment, and special exams (Table 1). This scoring system was previously validated [19]. The degree of KOA is divided into three levels: mild <5 scores; moderate 5~9 scores; severe >9 scores. In the terms of swelling knee, knee circumference was assessed at each time point. The parameter was measured in centimeters across the middle of a patella, with ordinary tape measure [20].

Therapeutic effect was evaluated by comparing baseline and final conditions reported by the patient. This trial also recorded adverse effects reported by patients during treatment. The outcome measures above were assessed before the treatment (month 0), at the end of the treatment period (month 1), and 6 months after the end of the treatment period (month 7).

2.7. Statistical Methods. Statistical analyses were based on the intention-to-treat (ITT) principle, including all patients with baseline values to receive treatment. All tests were exploratory and two sided with a level of significance of 5%. The statistician who conducted the analyses remained blind to treatment group, and data were only unblended once all data were summarized, and analyses were completed. Statistical analyses were performed according to a predefined statistical analysis plan using SAS for Windows, version 9.2 (SAS Institute, Cary, NC, USA). We adopted multilevel models analysis of covariance (ANCOVA) or generalized estimating equations (GEE). In these models, physicians considered random effects, and fixed effects were GPCRND-KOA (continuous), patient's age and gender, Body Mass Index (BMI), knee circumference (continuous), and previous treatment. Results are presented as adjusted mean or proportioned with a standard error (SE) and/or 95% confidence interval (CI).

2.8. Adverse Events. We defined adverse events as unfavorable or unintended signs, symptoms, or disease presenting after treatment; however, they were not necessarily related to the moxibustion intervention. Adverse events were analyzed descriptively by frequencies, percentages, and by chi-squared or Fisher's exact test (if feasible).

3. Results

3.1. Population and Baseline. Among 266 screened patients, 106 could not be included in the study, mainly because they did not meet all eligibility criteria (Figure 1). Patients were recruited by 28 physicians experienced in the treatment of KOA (15 acupuncture doctors and 13 conventional doctors). After the search of the Deqi, 160 patients experienced heat-sensitive moxibustion sensation; 51 patients had no Deqi sensation. Since a sample of 90 people was calculated in our trial, we selected 45 patients from each queue separately by random drawing.

After seven months, 2 patients missed. Reasons for missing follow-up data were not contactable.

Patients' preferences resulted in the following baseline differences: patients in the trial group showed lower severe BMI scores, while the GPCRND-KOA score was higher in

TABLE 1: List of GPCRND-KOA.

Item	Grade/classification	Score
	No	0
Pain or discomfort in night when lying in bed	Pain in activity or some position	1
	Pain in nonactivity	2
	No	0
Morning stiffness or pain worse when getting out of bed	<30 minutes	1
	≥30 minutes	2
	No	0
Pain or discomfort in walk	After walking in some distance	1
	Pain at beginning of walk or worse	2
Arise from seat	Independent	0
	Need assistance	1
	Unrestricted	0
The maximum walk distance (accompanied with pain)	Restricted, >1 km	1
	300 m~1 km	2
	<300 m	3
	Board standard airstairs	
	Independent	0
	Difficulty	1
	Unable	2
	Step down standard airstairs	
	Independent	0
	Difficulty	1
Daily activities	Unable	2
	Squat or bend knees	
	Independent	0
	Difficulty	1
	Unable	2
	Walk over rough terrain	
	Independent	0
	Difficulty	1
	Unable	2

the control group. The males of the trial group were more than those of control group. In the previous treatment, there were obviously differences among the two treatment groups, as well as gender (Table 2).

3.2. Outcome Parameters

3.2.1. Total GPCRND-KOA Score. After 1 month the primary outcome parameter GPCRND-KOA showed significant differences between groups: trial group 5.23 ± 2.65 (adjusted mean $\pm$ SE) 95% CI [4.44~6.01] versus control group 7.43 ± 2.80 [6.59~8.26], $P = 0.0001$ (Table 3). Significant differences in total M-JOA score were also evident during the follow-up period ($P = 0.0006$).

3.2.2. Knee Circumference. Reductions in mean knee circumference at months 1 and 7 compared with control group were observed, and they were significant. Significant differences presented between the groups ($P < 0.05$) were shown in Table 4.

3.3. Safety. No adverse events were reported in the 90 participants.

4. Discussions

In this observational comparative effectiveness study, patients with KOA who presented heat-sensitive moxibustion sensation significantly reduced pain and possessed better function after one month than the ones who received conventional local superficial heat sensation, according to the total GPCRND-KOA score. Both of the groups substantially improved during the observation period. After 7 months, exploratory analysis indicated that the differences between the two groups were still significant. Significant differences were also evident for knee circumference.

The design of the study (observational and multicenter setting) allows evaluation of a therapy's comparative effectiveness considering the acupuncture point's own reactions and the Deqi sensation. Both the evaluation of the results and the statistical analysis were carried out in a blind fashion to improve the objectivity and validity of the study outcomes.

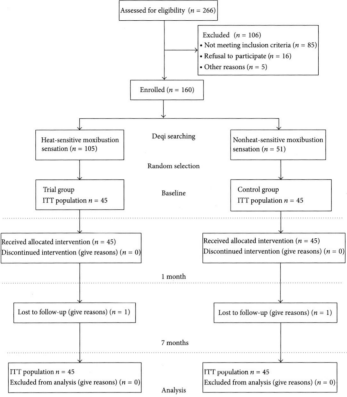

FIGURE 1: Flow diagram.

The aim of this study was to compare the Deqi effect and non-Deqi effect stimulated by suspended moxibustion and to confirm that heat-sensitive moxibustion sensation simulated by moxibustion is a sign of the Deqi. Thus, Deqi sensation occurrence preferences were chosen to take it into account, and it made randomization not possible. The observational design resulted in relevant baseline differences of the two groups. In the trial group GPCRND-KOA appeared higher compared with the conventional group. In the previous treatment, there were obvious differences between the two groups. To take baseline differences into account, we adjusted our analyses of these factors. However, it is possible that other unknown and unmeasured factors might have influenced the results. Therefore, the nonrandomized design is a clear limitation of our study considering the internal validity of our results.

In this study, we investigated the relationship between the Deqi sensation and therapeutic effect according to moxibustion stimulation. Previous studies manifested that the Deqi (heat-sensitive moxibustion sensation) was elicited in 70% of the moxibustion procedures of patients [21]. The frequency and intensity of individual sensations were significantly higher in KOA. Among the sensations typically associated with the Deqi, penetrating heat, expanding heat, and transmitting heat were most common [22]. Being consistent with their prominent roles in TCM, bilateral Xi Yan (EX-LE5) and He Ding (EX-LE2) showed the most prominent sensations [13, 21].

In terms of the Deqi sensation of acupuncture needle, it has been demonstrated that most of the Deqi sensations are conveyed by different nerve fiber systems. Aching, soreness, distension, heaviness, warmth, and dull pain are conveyed by the slower conducting $A\delta$ and C fibers, whereas numbness is conveyed by the faster conducting $A\beta$ fibers [23, 24]. However, there is lack of experimental data to indicate the basic substances that contribute to the Deqi sensation of moxibustion. Further research is required to discover the underlying mechanisms of the Deqi in moxibustion.

TABLE 2: Baseline characteristics of study patients.

Items	Trial group	Control group	P value
Age, mean (SD), years	56.13 (7.55)	59.34 (7.21)	0.04
Sex n (%)			0.0002
Female	12 (26.67)	32 (71.11)	
Male	33 (73.33)	13 (28.89)	
Duration of knee pain n (%)			0.67
<5 years	33 (73.33)	30 (66.67)	
5–10 years	9 (20.00)	11 (24.44)	
>10 years	3 (6.67)	4 (8.89)	
BMI, mean (SD), kg/m$'$	22.12 (3.12)	24.22 (3.30)	0.002
GPCRND-KOA grade n (%)			0.51
Severe	31 (68.89)	28 (62.22)	
Moderate	14 (31.11)	17 (37.78)	
Knee circumference, mean (SD), cm	40.26 (3.31)	42.21 (3.25)	0.005
GPCRND-KOA score, mean (SD)	13.45 (3.28)	11.12 (3.13)	0.0006
Previous treatment (past half year, %)			0.041
Pharmaceutical intervention	31 (68.89)	18 (40.00)	
Physiotherapy	11 (24.44)	20 (44.44)	
Previous acupuncture treatment	3 (6.67)	5 (11.11)	

BMI: Body Mass Index; GPCRND-KOA: guiding principle of clinical research on new drugs in the treatment of KOA score; SD: standard deviation; KOA: knee osteoarthritis.

TABLE 3: Comparison of GPCRND-KOA scores.

Variable	Month 1		Month 7	
	Mean	95% CI	Mean	95% CI
Trial group	5.23	4.44~6.01	4.78	4.37~5.18
Control group	7.43	6.59~8.26	6.11	5.45~6.76
P value	0.0001		0.0006	

*Adjusted means or proportions and confidence intervals (CI) from multi-level models (ANCOVA or GEE) with fixed effects. All data are intended to treat. Both groups $n = 45$. SD: standard deviation; GPCRND-KOA: guiding principle of clinical research on new drugs in the treatment of KOA score; KOA: knee osteoarthritis.

TABLE 4: Comparison of knee circumference.

Variable	Month 1		Month 7	
	Mean	95% CI	Mean	95% CI
Trial group	38.32	37.07~39.56	37.22	36.24~38.19
Control group	40.30	39.95~41.64	39.10	38.39~40.19
P value	0.03		0.007	

*Adjusted means or proportions and confidence intervals (CI) from multi-level models (ANCOVA or GEE) with fixed effects. All data are intended to treat. Both groups $n = 45$. SD: standard deviation; GPCRND-KOA: guiding principle of clinical research on new drugs in the treatment of KOA score; KOA: knee osteoarthritis.

Both the total GPCRND-KOA score and reduction in knee circumference were evident in the Deqi sensation of heat-sensitive phenomenon and conventional local superficial heat sensation by applying suspended moxibustion. What is more important is that our trial result conforms to the theory of TCM, "the arrival of meridian Qi ensures the therapeutic effects." The effectiveness of the Deqi sensation group might be more superior than the non-Deqi sensation

one in the treatment of KOA. In a word, this study is aimed at providing scientific evidence for the Deqi sensation of moxibustion and at showing that heat-sensitive moxibustion sensation is essential to achieve the preferable treatment effects for KOA.

Authors' Contribution

Rixi Chen and Mingren Chen obtained fund of the research project. Jun Xiong wrote the final paper. Tongsheng Su, Jianhua Sun, Meiqi Zhou Zhenhai Chi, Dingyi Xie, and Bo Zhang contributed to the trial implement. All authors read and approved the final paper.

Acknowledgment

This study was supported by the Major State Basic Research Development Program of China (Grant no. 2009CB522902).

References

[1] C. Xinnong, *Chinese Acupuncture and Moxibustion*, Foreign Languages Press, Beijing, China, 1999.

[2] A. Tiplt, H. Tessenow, and D. Irnich, "Lingshu research and the interpretation of clinical trials in acupuncture," *Deutsche Zeitschrift für Akupunktur*, vol. 52, no. 1, pp. 12–18, 2009.

[3] K. K. S. Hui, E. E. Nixon, M. G. Vangel et al., "Characterization of the "deqi" response in acupuncture," *BMC Complementary and Alternative Medicine*, vol. 7, article 33, 2007.

[4] H. M. Langevin, D. L. Churchill, J. R. Fox, G. J. Badger, B. S. Garra, and M. H. Krag, "Biomechanical response to acupuncture needling in humans," *Journal of Applied Physiology*, vol. 91, no. 6, pp. 2471–2478, 2001.

[5] R.-X. Chen and M.-F. Kang, "Key point of moxibustion, arrival of qi produces curative effect," *Zhongguo Zhen Jiu*, vol. 28, no. 1, pp. 44–46, 2008.

[6] H. Park, J. Park, H. Lee, and H. Lee, "Does Deqi (needle sensation) exist?" *American Journal of Chinese Medicine*, vol. 30, no. 1, pp. 45–50, 2002.

[7] J. Kong, R. Gollub, T. Huang et al., "Acupuncture De Qi, from qualitative history to quantitative measurement," *Journal of Alternative and Complementary Medicine*, vol. 13, no. 10, pp. 1059–1070, 2007.

[8] M. Fink and M. Karst, "Needling sensations following real and placebo acupuncture—a randomised single-blinded two-period cross-over pilot study," *Deutsche Zeitschrift für Akupunktur*, vol. 48, no. 2, pp. 6–10, 2005.

[9] C. Siedentopf, I. A. Haala, and F. Koppelstätter, "Placebo-laser kontrollierte, computer gesteuerte doppelblind-untersuchung—neue ansätze für die akupunktur-grund-lagenforschung," *Deutsche Zeitschrift für Akupunktur*, vol. 48, no. 1, pp. 18–23, 2005.

[10] M. Weber, "Nadeln aus Licht—vorstellung einer neuen thera-piemethode," *Deutsche ZeitschRiFt für Akupunktur*, vol. 48, no. 1, pp. 24–32, 2005.

[11] R. X. Chen and M. F. Kang, *Acupuncture Point Heat-Sensitization Moxibustion: A New Therapy*, People's Medical, Beijing, China, 1st edition, 2006.

[12] R. X. Chen, M. R. Chen, and M. F. Kang, *A Practical Textbook of Heat-Sensitive Moxibustion Therapy*, People's Medical, Beijing, China, 1st edition, 2009.

[13] R.-X. Chen and M.-F. Kang, "Clinical application of acupoint heat-sensitization," *Zhongguo Zhen Jiu*, vol. 27, no. 3, pp. 199–202, 2007.

[14] M. F. Kang, R. X. Chen, and Y. Fu, "Observation on cura-tive effect of moxibustion on heat-sensitive points on knee osteoarthritis," *Jiangxi Journal of Traditional Chinese Medicine and Pharmacy*, vol. 18, pp. 27–28, 2006.

[15] S. H. Huang, B. J. Feng, P. Yu, L. Fan, and Z. H. Xu, "Therapeutic effect of heat-sensitive moxibustion knee osteoarthritis: an observation of 35 cases," *Journal of New Chinese Medicine*, vol. 41, pp. 86–89, 2009.

[16] S. Q. Mo, "Observation of heat-sensitive moxibustion plus abdomen acupuncture on knee osteoarthritis," *Journal of External Therapy of Traditional Chinese Medicine*, vol. 18, pp. 44–45, 2009.

[17] J. J. Peng, "Clinical research of the treatment of Bushen Huoxue formula combined with heat-sensitive moxibustion for patients with knee osteoarthritis," *Youjiang Medical Journal*, vol. 38, pp. 260–262, 2010.

[18] X. Y. Zhen, Ed., *The Guideline of the Latest Chinese Herbs to Clinical Research*, Medicine Science and Technology Press of China, Beijing, China, 1st edition, 2002.

[19] X. J. Wang, J. C. Liu, Y. Y. Zhou, Y. Zhao, Y. J. Wang, and X. J. Zhang, "The establishment and evaluation of knee osteoarthritis and function assessment scale," *Yunnan Journal of Traditional Chinese Medicine*, vol. 28, no. 8, pp. 34–36, 2011.

[20] J. J. Nicholas, F. H. Taylor, R. B. Buckingham, and D. Ottonello, "Measurement of circumference of the knee with ordinary tape measure," *Annals of the Rheumatic Diseases*, vol. 35, no. 3, pp. 282–284, 1976.

[21] R. X. Chen, C. Mingren, and M. F. Kang, *Heat-Sensitive Mox-ibustion Therapy*, People's Medical, Beijing, China, 1st edition, 2013.

[22] G. W. Lu, "Characteristics of afferent fiber innervation on acupuncture points zusanli," *The American Journal of Physiol-ogy*, vol. 245, no. 4, pp. R606–612, 1983.

[23] K. M. Wang, S. M. Yao, Y. L. Xian, and Z. L. Hou, "A study on the receptive field of acupoints and the relationship between characteristics of needling sensation and groups of afferent fibres," *Scientia Sinica B*, vol. 28, no. 9, pp. 963–971, 1985.

[24] W. Lin and P. Wang, *Experimental Acupuncture*, Shanghai Scientific and Technology, Shanghai, China, 1999.

Hindawi Publishing Corporation
Evidence-Based Complementary and Alternative Medicine
Volume 2013, Article ID 718593, 6 pages
http://dx.doi.org/10.1155/2013/718593

Hindawi

Research Article

Influence of the Deqi Sensation by Suspended Moxibustion Stimulation in Lumbar Disc Herniation: Study for a Multicenter Prospective Two Arms Cohort Study

Rixin Chen,[1] Mingren Chen,[1] Jun Xiong,[1] Tongsheng Su,[2] Meiqi Zhou,[3] Jianhua Sun,[4] Zhenhai Chi,[1] Bo Zhang,[1] and Dingyi Xie[1]

[1] The Affiliated Hospital with Jiangxi University of TCM, No. 445 Bayi Avenue, Nanchang, China
[2] Shanxi TCM Hospital, Xi'an, China
[3] The First Affiliated Hospital with Anhui University of TCM, Hefei, China
[4] Jiangsu TCM Hospital, Nanjing, China

Correspondence should be addressed to Rixin Chen; chenrixin321@163.com

Received 10 May 2013; Accepted 24 June 2013

Academic Editor: Fan-Rong Liang

Moxibustion stimulates the Deqi (Qi arrival) phenomenon. Many clinical observations have documented that the character of the Deqi was a composite heat-sensitive moxibustion sensation. In this prospective multicentre comparative observational nonrandomized study, 92 patients with moderate to severe LDH were included. This study consisted of two parallel arms (A: heat-sensitive moxibustion sensation group; B: nonheat-sensitive moxibustion sensation group). Moxibustion was applied in the following three acupuncture points simultaneously: Da Changshu (BL25), Wei Zhong (BL40), and A-Shi acupuncture point (tenderness). The adjusted mean total Modified-JOA score showed significant differences between the groups in the first week (10.32 ± 4.27 95% CI [9.23 ~ 11.40] versus control group 12.42 ± 5.02 [11.62 ~ 13.69], $P = 0.03$). The outcome in the second week also presented significant differences in both groups (7.62 ± 4.80 [6.46 ~ 8.77] versus 10.56 ± 4.75 [9.35 ~ 11.76], $P = 0.005$). Significant differences were also manifested in the follow-up period ($P = 0.007$). It can be inferred that the existence of the Deqi (heat-sensitive moxibustion sensation) phenomenon in the process of suspended moxibustion is closely related to the curative effect, and arrival of heat-sensitive moxibustion sensation could improve the clinical curative effect of moxibustion.

1. Background

Lumbar disc herniation (LDH) is one of the major chronic musculoskeletal diseases that are highly prevalent. In China, about 10%~15% patients with low back pain were diagnosed with LDH [1]. It seriously affects patient's quality of life (QoL) and leads to economic burden [2, 3]. Epidemiological studies from several countries showed that the prevalence of LDH frequently appeared in adults at the age of 30~55 [4]. LDH causes symptoms of sciatica and possible foot pain, numbness, or weakness. In most of the cases, a conservative attitude with different types of physiotherapy is preferred as the first choice [5, 6]. Most of patients with low back pain responded well to conservative therapy [7]. Absolute indications for surgery include altered bladder function and progressive muscle weakness, but these are rare. Therefore, many studies have already reported encouraging results in the treatment of LDH by acupuncture and moxibustion [8].

Moxibustion is a traditional Chinese method of treatment, which applies the heat generated by burning moxa (it is also called Mugwort or Moxa) to stimulate on the acupuncture points. Suspended moxibustion is commonly used, and it refers to application of the burning moxa stick on the acupuncture points at a distance. The results of a recent meta-analysis of six randomized controlled trials (RCTs) on moxibustion for LDH manifested that moxibustion presented a favorable effect on LDH symptom scores compared with that of the drug [RR = 1.91, 95% CI (1.01, 3.60)] [9].

According to traditional Chinese medicine (TCM), the Deqi is the key point to the clinical efficacy of acupuncture and moxibustion [10]. The Deqi is a term originated from *Huangdi Neijing*, also known as "Qi arrival." In the part of *Miraculous pivot, the chapter of nine needles and twelve sources* said: "The key point of acupuncture is the arrival of Qi, it ensures therapeutic effect. It resembles the wind over blows the cloud, soon the sky is clear." [11]. The Deqi's primary connotation is the endogenous Qi of regulation stimulated by acupuncture and moxibustion, which is closely related to the curative effect [12]. When Qi arrives at one part of the body, it can treat the diseases nearby.

Numerous studies have now shown that moxibustion stimulation stimulated a unique Deqi, heat-sensitive moxibustion sensation [13, 14]. In the process of moxibustion treatment, the researchers discovered that, when human body is in morbid condition, related acupuncture points were quite sensitive to moxa's heat and produced nonlocal or nonsuperficial heat sensation, such as penetrating heat, expanding heat, and transmitting heat [15]. This phenomenon resembles the one that occurs when the Deqi appears after moxibustion rather than local heat sensation and surface glow of the skin. The researchers named the phenomenon as heat-sensitive phenomenon of moxibustion or acupuncture point's heat-sensitive phenomenon, and it belongs to the Deqi phenomenon of moxibustion therapy [16].

However, there is lack of experimental data to indicate the difference of heat-sensitive moxibustion sensation (the Deqi stimulated by moxibustion) compared with conventional local superficial heat sensation (non-Deqi by moxibustion stimulation). For LDH especially, is it necessary for moxibustion to produce the phenomenon of obtaining Qi in order to improve the curative effect? Therefore, it would be valuable to know whether there is difference between the moxibustion sensations in the treatment of LDH. Therefore, we planned the rigorous multi centre prospective cohort study trial to investigate the difference.

2. Methods

2.1. Objective.
The aim of this study is to determine the effectiveness of heat-sensitive moxibustion sensation and non-heat-sensitive moxibustion sensation in the treatment of patients with moderate to severe LDH in China.

2.2. Sample Size.
The effective rate was used to determine sample size. There are few reports in the literature of clinical trials of control mode for LDH. Based on our earlier randomized controlled pretrial in the Affiliated Hospital of Jiangxi University of TCM, we believe that the effective rate for LDH is approximately 45% when adopting the non-heat-sensitive moxibustion sensation and should be increased to 75% when using the heat-sensitive moxibustion sensation. Based on 90% power at $P = 0.05$, 38 participants were included in each group to be calculated with the SPSS 13.0 programme. 20% loss was allowed to follow up a total of 46 participants were included in each group, with 92 participants in total.

Moreover,

$$n = \left\{ \frac{Z_{1-\alpha}\sqrt{2pq} + Z_{1-\beta}\sqrt{p_1(1-p_1) + p_2(1-p_2)}}{p_1 - p_2} \right\}^2,$$

$$p = \frac{(p_1 + p_2)}{2} \quad q = 1 - p. \tag{1}$$

2.3. Design.
The patients were referred by the doctors and acupuncturists from branch centers in Nanchang, Hefei, Nanjing, and Xian. Their patients were recruited at either outpatient service or inpatient department and had already made their own choice of moxibustion therapy. Thus, the acupuncture point's Deqi sensation towards manipulation of suspend moxibustion generated the groups to be compared. In trial group, patients felt the Deqi sensation when the acupuncture point was stimulated by moxibustion heat. In the control group, patients only felt local superficial heat sensation (non-Deqi sensation) when the acupuncture point was stimulated by moxibustion heat.

2.4. Participants

2.4.1. Recruitment.
Patients were recruited in China for this nonrandomized prospective multicentre open comparative cohort study from November 27, 2009, to December 27, 2010. This trial protocol has been approved by local institutional review boards and ethics committees (code issued is 2008(11)) and follows the principles of the Declaration of Helsinki (Edinburgh Version 2000). Oral and written informed consent was obtained after verbal information about the study was provided by the physician.

2.4.2. Inclusion Criteria.
Participants were included if they fulfilled the following conditions: (1) participants were diagnosed with LDH according to the guiding principles of clinical research on new drugs [17]; (2) participants were at the age of 18 to 65; participants suffered from moderate to severe LDH, according to the Modified-JOA criteria (>10 score). Standards of diagnosis were listed as follows: (1) pain occurred in lower back and radiated to the lower limb; (2) limitations of tender point; straight leg raising test and it's strengthen test are positive; (3) skin sensation, muscle strength, and tendon reflex had some changes; (4) changes in spinal posture; (5) X-lateral lumbar spine films showed scoliosis or lumbar lordosis; (6) CT suggestive of disc herniation. Participants were instructed to stop LDH symptomatic relief medication during the run-in and treatment periods and provided the usual care instruction for LDH.

2.4.3. Exclusion Criteria.
Patients with any of the following conditions were excluded: (1) patients suffered from serious life-threatening disease, such as the heart disease and disease of brain blood vessels, liver, kidney, or hematopoietic system, and psychotic patients; (2) pregnant women or women in lactation; (3) patients suffered from a single nerve palsy or cauda

Evidence-Based Complementary and Alternative Medicine

3

equina nerve palsy, patients suffered from muscle paralysis or rectum, and Patients presented bladder symptoms; (4) patients complicated with lumbar spinal canal stenosis and space-occupying lesions for other reasons; (5) patients complicated with lumbar spine tumors, infections, tuberculosis, and so forth; (6) patients complicated with moxibustion syncope and unwilling to be treated with moxibustion; (7) patients signed no informed consent.

2.4.4. Interventions and Comparison. Qualified specialists of acupuncture in TCM with at least five years of clinical experience performed the moxibustion in this study. All treatment regimens were standardized between four centers practitioners by means of video, hands-on training, and internet workshops. Both groups of patients were requested to receive no other treatments such as physical therapies, pain-killing medicines, or acupuncture treatment from other places.

In the two groups, 22 millimeter (diameter) × 120 millimeter (length) moxa sticks (made by Jiangxi Provincial TCM Hospital, China) were adopted. The patient usually lied in the comfortable supine position for treatment, with room temperature of 24°C ~ 30°C. Moxibustion was applied simultaneously on the following three acupuncture points: Da Changshu (BL25), Wei Zhong (BL40), and A-Shi Xue (tenderness). The suspended moxibustion was applied 3 centimetre, far from the surface of skin to search for the heat-sensitive moxibustion sensation.

2.4.5. The Heat-Sensitive Moxibustion Sensation Group. In this group, the three acupuncture points were brought mild warmth without burning by moxa sticks and manipulated until the patient reported the characteristic heat sensitization sensation that is commonly called Deqi. Patients felt comfortable in the moxibustion manipulation.

The following patients' sensation suggested the Deqi: penetrating heat sensation due to moxa heat, defined as the heat sensation conducted from the moxa local skin surface into deep tissue, or even into the joint cavity; expanding heat sensation due to moxa heat, defined as the heat sensation spreading the surrounding little by little around the moxa point; transmitting heat sensation due to moxa heat, defined as the heat sensation transferring along some pathway or direction, even to the ankle or hip conduction. In the course of manipulation, the therapist continued for 15 minutes in pertreatment session. Patients received the treatment two times/day in the 1st week (one time/day from the 2nd week) for a total of 18 sessions over 14 days.

2.4.6. The Non-Heat-Sensitive Moxibustion Sensation Group. Common practices were similar to the first group. Only one difference was that patients in this group felt local superficial heat sensation. No Deqi sensations were stimulated in this group.

2.4.7. Outcome Measure. The primary outcome in this trial was measured by Modified-JOA scale. The scale was proposed by Improvement Japanese Orthopaedic Association and was

known as the modified edition of JOA Back Pain Evaluation Questionnaire [18]. This scoring system was previously validated [19]. The degree of LDH was divided into three levels: mild: <10, moderate: 10 to 20, and severe: >20. The outcome measured above was assessed before the treatment, 14 days of the last moxibustion session, and 6 months after the last moxibustion session.

2.4.8. Statistical Methods. The statistician was blinded from the allocation of groups. SPSS13.0 and SAS9.0 statistical software packages were used to analyze the data. Statistical analyses were based on the intention-to-treat (ITT) principle, including all patients with baseline values to receive treatment. All tests were exploratory and two-sided with a level of significance of 5%.

We used multilevel models in analysis of covariance (ANCOVA) or generalized estimating equations (GEE). In these models, physicians were considered random effect, and fixed effects were baseline value (continuous), duration of low back pain, patient's age and gender, body mass index (BMI), and Modified-JOA score (continuous). Results are presented as adjusted mean or proportioned with a standard error (SE) and/or 95% confidence interval (CI).

2.4.9. Adverse Events. We defined adverse events as unfavorable or unintended signs; however, symptoms or disease occurred after treatment was not necessarily related to the moxibustion intervention. Adverse events were analyzed descriptively by frequencies, percentages, and Chi-squared or Fisher's exact test (if feasible).

3. Results

3.1. Population and Baseline. Of 290 screened patients, 120 could not be included in the study, mainly because they did not meet all eligibility criteria (Figure 1). After searching for the Deqi, 112 patients experienced heat-sensitive moxibustion sensation; 58 patients had no Deqi sensation. Since a sample of 92 people was calculated in our trial, we selected 46 patients from each queue separately by random drawing.

After six months, data from 89 participants (44 in the trial group and 45 in the control group) were available. Reasons for missing follow-up data included refusal of further participation or being not contactable.

Patient preferences resulted in the following baseline differences: patients in the trial group showed more severe BMI scores, while the Modified-JOA score was higher in the control group. The females of the trial group were more than those of control group. For duration of low back pain, there were obviously differences among the two treatment groups (Table 1). These differences of baseline characteristics were similar to the patients who were still available to be assessed at the 7th month.

3.2. Outcome Parameters. After one week, the primary outcome parameter Modified-JOA score showed significant differences between groups: trial group 10.32±4.27 ((adjusted mean ± SE) 95% CI [9.23 ~ 11.40] versus control group

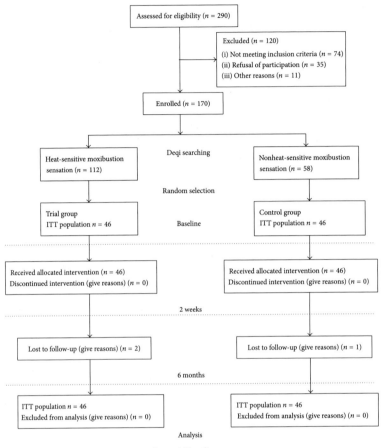

FIGURE 1: Flow diagram.

12.42 ± 5.02 [11.62 ~ 13.69], P = 0.03) (Table 2). Total Modified-JOA score was significantly lower in the trial group in the second week (7.62 ± 4.80 [6.46 ~ 8.77 versus 10.56 ± 4.75 [9.35 ~ 11.76], P = 0.005). Significant differences in total Modified-JOA score were observed between the groups, also evident during the follow-up period (P = 0.007).

3.3. *Safety.* No adverse events were reported for the 92 participants.

4. Discussions

The comparison of the trial group and control group in this study revealed differences that were statistically significant and clinically relevant in terms of efficacy in reducing Modified-JOA score. The relative change in the mean Modified-JOA score among the heat-sensitive moxibustion sensation group was 10.32 (SE 4.27), compared with 12.42 (SE 5.02) among the non-heat-sensitive moxibustion sensation group in the first week. In the second week, the trend of the differences was enlarged. In addition, significant differences in total Modified-JOA score were observed between the groups, which were also evident during the follow-up period.

To make the most of our knowledge, our study is the largest reported cohort study that compared effectiveness of heat-sensitive moxibustion sensation group with the non-heat-sensitive moxibustion sensation one in the treatment of patients with LDH. Both the evaluation of the results and

Hindawi Publishing Corporation
Evidence-Based Complementary and Alternative Medicine
Volume 2012, Article ID 696498, 7 pages
doi:10.1155/2012/696498

Research Article

Is There Difference between the Effects of Two-Dose Stimulation for Knee Osteoarthritis in the Treatment of Heat-Sensitive Moxibustion?

Rixin Chen,[1] Mingren Chen,[1] Jun Xiong,[1] Zhenhai Chi,[1] Meiqi Zhou,[2] Tongsheng Su,[3] Jianhua Sun,[4] Fan Yi,[1] and Bo Zhang[1]

[1] *Acupuncture and Rehabilitation Department, The Affiliated Hospital, Jiangxi University of TCM, 445 Bayi Avenue, Nanchang 330006, China*
[2] *Acupuncture Department, The First Affiliated Hospital, Anhui University of TCM, Hefei 330006, China*
[3] *Acupuncture Department, Shanxi TCM Hospital, Xian 330006, China*
[4] *Acupuncture Department, Jiangsu TCM Hospital, Nanjing 330006, China*

Correspondence should be addressed to Rixin Chen, chenrixin123@yahoo.com.cn

Received 29 January 2012; Revised 27 March 2012; Accepted 3 April 2012

Academic Editor: Wolfgang Weidenhammer

Considering that the dosage of manipulating Moxa plays an important role in obtaining good effects for heat-sensitive moxibustion, it would be valuable to know whether the use of fixed dosage is as effective as the use of an individual one. The paper carried out a rigorous multi-centre randomized controlled trial, and its result demonstrated that the effectiveness of individual eliminate-sensitive dosing regimen might more superior to the stable conventional dosing regimen in the treatment of KOA. According the record of individual moxibustion time, the dosage differed in the terms of patients' conditions and moxibustion sensation, which had been measured about 47.30 ± 6.20 minutes ($28 \sim 65$ minutes).

1. Background

Suspended moxibustion is a traditional Chinese medical intervention that involves the burning of moxa indirectly at the acupoints. Moxibustion has anti-inflammatory or immunomodulatory effects against chronic inflammatory conditions in humans [1]. Heat-sensitive moxibustion therapy is one of common suspended moxibustion treatments in China [2]. A great deal of physicians utilized heat-sensitive moxibustion therapy in different kinds of diseases in China. Moreover, several articles and research reports have reported the effectiveness and safety of heat-sensitive moxibustion for KOA [3–8].

Moxibustion uses heat stimulation at various temperature levels from mild skin warming to tissue damage from burning. Therefore, the dose of manipulating Moxa plays an important role in obtaining good effects. The regimen of moxibustion used for treatment of KOA has varied between studies.

To sum up, two main regimens were carried out in these papers. One selected the stable conventional dose, which was recommended by the universal text book [1]. The therapy was executed for 15 minutes per acupoint. The other one held that the dose differed in the terms of patients' conditions and moxibustion sensation. Treatment sessions should be ended when patients felt the acupoint heat-sensitization phenomenon disappeared. We called it individual eliminate-sensitive dose. Therefore, it would be valuable to know whether there is difference between the effects of two-dose stimulation for KOA in the treatment of heat-sensitive moxibustion. We planned the rigorous multicentre randomized controlled trial, in order to seek for optimal dose of the best therapeutic effect.

2. Methods

2.1. Objective. The aim of this study is to compare the effectiveness of an individual eliminate-sensitive dose and a stable conventional dose in the treatment of patients with moderate to severe swelling KOA in China.

2.2. Sample Size. The sample size for testing the difference between means was calculated with the SPSS 13.0 programme, by setting the standard deviation of the guiding principle of clinical research on new drugs in the treatment of KOA (GPCRND-KOA) [9] score of 2.55 and 3.39 [5, 6] and mean difference of total GPCRND-KOA score between groups of 2.50, power of 0.9, and a level of significance at 0.05. Allowing for a 20% loss to follow up, a total of 36 participants were required in each group, with 72 participants in total.

2.3. Design. A multicentre (four centers in China), randomized, and assessor blinded, controlled trial was conducted at the Affiliated Hospital with Jiangxi University of Traditional Chinese Medicine (TCM) in Nanchang, The first Affiliated Hospital with Anhui University of TCM in Hefei, Jiangsu TCM Hospital in Nanjing, and Shanxi TCM Hospital in Xian. The study was sequentially conducted as follows: a run-in period of one week prior to randomization, a treatment period of 30 days, and a follow-up period of six months. At the end of the run-in period, participants were randomized to the individual eliminate-sensitive dose group or the stable conventional dose group by the central randomization system. This system was provided by China Academy of Chinese Medical Sciences, which adopted the computer telephone integration (CTI) technology to integrate computer, internet, and telecom. The random number list was assigned by interactive voice response (IVR) and interactive web response (IWR) [10]. The success of blinding was assessed at each participant's last visit. Data collection staff, and data analysts were blinded to treatment group.

2.4. Participants

2.4.1. Recruitment. A total of 72 eligible patients were enrolled in the study between December 30, 2009, and March 18, 2010, from this multisite. The ethics committees of the Affiliated Hospital with Jiangxi University of TCM approved the study.

2.4.2. Inclusion Criteria. Eligible participants were those previously diagnosed with moderate to severe swelling KOA, according to the GPCRND-KOA criteria (>5 score). Patients were required to complete the baseline KOA diary. Written informed consent was obtained from each participant. The inclusion criteria restricted the following conditions. According with the below KOA diagnosis standard, meanwhile, knee joints appeared swell; Floating patella test was negative; patients accepted the treatment protocol in this trial; acupoint heat-sensitization phenomenon existed in the region consisting of Yin Lingquan (SP9), Yang Lingquan (GB34), Liang Qiu (ST34), and Xue Hai (SP10). Patients had been stopped receiving previous intervention before recruitment for two weeks.

2.4.3. Exclusion Criteria. Participants were excluded if they suffer from serious life-threatening disease, such as disease of the heart and brain blood vessels, liver, kidney, and hematopoietic system, and psychotic patients. We excluded patients with diabetes, diabetic polyneuropathy, and polyneuropathic disturbances. Participants were not being eligible if the females are in the duration of pregnancy or lactation. The following conditions were also excluded items: acute knee joint trauma or ulceration in its local skin, complicated with serious genu varus/valgus and flexion contraction.

2.5. Study Interventions. Qualified specialists of acupuncture in TCM with at least five years of clinical experience performed the moxibustion in this study. All treatment regimens were standardized between four centers practitioners via video, hands-on training, and internet workshops. Both groups of patients were requested not to receive other treatments including any physical therapies, any pain-killing medicines, and acupuncture treatment from another place.

In the two groups, 22 mm (diameter) × 120 mm (length) moxa-sticks (Jiangxi TCM Hospital, China) were used. The patient was usually in the comfortable supine position for treatment, with 24°C~30°C temperature in the room. He should be wearing loose trousers, especially making his knee joints exposed.

2.5.1. The Individual Eliminate-Sensitive Dose Group. For the group, the moxa-sticks were lit by the therapist and held over the region consisting of Yin Lingquan (SP9), Yang Lingquan (GB34), Liang Qiu (ST34), and Xue Hai (SP10). The warming suspended moxibustion lied 3 cm far from the surface of skin was used to search the acupoint heat-sensitization phenomenon. The areas were brought mild warmth without burning by moxa-sticks and manipulated until the patient reported the characteristic heat sensitization sensation, said to indicate effective moxibustion, that is commonly called De Qi. Patients felt comfortable in the moxibustion manipulation.

The following patients sensation suggested the special heat sensitization acupoint: diathermanous sensation due to moxa-heat, defining as the heat sensation conducting from the moxa local skin surface into deep tissue, or even into the joint cavity; expand heat sensation due to moxa-heat, defining as the heat sensation spreading the surrounding little by little around the moxa point; transfer heat sensation due to moxa-heat, defining as the heat sensation transferring along some pathway or direction, even to the ankle or hip conduction. When some acupoint existed one below sensation at least, the therapists marked the point as heat-sensitive acupoint. We tried our best to seek all the special acupoints in each patient by the repeated manipulation.

After obtaining the heat sensitization sensation, the therapists began to treat patient's at these heat-sensitive acupoints. There was a therapist working on the patient for the whole time of moxibustion. For moxibustion manipulation, the intensity of the given stimulation was varied with heat-sensitive sensation. Treatment sessions ended when patients felt the acupoint heat-sensitization phenomenon disappeared.

In the course of manipulation, the therapist recorded the time length of every patient from the beginning to the end in per treatment session. Patients received the treatment two times/day in the 1st week (one time/day from the 2nd week) for a total of 35 sessions over 30 days.

2.5.2. The Stable Conventional Dose Group. Common practices were similar with the first group. Only one difference was that patients in this group received the identical dose (15 minutes).

2.6. Outcome Measures. Ministry of Health of the People's Republic of China (MHPRC) has proposed the guiding principle of clinical research on new drugs (GPCRND) [9]. In this criteria, a patient with KOA was assessed including pain, the relation between activity and pain, function impairment, and special exams. This scoring system was previously validated. The degree of KOA is divided into three levels: mild—<5 scores; moderate—5~9 scores; severe—>9 scores. In the terms of swelling knee, knee circumference was assessed at each time point. The parameter was measured in centimeters across the middle of a patella, with ordinary tape measure [11].

Therapeutic effect was assessed by comparing baseline and final conditions reported by the patient. This trial also recorded adverse effects reported by patients during treatment. The outcome measures above were assessed before the treatment (month 0), at the end of the treatment period (month 1), and 6 months after the end of the treatment period (month 7).

2.7. Statistical Methods. We conducted analysis on an intention-to-treat basis, including all randomized participants with at least one measurable outcome report. Analyses will be conducted using 2-sided significance tests at the 5% significance level. The statistician conducting the analyses remained blind to treatment group and data was only unblended once all data summarized and analyses were completed. All analyses were conducted in the SAS statistical package program (ver.9.1.3).

Baseline characteristics were shown as mean standard deviation (SD) for continuous data including age, previous duration, and others. As for participants' gender, n (%) of male and female in each group were shown as baseline characteristics. We will consider $P < 0.05$ as statistically significant.

Outcome measures were summarized descriptively (mean, SD, median, minimum, and maximum) at each time point by treatment group. The t-test, Mann-Whitney U, and Wilcoxon test were used for comparison of variables, as appropriate. All adverse events reported during the study were included in the case report forms; the incidence of adverse events were calculated. Missing data was replaced according to the principle of the last observation carried forward.

2.8. Adverse Events. We defined adverse events as unfavorable or unintended signs, symptoms, or disease occurring after treatment that were not necessarily related to the moxibustion intervention.

2.9. Ethics. Written consent was obtained from each participant. The study was conducted by a coordination center at the Affiliated Hospital with Jiangxi University of TCM in Nanchang and was approved by the Ethics Committee of the Affiliated Hospital of Jiangxi University of TCM.

3. Results

3.1. Recruitment and Baseline. Participants 42~70 years of age were recruited from outpatient and inpatient in four centers. Of 288 screened patients, 216 could not be included in the study, mainly because they did not meet all eligibility criteria (Figure 1). Thus, 72 patients were randomly assigned into 2 treatment groups by 30 investigators. In follow-up visit, two patients dropped out of the study. One was in the individual eliminate-sensitive dose: because of falling injury of Legs. One patient in the stable conventional dose group was lost because of requiring another treatment in other hospitals. We also questioned patients about the intake of medication. Of 34 patients receiving pharmaceutical intervention before recruitment, 20 took NSAIDS such as ibuprofen, and Naprosyn; 14 were treated by glucosamine/chondroitin. There were no pretreatment differences among the two treatment groups at baseline (Table 1).

3.2. Outcome

3.2.1. Total GPCRND-KOA Score. Reductions in mean total GPCRND-KOA score at months 1 and 7 compared to baseline were observed and were highly significant ($P < 0.001$ for all comparisons). At both time points, there was highly significant difference between the groups ($P < 0.01$) as shown in Table 2. Figure 2 shows that the mean total GPCRND-KOA score of both groups reduced sharply at the first month then remained decreasing to the end of month 7.

3.2.2. Knee Circumference. Reductions in mean knee circumference at months 1 and 7 compared to baseline were observed and were significant ($P < 0.05$ for all comparisons). At both time points, there was significant difference between the groups ($P < 0.05$) as shown in Table 3. Figure 3 shows that the mean knee circumference of both groups reduced a few at the first month then remained decreasing to the end of month 7.

3.3. Moxibustion Time in the Experimental Group. Different from the control group, moxibustion dose was individual in the experimental group. According the record of individual moxibustion time, the dose differed in the terms of patients' conditions and moxibustion sensation, which had been measured about 28~65 minutes in the treatment of KOA.

TABLE 1: Baseline characteristics of KOA patients.

	Individual group	Stable group
Age, mean (SD), years	58 (8.03)	59 (6.94)
Age, min-max, years		
Age, min-max, years	42~70	45~70
Age >60 year n (%)	14 (38.89%)	12 (33.33%)
Sex n (%)		
Male	8 (22.22%)	6 (16.67%)
Female	28 (77.78%)	30 (83.33%)
Duration of knee pain n (%)		
<5 year	24 (66.67%)	30 (83.33%)
5–10 year	4 (11.11%)	3 (8.33%)
>10 year	8 (22.22%)	3 (8.33%)
BMI, mean (SD), kg/m'	23.08 (2.71)	21.52 (2.43)
BMI, min-max, kg/m'	15.64~31.08	14.98~28.11
GPCRND-KOA grade n (%)		
Severe	24 (67%)	21 (58%)
Moderate	12 (33%)	15 (42%)
Knee circumference at baseline(SD), cm	39.32 (3.43)	39.01 (2.41)
GPCRND-KOA score at baseline		
Total score mean (SD)	11.22 (3.06)	10.14 (3.00)
Pain or discomfort in night score mean (SD)	1.33 (0.68)	1.25 (0.73)
Morning stiffness score mean (SD)	0.97 (0.56)	1.16 (0.51)
Pain or discomfort in walk score mean (SD)	1.67 (0.53)	1.55 (0.64)
Arise from seat score mean (SD)	0.64 (0.49)	0.58 (0.50)
The maximum walk distance score mean (SD)	1.86 (0.90)	1.50 (0.85)
Board standard airstairs score mean (SD)	1.08 (0.55)	1.14 (0.35)
Step down standard airstairs score mean (SD)	1.19 (0.52)	1.05 (0.41)
Squat or bend knees score mean (SD)	1.36 (0.59)	1.17 (0.61)
Walk over rough terrain score mean (SD)	1.06 (0.53)	0.86 (0.42)
Previous treatment (past-half year)		
Pharmaceutical intervention	18 (50.00%)	16 (44.00%)
Physiotherapy	7 (19.44%)	8 (22.22%)
Previous acupuncture treatment	2 (5.56%)	3 (8.33%)

BMI: body mass index; GPCRND-KOA: guiding principle of clinical research on new drugs in the treatment of KOA score; SD: standard deviation; KOA: knee osteoarthritis.

TABLE 2: Comparison of GPCRND-KOA scores at baseline, end of treatment (month 1), and followup (month 7), together with between-group statistical test.

Variable	Baseline			Month 1			Month 7		
	Mean	SD	t-test*	Mean	SD	t-test*	Mean	SD	t-test*
Total									
Individual group	11.22	3.06	1.51	3.44	1.93	4.51	2.19	1.85	6.31
	95% CI = (10.50~11.94)			95% CI = (2.99~3.89)			95% CI = (1.76~2.62)		
Stable group	10.14	3.00		6.13	3.01		5.11	2.07	
	95% CI = (9.44~10.84)			95% CI = (5.42~6.84)			95% CI = (4.62~5.60)		

*t-test of group differences at time period, using independent t-test. All data are intention to treat. Both groups n = 36. SD: standard deviation; GPCRND-KOA: guiding principle of clinical research on new drugs in the treatment of KOA score; KOA: knee osteoarthritis.

Evidence-Based Complementary and Alternative Medicine 5

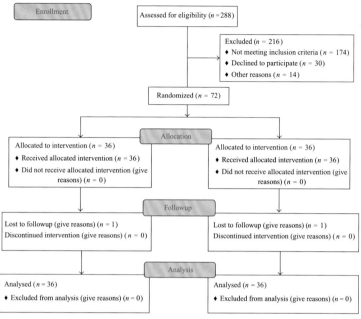

FIGURE 1: Flow diagram.

The range of mean moxibustion dose was about 47.30 ± 6.20 minutes in the experimental group.

3.4. Safety. No adverse events were reported for the 72 participants.

4. Discussions

The results of our study extended those previous trials and demonstrated that patients with KOA who received individual eliminate-sensitive dose had significantly less pain and better function after 1 month than did patients who received stable conventional dose, according to the total GPCRND-KOA score.

After 7 months, exploratory analysis indicated that the differences between the two groups were still significant. Significant differences were also evident for knee circumference.

The side-effects of heat-sensitive moxibustion were not observed. Several large surveys have also provided evidence that moxibustion is a relatively safe treatment [12–14]. To our knowledge, our study is the largest reported randomized controlled trial in this regard. Its strengths included interventions based on expert consensus by qualified and experienced medical acupuncturists, outcome measurements as

recommended in guidelines for trials on KOA, and very high follow-up rates. Our study used central randomization to ensure adequate concealment in group assignment. However, one could argue that our results might have been biased by a lack of sufficient blinding. Due to the nature of the intervention, it was not possible to blind therapists to treatment. Both the evaluation of the results and the statistical analysis were carried out in a blind fashion.

Our results lent support to the findings of two previous smaller trials, one of which were randomized [5] and one was not [6]. The differences in findings might be due to low statistical power in the early trials, use of different measurement instruments and a short-term followup.

Traditionally, different moxibustion techniques were used and suspended moxibustion is the main therapy resulting from the burning of moxa produces the radiant heat and drug effects to acupoints. Heat-sensitive moxibustion is different from other conventional suspended moxibustion treatments. Generally speaking, the conventional suspended moxibustion manipulates a moxa stick in which the moxa stick is placed 2-3 cm from the skin with the intention of mildly warming local sites. Facing different patients, it selects a series of identical and fixed acupoints to treat. And the moxa stick isusually lighted around the acupoints to bring mild warmth to the area without burning, until

Evidence-Based Complementary and Alternative Medicine

TABLE 3: Comparison of Knee circumference scores at baseline, end of treatment (month 1), and followup (month 7), together with between-group statistical test.

Variable	Baseline			Month 1			Month 7		
	Mean	SD	t-test*	Mean	SD	t-test*	Mean	SD	t-test*
Knee circumference, cm									
Individual group	39.32	33.42	0.44	36.21	3.40	2.51	35.81	3.63	2.78
	95% CI = (38.52~40.12)			95% CI = (35.41~37.01)			95% CI = (34.96~36.66)		
Stable group	39.01	2.41		38.03	2.72		37.92	2.74	
	95% CI = (38.44~39.58)			95% CI = (37.39~38.67)			95% CI = (37.28~38.56)		

*t-test of group differences at time period, using independent t-test. All data are intention to treat. Both groups $n = 36$. SD: standard deviation.

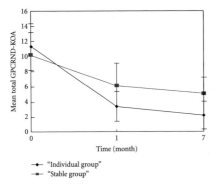

FIGURE 2: Mean total GPCRND-KOA (ITT, intention to treat analysis) at each time point.

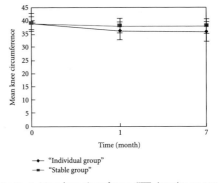

FIGURE 3: Mean knee circumference (ITT, intention to treat analysis) at each time point.

the skin becomes slightly red. In this traditional mode, therapists consider that moxibustion can take effect when the patients feel local and surface heat sensation. Time consumed in this regimen is identical length for various patients. Namely, moxibustion time per acupoint is uniform but not individual. We believe that the potential clinical efficacy of moxibustion cannot be produced by conventional suspended moxibustion treatment. A number of evidences proved heat-sensitive moxibustion were superior to needle acupuncture and conventional suspended moxibustion in clinical practice [2]. The reason is that moxibustion dose in heat-sensitive moxibustion is different from that in conventional sus-pended moxibustion.

Theoretically, three factors have an impact on moxi-bustion dose, including intensity, area, and time. The two former factors are routine as a result of the standard size of moxa stick in practice. Hence, time becomes a variable parameter and plays a quite important part in moxibustion dose. We wonder how long the optimum dose should be obeyed in heat-sensitive moxibustion. The simplest method refers to the stable 15 minutes, which was recommended by the universal text book. In the book of Method of Needling and Moxibustion, which was considered as authoritative

teaching material in moxibustion technique in China [1], a practitioner should light one end of a moxa stick and hold it an inch or two away from the skin, usually around the inserted needles to bring mild warmth to the area without burning, until the skin becomes slightly red. The moxibustion is recommended as 15 minutes in this book. Practitioners use moxa to warm regions and acupuncture points with the intention of stimulating circulation through the points and inducing a smoother flow of blood and qi. It is claimed that moxibustion takes, effect in the body with 15 minutes moxibustion.

In this study, our result supported that the individual eliminate-sensitive dose was likely to become an optimum selected regimen in heat-sensitive moxibustion. The amount of moxibustion per acupoint was not fixed, according to the patient condition and moxibustion sensation. Treat-ment sessions ended when patients felt the acupoint heat-sensitization phenomenon disappeared. Thus, the dose is individual and fit for every patient. It reflects the requirement from patients' bodies. We termed it as individual eliminate-sensitive dose. In our study, the range of mean moixbustion dose was about 47.30 ± 6.20 minutes in the experimental group. The maximum length was 65 minutes, while the

Evidence-Based Complementary and Alternative Medicine

7

shortest one was 28 minutes. As far as we know, the feasibility of such a time intensive treatment can be carried out by normal acupuncture-practitioner's office in China. Many TCM hospitals possessed qualified specialized moxibustion technicians. Meanwhile, various moxibustion devices were used to fix the moxa-sticks and reduced manual labour.

As we all know, KOA is an incurable complaint of musculoskeletal system disease. The aim of initial design was to explore a better dose of heat-sensitive moxibustion in the treatment of KOA. Special theory penetrated in our thought and design, which is the presupposition and basis in this trial. In the human nature, there are two states of acupoints, the stimulated or awake state and the rest state. When the human body suffers form disease, the acupoints on the surface of the body are stimulated and sensitized. These sensitized acupoints are changed into rest ones in the course of treatment. The elimination of heat-sensitization phenomenon is the indication to examine clinical efficacy. Our final results confirmed the theory involving with heat-sensitive moxibustion to some extent. We also found an approach to quantify moxibustion dose individually in clinical practice.

In a word, the result demonstrated that the effectiveness of individual eliminate-sensitive dose might be more superior to the stable conventional dose in the treatment of KOA. Obviously, only 15 minutes in the moxibustion dose was very difficult to show and uncover the real clinical effects of suspend moxibustion therapy. According to the record of individual moxibustion time, the dose differed in the terms of patients' conditions and moxibustion sensation, which had been measured about 28~65 minutes in the treatment of KOA. In future, if we can confirm this conclusion in other diseases. Through more rigorous and scientific evidences, it will be helpful to disclose inherent law of moxibustion.

Conflict of Interests

The authors declare that they have no competing interests.

Authors' Contribution

R. Chen and, M. Chen obtained funding for the research project. J. Xiong, Z. Chi, and B. Zhang drafted the protocol, and J. Xiong wrote the final paper. Z. Chi, S. Tongsheng, S. Jianhua, and Z. Meiqi contributed to the research design and made critical revisions. B. Zhang was responsible for the statistical design of the trial and wrote portions of the statistical methods, data handling, and monitoring sections. All authors read and approved the final paper.

Acknowledgments

This study was supported by the National Natural Science Foundation of China and the Major State Basic Research Development Program of People's Republic of China (Grant no. 2009CB522902) and Jiangxi Key R & D Project.

References

[1] S. K. Lu, *Method of Needling and Moxibustion*, China Publishing House of Traditional Chinese Medicine, Beijing, China, 1st edition, 2002.

[2] R. X. Chen and M. F. Kang, *Acupoint Heat-Sensitive Moxibustion a New Therapy*, People's Medical Publishing House, Beijing, China, 1st edition, 2006.

[3] R. Chen, M. Chen, M. Kang et al., "The design and protocol of heat-sensitive moxibustion for knee osteoarthritis: a multicenter randomized controlled trial on the rules of selecting moxibustion location," *BMC Complementary and Alternative Medicine*, vol. 10, article 32, 2010.

[4] R. Chen, M. Chen, J. Xiong, F. Yi, Z. Chi, and B. Zhang, "Comparison of heat-sensitive moxibustion versus fluticasone/salmeterol (seretide) combination in the treatment of chronic persistent asthma: design of a multicenter randomized controlled trial," *Trials*, vol. 11, article 121, 2010.

[5] M. F. Kang, R. X. Chen, and Y. Fu, "Observation on curative effect of moxibusting on heat-sensitive points on knee osteoarthritis," *Jiangxi Journal of Traditional Chinese Medicine and Pharmacy*, vol. 18, pp. 27–28, 2006.

[6] S. H. Huang, B. J. Feng, P. Yu et al., "Therapeutic effect of heat-sensitive moxibustion knee osteoarthritis: an observation of 35 cases," *Journal of New Chinese Medicine*, vol. 41, pp. 86–89, 2009.

[7] S. Q. Mo, "Observation of heat-sensitive moxibustion plus abdomen acupuncture on knee osteoarthritis," *Journal of External Therapy of TCM*, vol. 18, pp. 44–45, 2009.

[8] J. J. Peng, "Clinical research of the treatment of Bushen Huoxue formula combined with heat-sensitive moxibustion for patients with knee osteoarthritis," *Youjiang Medical Journal*, vol. 38, pp. 260–262, 2010.

[9] X. Y. Zhen, Ed., *The Guideline of the latest Chinese herbs to Clinical Research*, Medicine Science and Technology Press of China, Beijing, China, 1st edition, 2002.

[10] B. Liu, T. Wen, C. Yao et al., "The central randomization system in multi-center clinical trials," *Chinese Journal of New Drugs and Clinical Remedies*, vol. 12, pp. 931–935, 2006.

[11] J. J. Nicholas, F. H. Taylor, R. B. Buckingham, and D. Ottonello, "Measurement of circumference of the knee with ordinary tape measure," *Annals of the Rheumatic Diseases*, vol. 35, no. 3, pp. 282–284, 1976.

[12] A. White, S. Hayhoe, A. Hart, and E. Ernst, "Survey of adverse events following acupuncture (SAFA): a prospective study of 32,000 consultations," *Acupuncture in Medicine*, vol. 19, no. 2, pp. 84–92, 2001, Department of Complementary Medicine, University of Exeter, Exeter, UK.

[13] D. Melchart, W. Weidenhammer, A. Streng et al., "Prospective investigation of adverse effects of acupuncture in 97733 patients," *Archives of Internal Medicine*, vol. 164, no. 1, pp. 104–105, 2004.

[14] H. Yamashita, H. Tsukayama, N. Hori, T. Kimura, and Y. Tanno, "Incidence of adverse reactions associated with acupuncture," *Journal of Alternative and Complementary Medicine*, vol. 6, no. 4, pp. 345–350, 2000.

Original paper

Evaluation of different moxibustion doses for lumbar disc herniation: multicentre randomised controlled trial of heat-sensitive moxibustion therapy

Mingren Chen,[1] Rixin Chen,[1] Jun Xiong,[1] Zhenhai Chi,[1] Jianhua Sun,[2] Tongsheng Su,[3] Meiqi Zhou,[4] Fan Yi,[1] Bo Zhang[1]

► An additional supplementary data is published online only. To view these files please visit the journal online (http://dx.doi.org/10.1136/acupmed-2012-010142).

[1]Department of Acupuncture, Affiliated Hospital with Jiangxi University of Traditional Chinese Medicine, Nanchang, People's Republic of China
[2]Department of Acupuncture, Jiangsu Traditional Chinese Medicine Hospital, Nanjing, People's Republic of China
[3]Department of Acupuncture, Shanxi Traditional Chinese Medicine Hospital, Xian, People's Republic of China
[4]Department of Acupuncture, First Affiliated Hospital with Anhui University of Traditional Chinese Medicine, Hefei, People's Republic of China

Correspondence to
Professor Rixin Chen, Department of Acupuncture, Affiliated Hospital with Jiangxi University of Traditional Chinese Medicine, No. 445 Bayi Avenue, Nanchang City 330006, People's Republic of China; chenrixin123@yahoo.com.cn

Accepted 11 July 2012
Published Online First
1 August 2012

Abstract

Background There is some evidence for the effectiveness of moxibustion for the treatment of lumbar disc herniation (LDH), but it remains unclear what dose is optimal.

Objective To compare the effectiveness of a new technique of individualised 'sensitivity elimination' dose versus a standardised 15 min dose in the treatment of LDH.

Methods This study was a multicentre (four centres in China), randomised, controlled trial with two parallel arms (group A, individualised sensitivity elimination dose; group B, standardised dose). The most heat-sensitised acupuncture point from the triangle bound by BL25 and GV2 was selected. Both groups received 18 sessions over 2 weeks. The outcome was evaluated by Modified Japanese Orthopaedic Association scale (M-JOA) score before and after treatment and at 6-month follow-up examination. All main analyses were by intention to treat.

Results A total of 96 patients were included. A significant difference of total M-JOA score was noted between the groups at weeks 1 and 2 (p<0.05). Significant differences were also evident during the follow-up period (p<0.01). The mean duration of moxibustion was 42.7±5.4 (range, 22–58) minutes in the experimental group.

Conclusions The effectiveness of the individualised sensitivity elimination dose appears superior to the standardised dose in the treatment of LDH. Only 15 min moxibustion in the conventional dose group seemed insufficient to elicit the satisfactory clinical effects obtained by heat-sensitive moxibustion therapy. However, in view of some limitations of this study further research is necessary before this can be stated conclusively.

Trial Registration Controlled Clinical Trials: ChiCTR-TRC-09000602.

BACKGROUND

Heat-sensitive moxibustion therapy is a common method of 'suspended moxibustion' treatment in China.[1] Suspended moxibustion is a traditional Chinese medical intervention that involves burning of moxa indirectly at the acupuncture points. Moxibustion has anti-inflammatory and immunomodulatory effects against chronic inflammatory conditions in humans.[2] Moxibustion as treatment of lumbar disc herniation (LDH) exerts diverse therapeutic effects and its mechanisms are suggested by the observations that moxibustion can improve local blood circulation, eliminate nerve root inflammation and oedema, soften adhesions and reduce protrusion of the nerve root, thereby promoting nerve injury repair.[3] Moreover, the heat of moxa treatment improves microcirculation in the lumbar vertebrae.[4]

The treatment may be used for various diseases in one particular way, at 'heat-sensitised' acupuncture points. In humans, it is believed that there are two states of acupuncture points, that is, the sensitised or 'awake' state and the resting state. According to this theory, in the presence of disease, acupuncture points on the body surface are stimulated and become sensitive. The sensitive areas are susceptible to heat stimulation and called 'heat-sensitised points'. One of the characteristics of these areas is that they are specific or closely related to acupuncture points, and behave similarly in clinical observations, that is, 'small stimulation induces a large response'.

Thus, according to the current theory of heat-sensitive moxibustion, disease within the body can be reflected in acupuncture points of the body surface.[1] We have identified this phenomenon in certain areas in patients with LDH. The triangular region bordered by bilateral *Dachangshu* (BL25) and *Yaoshu* (GV2) is the most common. Several articles have reported the effectiveness and safety of heat-sensitive moxibustion for LDH.[5–9]

Unlike acupuncture stimulation, which involves thrusting or twisting needles resulting in various biochemical reactions that can have effects throughout the body, moxibustion uses heat stimulation at various temperature levels from mild skin warming to tissue

Acupunct Med 2012;**30**:266–272. doi:10.1136/acupmed-2012-010142

damage from burning. The dose of moxa plays an important role in obtaining good effects. The regimen of moxibustion used for treatment of LDH has varied among studies, essentially in two main regimens. One uses a standardised dose, recommended by a widely accepted textbook[10]: moxa is applied for 15 min per acupuncture point. The other regime considers that the dose should differ according to patients' condition and moxibustion sensation. Treatment sessions only end when patients feel that the acupuncture point heat-sensitisation phenomenon has disappeared. We called this the 'individualised sensitivity elimination dose'.

It would be valuable to know whether the use of fixed dose is as effective as that of an individualised approach. We planned a rigorous multicentre, randomised controlled trial to seek for optimal dose model of the best therapeutic effect.

METHODS
Design
A multicentre, randomised, assessor blinded, controlled trial was conducted at four centres in China: the Affiliated Hospital with Jiangxi University of Traditional Chinese Medicine (TCM), Nanchang, First Affiliated Hospital with Anhui University of TCM, Hefei, Jiangsu TCM Hospital, Nanjing, and Shanxi TCM Hospital, Xian. The study was sequentially conducted as follows: a run-in period of 1 week prior to randomisation, a treatment period of 14 days and a follow-up period of 6 months. At the end of the run-in period, participants were randomised to the individualised sensitivity elimination dose group or the standardised dosage group by a central randomisation system (CRS) provided by China Academy of Chinese Medical Sciences, which adopted computer telephone integration technology to integrate computer, internet and telecom. The random number list was assigned by interactive voice response (IVR) and interactive web response.[11] The CRS is a web-based electronic system used to screen and enrol patients. The CRS presented a site status page that listed all screened patients. Each entered patient was assigned a unique screening number. Patients that were randomised and assigned a computer generated code from the CRS.

Researchers who did not participate in the treatment and who were blinded to the allocation results performed the outcome assessment.

Sample size
We wanted to estimate the sample size that would suffice to detect differences of Modified Japanese Orthopaedic Association scale (M-JOA; see website) between the two groups. On the basis of a pilot study, the SD of the M-JOA score was set at 4.24 and a mean difference between groups of 2.47 was considered relevant. It was calculated that 80 patients were needed to obtain statistical power >90% and a significance level 0.05 in both outcomes. We estimated a dropout rate of 20%; therefore we aimed to recruit 96 patients.

Participants
Recruitment
A total of 96 eligible patients were enrolled in the study between September 2009 and March 2010. Recruitment strategies included dissemination of information on the study through newspapers, television, advertisements, signs posted at university-affiliated hospitals, and letters to local LDH support groups and healthcare providers with large caseloads of patients with LDH. Potential participants were informed that they had an equal chance of being assigned to one of two moxibustion interventions.

Inclusion criteria
Eligible participants were those previously diagnosed as having moderate-to-severe LDH according to the M-JOA criteria (score, >10). Patients were required to complete the baseline LDH diary. Written informed consent was obtained from each participant. Diagnosis was made according to the following criteria: (1) pain occurring in lower back and radiating to lower limb; (2) straight leg raising test positive; (3) computed tomography (CT) suggestive of disc herniation; (4) skin sensation, such as tingling (a 'pins-and-needles' sensation) or numbness in a part of one leg; (5) muscle weakness or atrophy in later stages; (6) a loss of deep tendon reflexes in the lower extremities; (7) changes in spinal posture; (8) lateral lumbar spine x-ray films showing scoliosis or lumbar lordosis. The first three items were essential inclusion criteria, the other items were optional. The above criteria mainly derived from the guiding principles of clinical research on new drugs.[12 13] Because the research involved moderate-to-severe or severe LDH, the inclusion criteria also included the following: the triangle region formed by bilateral BL25 and GV2 (*Dachangshu-Yaoshu*-contralateral *Dachangshu* intraregion) had to reveal heat-sensitive points. Participants were instructed to stop LDH symptomatic relief medication during the run-in and treatment periods and provided usual care instruction for LDH.

Exclusion criteria
Participants were excluded if they had serious life-threatening disease such as disease of the heart and brain blood vessels, liver, kidney and haematopoietic system, and psychosis. Women participants who were pregnant or lactating were ineligible. The following conditions were also excluded: single nerve palsy or cauda equina nerve palsy manifested as muscle paralysis or rectum or bladder symptoms; complication with lumbar spinal canal stenosis and space-occupying lesions for other reasons; complication with lumbar spine tumours, infections, tuberculosis, and so on; moxibustion syncope and unwilling to be treated with moxibustion; no written informed consent.

Study interventions
Moxibustion was performed by certified acupuncture medical doctors at four centres. Qualified specialists of

Acupunct Med 2012;30:266–272. doi:10.1136/acupmed-2012-010142

267

381

Original paper

acupuncture in TCM with ≥5 years' clinical experience performed moxibustion in this study. All treatment regimens were standardised among practitioners at the four centres by video, hands-on training and internet workshops.

In the two groups 22 mm (diameter)×120 mm (length) moxa-sticks (Jiangxi TCM Hospital, China) were used. Patients were usually in the comfortable prone position for treatment, at a room temperature 24–30°C.

Individualised sensitivity elimination dose group

In the individualised sensitivity elimination dose group, moxa-sticks were lit by the therapist and held over the region comprising BL25 and GV2. The moxa-stick suspended at an approximate distance of 3 cm was used to search for acupuncture points showing the heat-sensitisation phenomenon. The areas were given mild warmth without burning by moxa-sticks, which was maintained until the patient reported the characteristic heat sensitisation sensation, said to indicate effective moxibustion, that is commonly called *de qi*. Patients felt comfortable throughout the moxibustion manipulation.

The following sensation indicated the presence of a heat sensitisation acupuncture point: 'diathermic' sensation due to moxa heat, defined as heat sensation conducting from the local skin surface into deep tissue, or even into the abdomen; 'expanding' sensation defined as the heat sensation spreading to surrounding area little by little around the moxa point; 'transferred' sensation defined as the heat sensation transferring along some pathway or direction. When such an acupuncture point was found, the therapists marked the point. We explored the whole area to find all heat-sensitive points.

After obtaining the heat sensitisation sensation, the therapists began to treat patients at the most heat-sensitive intensity acupuncture point. The moxibustion was continued as long as the patient reported heat sensitivity. One acupuncture point was stimulated during each session. The moxa stick also held steadily at the 3 cm distance using a device used to fix the moxa-sticks (figure 1).

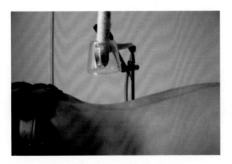

Figure 1 Device holding moxa stick at fixed location.

Treatment sessions ended when patients felt the acupuncture point heat-sensitisation phenomenon had disappeared. Heat sensitivity tended to reduce over the course of treatment, but could always be identified even at the end of treatment. After each treatment, the therapist recorded the duration of moxibustion. Patients received treatment twice/day in week 1 then once/day starting from week 2 for a total of 18 sessions over 14 days.

Standardised dose group

Patients in the standardised dose group received treatment identical to the individualised group except that the duration was 15 min. Likewise, patients received treatment twice/day in week 1 then once/day starting from week 2 for a total of 18 sessions over 14 days.

Outcome measures

The JOA has proposed a series of criteria to define patient response in the context of clinical trials of LDH. M-JOA scale is a modified edition of JOA Back Pain Evaluation Questionnaire.[13] According to these criteria, a patient with LDH is assessed for pain, the ability to conduct daily life and work, functional impairment and particular clinical examinations. This scoring system has been previously validated.[14] The degree of LDH severity was divided into three levels: mild (score, <0), moderate (10–20) and severe (>20).

Therapeutic effect was assessed by comparing baseline and final conditions reported by the patient. We also recorded adverse effects reported by patients during treatment. Outcome measures were assessed before treatment, after 7 and 14 days' treatment, and 6 months after the last moxibustion session.

Statistical methods
Statistical analysis

Data were analysed on an intention-to-treat (ITT) basis including all randomised participants with at least one measurable outcome report. The statistician conducting the analyses remained blinded to treatment groups. All analyses were conducted using SAS statistical package program (V.9.1.3; SAS, Cary, North Carolina, USA).

Baseline data

Baseline characteristics are shown as mean±SD for continuous data. We conducted between-group comparisons of baseline data using the two-sample t test or Wilcoxon rank sum test for continuous data and χ^2 test or Fisher's exact test for sex composition considering $p<0.05$ as statistically significant.

Outcome data

Between-group analysis of M-JOA score was performed using an unpaired t test and the 95% CI of the difference between groups. If M-JOA scores did not have normal frequency distribution, the data were modified before testing, and if not normal after transformation, we used the non-parametric Wilcoxon rank sum test. To check

Acupunct Med 2012;**30**:266–272. doi:10.1136/acupmed-2012-010142

whether the data had normal distribution frequency, we used Shapiro-Wilk or W tests. For the ITT analysis we adopted the principle of last observation carried forward (LOCF).

All adverse events reported during the study were included in the case report forms; the incidence of adverse events was calculated.

Dropouts and missing data
Reasons for dropouts or missing data were explored descriptively. Missing data were replaced according to the principle of LOCF.

Follow-up data
The primary outcome was M-JOA score. The primary analysis compared the two groups at 2 weeks. A secondary analysis compared the two groups at 6 months to assess whether any differences between groups were maintained over time.

Data integrity
The integrity of trial data was monitored by regularly scrutinising data sheets for omissions and errors. Data were double entered and the source of any inconsistencies was explored and resolved.

Adverse events
We defined adverse events as unfavourable or unintended signs, symptoms, or disease occurring after treatment that were not necessarily related to the moxibustion intervention. In each visit, adverse events were reported by participants and examined by the practitioner.

Ethics
Written consent was obtained from each participant. This study was approved by all relevant local ethics review boards. Ethics Committee of the Affiliated Hospital of Jiangxi University of TCM approved this trial (code no. 2008[10]).

RESULTS
Recruitment
Participants aged 18–65 years were recruited from outpatients and inpatients in the four study centres. A total of 306 persons underwent screening; of these, 96 met inclusion criteria and received allocated interventions (figure 2). Among the 210 excluded patients, 173 did not meet inclusion criteria, 25 refused to participate because they were wary of the treatment, 12 refused to be randomised because they wanted to be treated by moxibustion plus acupuncture (8 cases) or might go abroad before the end point (4 cases). Thus 96 patients were randomly assigned into 2 treatment groups by 30 investigators. During the follow-up visits, two patients dropped out of the study. In the experimental group, one patient left the study prematurely because of a medical emergency. In the control group, one patient left prior to study completion because of a fall injury. The M-JOA score at baseline was carried

forward to all time points. All patients receiving the full course of treatment attended follow-up at 6 months. None of these patients dropped out of the study due to adverse events.

Baseline
At baseline, men and women were equally represented. Most (81%) patients were aged <60 years. Mean total M-JOA score at baseline of both groups showed no significant difference (p>0.05). All subordinate scores had similar tendency in accordance with the total score. Demographic and clinical features at baseline did not differ across the two treatment groups (table 1).

Assessor blinded
We ensured assessor blinding in this trial. Patients were informed not to tell outcome assessors the treatment they were received. The outcome assessor was not involved in treatment administration.

Outcome
After intervention the two groups showed a significant improvement from baseline, measured as difference in total M-JOA score after 1 week of starting treatment (table 2). Total M-JOA score was significantly lower in the individualised dose group at weeks 1 and 2 (p<0.05). The effect already shown in the first week was maintained ≤6 months after finishing treatment. Mean total M-JOA score of both groups reduced sharply at the first 1 week then remained decreased to the end of 6 months (Figure 3).

Moxibustion time in the experimental group
The moxibustion dose was individualised in the experimental group, not in the control group. The duration ranged between 22–58 min, with a mean moxibustion duration of 42.7±5.4 min. We used a linear correlation to measure the strength of a relationship between change in M-JOA score and stimulation duration in the test group. The Pearson coefficient r=0.003, showing a poor correlation between the two values.

Safety
No adverse events were reported for the 96 participants.

DISCUSSION
Patients in the two groups showed marked improvements in pain and function parameters for ≤6 months of follow-up. Significant differences in total M-JOA score were observed between the groups, also evident during the follow-up period. Our results suggest that an individualised sensitivity elimination dose of heat-sensitive moxibustion treatment showed superior long-term effects.

In our study, no unwanted side effects of heat-sensitive moxibustion were observed. Several large surveys have also provided evidence that indirect moxibustion is a relatively safe treatment.[15–17]

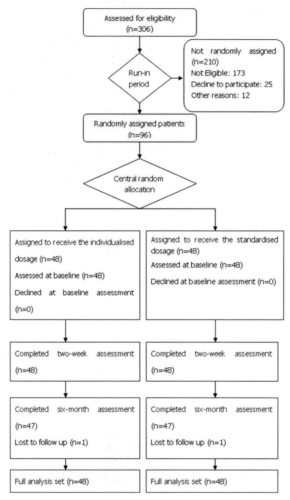

Figure 2   Study flow chart.

To the best of our knowledge, our study is the largest reported randomised, controlled trial that compared effectiveness of an individualised sensitivity elimination dose with a standardised dose in the treatment of patients with LDH. The studies published to date had certain methodological deficiencies in the description and application of the method chosen for randomisation, concealment of the treatment assignation scheme and homogeneity of comparator groups; moreover, heterogeneity of follow-up periods was high.[10–12] Unlike most previous studies of moxibustion, our study required participating therapists to fulfil a number of rigorous standards with regard to their medical education and practical training in TCM. In addition, our study used central randomisation to ensure adequate concealment in group assignment. The evaluation of the results and the statistical analysis were both carried out in blinded fashion. High follow-up rates were another factor for quality assurance.

Acupunct Med 2012;**30**:266–272. doi:10.1136/acupmed-2012-010142

Table 1   Baseline characteristics of patients with LDH

	Individualised group	Standardised group
Age, mean (SD), years	46.8±11.5	47.9±11.2
Age, years		
Minimum–maximum	18–58	28–67
>60, n (%)	8(16.7%)	10(20.8%)
Sex n (%)		
Male	21(43.8%)	25(52.1%)
Female	27(56.3%)	23(47.9%)
Duration of low back pain n (%)		
<1 months	10(20.8%)	15(31.3%)
2–6 months	13(27.1%)	10(20.8%)
7–12 months	13(27.1%)	12(25.0%)
1–5 years	10(20.8%)	10(20.8%)
>5 years	2(4.2%)	1(2.1%)
BMI, mean (SD), kg/m²	22.1 (2.7)	23.5 (2.4)
BMI, minimum–maximum, kg/m²	14.6–30.1	16.0–27.1
M-JOA grade n (%)		
Severe	32(66.7%)	30(62.5%)
Moderate	16(33.3%)	18(37.5%)
M-JOA score at baseline (SD)		
Total score mean	16.1±4.7	16.5±4.8
Lumbar and leg pain score mean	2.0±0.8	2.2±0.5
Numbness score mean	1.5±1.0	1.6±0.9
Paravertebral tenderness score mean	1.7±0.9	1.6±0.7
Myodynamia score mean	0.8±0.7	1.1±0.7
Straight leg raising test score mean	1.3±0.8	1.2±0.9
Radiating pain score mean	1.7±0.8	1.9±0.9
Stoop and lift heavy things score mean	1.9±0.9	1.5±0.9
Walk distance/time score mean	1.6±0.9	1.5±0.9
Daily time in bed score mean	1.3±1.1	1.4±1.0
Ability to work score mean	2.2±0.8	2.1±0.8

BMI, body mass index; LDH, lumbar disc herniation, M-JOA, Modified Improvement Japanese Orthopaedic Association scale.

Nonetheless, our study had some limitations, including a lack of blinding to moxibustion. A blinded study of moxibustion is challenging to conduct because it is almost impossible to blind therapists to the treatments they were delivering.

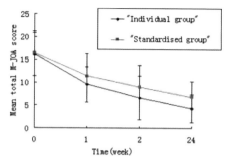

Figure 3   Mean total Modified Japanese Orthopaedic Association (M-JOA) scale (intention-to-treat analysis) at each time point.

Theoretically, three factors may impact on moxibustion dose: intensity, area and time. The two former factors are constant as a result of the standard size of moxa stick used in practice. Hence time is the variable parameter and plays an important part in moxibustion dose. We wondered how long the optimum dose should be for heat-sensitive moxibustion. The simplest and most obvious method refers to a standard 15 min as recommended by the universal textbook. Other proposed methods consider flushing of skin in the local region as indication of optimum dose regimen. However, our team's experimental evidence suggests that this regimen may not be superior. In this study, our results support the notion that individualised sensitivity elimination dose is likely to be optimal in heat-sensitive moxibustion.

The aim of our study was to explore the best dose of heat-sensitive moxibustion for the treatment of LDH. In summary, our results suggested that the effectiveness of individualised sensitivity elimination dose appears superior to standardised dose in the treatment of LDH. The application of only 15 min of moxibustion was insufficient to exert maximum clinical effects. A mean moxibustion dose of 42.70±5.40 min (range 22–58 min) was superior.

Table 2   Comparison of M-JOA scores at week 1, end of treatment (week 2) and follow-up (month 6), together with between group statistical tests

	Week 1			Week 2			Month 6		
Variable	Mean	SD	t Test	Mean	SD	t Test	Mean	SD	t Test
Totals									
Individualised group	9.5	3.9	2.0*	6.6	4.8	2.4*	4.4	3.1	3.7**
Standardised group	11.4	5.0		9.0	4.7		6.8	3.4	

*p<0.05.
**p<0.01.
M-JOA, Modified Improvement Japanese Orthopaedic Association scale.

Acupunct Med 2012;**30**:266–272. doi:10.1136/acupmed-2012-010142

271

Original paper

Summary points

▶ Moxibustion can elicit *de qi* in certain locations in low back pain.
▶ This sensation can be abolished by prolonging the moxibustion.
▶ We found this more effective than standard duration of moxibustion.

Contributors RC and MC obtained funding for the research project. JX, ZC and BZ drafted the protocol; JX wrote the final manuscript. ZC contributed to the research and made critical revisions. BZ was responsible for the statistical of the trial and wrote portions of the statistical methods, data handling and monitoring sections. All authors read and approved the final manuscript.

Funding This study was supported by the National Natural Science Foundation of China and Major State Basic Research Development Programme of People's Republic of China (grant no.: 2009CB522902) and Jiangxi Key R&D Project.

Competing interests The authors declare that they have no competing interests.

Patient consent Obtained.

Ethics approval Ethics Committee of the Affiliated Hospital of Jiangxi University of TCM.

Provenance and peer review Not commissioned; externally peer reviewed.

REFERENCES

1. **Chen RX,** Kang MF. *Acupuncture point heat-sensitive moxibustion an new therapy.* 1st edn. Beijing in China: Press by People's Medical Publishing House, 2006.
2. **Cho ZH,** Hwang SC, Wong EK, *et al.* Neural substrates, experimental evidences and functional hypothesis of acupuncture mechanisms. *Acta Neurol Scand* 2006;113:370–7.
3. **Xu GJ,** Ai BW. An overview of experimental study of lumbar disc herniation in the treatment of acupuncture and moxibustion. *Shan Xi TCM* 2010;26:36–8.
4. **Huang HL,** Lin WR, Huang Y, *et al.* Current status for lumbar disc herniation treated by acupuncture and moxibustion. *Mod Chinese J Integr* 2012;10:6–9.
5. **Tang FY,** Huang CJ, Chen RX, *et al.* Observation on therapeutic effect of heat-sensitive moxibustion for lumbar disc herniation. *Zhongguo Zhen Jiu* 2009;29:382–4.
6. **Tang FY,** Huang CJ, Chen RX, *et al.* Clinical study of heat-sensitive moxibustion for lumbar disc herniation. *J Jiangxi Univ TCM* 2009;21:25–7.
7. **He JP,** Huang YH. Clinical trial of heat-sensitive moxibustion in the treatment of lumbar disc herniation. *Asia-Pac Tradit Med* 2008;4:69–70.
8. **Kang MF,** Ren YL. Observation on therapeutic effect of heat-sensitive moxibustion plus acupuncture for lumbar disc herniation: 31 cases. *J Zhejiang TCM* 2009;44:289–90.
9. **Wang ZL.** Observation on therapeutic effect of heat-sensitive moxibustion plus acupuncture for lumbar disc herniation. *China Med Health* 2009;22:228.
10. **Lu SK.** *Method of needling and moxibustion.* 1st edn. Beijing in China: Press by China Publishing House of Traditional Chinese Medicine, 2002.
11. **Liu B,** Wen T, Yao C, *et al.* The central randomization system in multi-center clinical trials. *Chin J New Drugs Clin Rem* 2006;12:931–5.
12. **Zhen XY.** *The guideline of the latest Chinese herbs to clinical research.* 1st edn. Beijing: Medicine Science and Technology Press of China, 2002.
13. **JOA Back Pain Evaluation Questionnaire.** Janpanese Orthopaedic Association. http://www.joa.or.jp/english/english_frame.html
14. **Suzukamo Y,** Fukuhara S, Kikuchi S, *et al.* Committee on Science Project, Japanese Orthopaedic Association. Validation of the Japanese version of the Roland-Morris Disability Questionnaire. *J Orthop Sci* 2003;8:543–8.
15. **Nicholas JJ,** Taylor FH, Buckingham RB, *et al.* Measurement of circumference of the knee with ordinary tape measure. *Ann Rheum Dis* 1976;35:282–4.
16. **White AR,** Hayhoe S, Hart A, *et al.* Survey of Adverse events following Acupuncture (SAFA): a prospective study of 32 000 consultations. Exeter, UK: Department of Complementary Medicine, University of Exeter, 2001:1–20.
17. **Melchart D,** Weidenhammer W, Streng A, *et al.* Prospective investigation of adverse effects of acupuncture in 97733 patients. *Arch Intern Med* 2004;164:104–5.

Chen *et al. Trials* 2010, **11**:121
http://www.trialsjournal.com/content/11/1/121

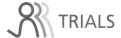 TRIALS

STUDY PROTOCOL　　　　　　　　　　　　　　　　　　　　　　　　**Open Access**

Comparison of heat-sensitive moxibustion versus fluticasone/salmeterol (seretide) combination in the treatment of chronic persistent asthma: design of a multicenter randomized controlled trial

Rixin Chen[1*], Mingren Chen[1], Jun Xiong[1], Fan Yi[2], Zhenhai Chi[1], Bo Zhang[1]

Abstract

Background: Asthma is a major health problem and has significant mortality around the world. Although the symptoms can be controlled by drug treatment in most patients, effective low-risk, non-drug strategies could constitute a significant advance in asthma management. An increasing number of patients with asthma are attracted by acupuncture and moxibustion. Therefore, it is of importance that scientific evidence about the efficacy of this type of therapy is regarded. Our past researches suggested heat-sensitive moxibustion might be effective in treatment of asthma. Our objective is to investigate the effectiveness of heat-sensitive moxibustion compared with conventional drug treatment.

Methods/Design: This study is comprised of a multi-centre (12 centers in China), randomized, controlled trial with two parallel arms (A: heat-sensitive moxibustion; B: conventional drug). Group A selects heat- sensitive acupoints from the rectangle region which consist of two outer lateral lines of dorsal Bladder Meridian of Foot-Taiyang, and two horizontal lines of BL13(Fei Shu) and BL17 (Ge Shu);6 inch outer the first and second rib gap of anterior chest. Group B treats with fluticasone/salmeterol (seretide). The outcome measures will be assessed over a 3-month period before each clinic visit at days 15, 30, 60, and 90. Follow-up visit will be at 3, 6 months after the last treatment session. Adverse event information will be collected at each clinic visit.

Discussion: This trial will utilize high quality trial methodologies in accordance with CONSORT guidelines. It may provide evidence for the effectiveness of heat-sensitive moxibustion as a treatment for chronic moderate persistent asthma. Moreover, the result may propose a new type moxibustion to control asthma.

Trial Registration: The trial is registered at Chinese Clinical Trials Registry: ChiCTR-TRC-09000599

Background

Asthma is a common chronic inflammatory disease of the airways characterized by variable and recurring symptoms, airflow obstruction, and bronchospasm [1]. It is also a complex disease involving many cells and mediators [2]. Asthma affects 300 million people worldwide [3], with an increasing prevalence in Western Europe (5%) and the USA(7%) in particular [4,5]. Despite the fact that there is still no cure for asthma, it has been established in a great number of small and large studies

that many patients can reach a good asthma control with controller treatment [6]. Generally speaking, Medications used to treat asthma are divided into two general classes: quick-relief medications used to treat acute symptoms and long-term control medications used to prevent further exacerbation [7]. The therapeutic options available for patients with asthma depend on the severity of the condition. Although the symptoms can be controlled by drug treatment in most patients, effective low-risk, non-drug strategies could constitute a significant advance in asthma management [1-3]. Therefore, an increasing number of patients with asthma are attracted by complementary and alternative medicine

* Correspondence: chenrixin123@yahoo.com.cn
[1]The Affiliated Hospital of Jiangxi University of TCM, Nanchang, PR China
Full list of author information is available at the end of the article

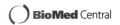

Chen *et al. Trials* 2010, **11**:121
http://www.trialsjournal.com/content/11/1/121

(CAM) [8]. A survey showed that roughly 50% of asthma patients used some form of unconventional therapy [9].

Acupuncture has traditionally been used in asthma treatment in China and is increasingly applied for this purpose in Western countries. Moxibustion is a traditional Chinese method of acupuncture treatment, which utilizes the heat generated by burning Moxa (it is also called Mugwort or Moxa) to stimulate the acupuncture points. The technique consists of lighting a moxa-stick and bringing it close to the skin until it produces hyperemia due to local vasodilatation. The intensity of moxibustion is just below the individual tolerability threshold. Moxibustion has anti-inflammatory or immunomodulatory effects against chronic inflammatory conditions in humans [10]. Moxibustion method for treatment of asthma diverse curative effect and its mechanism may be due to improve lung function, antagonize of inflammatory mediators, modulate of immune function, regulate the role of cyclic nucleotide levels, and can also affect the neuroendocrine network and inflammatory cells [11-14]. Therefore, these inflammatory substances may be reduced and weakened by moxibustion. Especially for chronic persistent asthma, moxibustion may get a better effect.

Although firm evidence has not been established, the results of some clinical trials suggest that acupuncture and moxibustion may effective in the treatment of asthma [15-18]. However, these researches do not confirm the efficacy of acupuncture and moxibustion. This may be because all relevant RCTs were limited by methodological defects, including inappropriate sample size, variability of acupuncture and sham protocols, and missing information. Therefore, rigorous high-quality randomized controlled trials are needed.

Thinking about moxibustion itself, the selection of location for manipulating Moxa plays an important role in obtaining good effects [19]. The moxibustion point location may be connected with the changes in the condition of the disease. Our team of experts were astonished to find that the main factor in selecting the location of acupuncture points is link with the area which is affected by disease, not only the standardized fixed position.

In the human nature, there are two state of being in acupuncture points, the sensitized or awake state and the rest state. When the human body suffers form disease, the acupoints on the surface of the body are stimulated and sensitive by various stimulants including heat. The specific areas stimulated by heat are then called "heat-sensitive points". One of the characteristics of these areas is that they are specific or closely related to acupuncture points and have the same clinical effect as "a small stimulation induces a large response". The *Inner Canon of Huangdi* or *Yellow Emperor's Inner Canon* is an ancient Chinese medical text that has been treated as the fundamental doctrinal source for Chinese medicine for more than two millennia and until today. According with its core viewpoint and theory, acupoint is described and understood with the state, which is certain area of the body surface in the course of diseases. Among the changes, sensitized status is the common one, described that acupoints on the body surface may be sensitized in the course of diseases. Acupoint heat-sensitization is a type of acupoint sensitization. Our research found that the heat-sensitive phenomenon to a point or an area is a new type of reaction featured in a pathological state [20-23]. We applicated the acupoint heat-sensitization phenomenon and rule in the past twenty years. Our team experimental evidence indicates that the state of a point might change from the rest state to the heat sensitized state while suffering from diseases. Its characteristic was thought that these special acupoints might produce heat response and farther warm sensation, as a result of stimulation of moxibustion heat. If we can search out these heat-sensitized acupoints associating with pathological state, good effect will be achieved. Therefore, selecting the heat-sensitized acupoint may obtain therapeutic effect far better than acupuncture and moxibustion at acupoints of routine rest state. So we defined the approach which treated various diseases through heat-sensitized acupoint, as heat- sensitive moxibustion therapy. We carried out many clinical trials to test and verify the efficacy of heat-sensitized acupoint, such as myofascial pain syndrome [22], lumbar disc herniation [24], pressure sores [25] and knee osteoarthritis [26]. The result of clinical trials almost suggested superiority effect of heat-sensitized acupoint and encouraged us to proceed. Hence, we planned a rigorous multi-centre randomized controlled trial with a large sample size.

Method/design
Objective
The aim of this study is to investigate the effectiveness of heat-sensitive moxibustion compared with fluticasone/salmeterol (seretide) in patients with chronic moderate persistent asthma in China.

Outcome measures
Primary outcome
At present, the goal of asthma care is to achieve and maintain control of clinical manifestation of the disease [27,28]. Hence, we use Asthma Control Test (ACT) to quickly access asthma control, a simple 5-question tool that is completed by the patient and parents/caregivers and recognized by the National Institutes of Health (Table 1) [29,30]. Patients should write the number of each answer in the score box provided, and then add up

Chen *et al. Trials* 2010, **11**:121
http://www.trialsjournal.com/content/11/1/121

Table 1 Asthma Control Test (ACT) for people 12 yrs and older.

1. In the past 4 weeks, how much of the time did your asthma keep you from getting as much done at work, school or at home?				Score
All of the time ①	Most of the time ②	Some of the time ③	A little of the time ④	None of the time ⑤

2. During the past 4 weeks, how often have you had shortness of breath?				
More than once a day ①	Once a day ②	3 to 6 times a week ③	Once or twice a week ④	Not at all ⑤

3. During the past 4 weeks, how often did your asthma symptoms (wheezing, coughing, shortness of breath, chest tightness or pain) wake you up at night or earlier than usual in the morning?				
4 or more nights a week ①	2 or 3 nights a week ②	Once a week ③	Once or twice ④	Not at all ⑤

4. During the past 4 weeks, how often have you used your rescue inhaler or nebulizer medication (such as albuterol)?				
3 or more times per day ①	1 or 2 times per day ②	2 or 3 times per week ③	Once a week or less ④	Not at all ⑤

5. How would you rate your asthma control during the past 4 weeks?				
Not controlled at all ①	Poorly controlled ②	Somewhat controlled ③	Well controlled ④	Completely controlled ⑤

each score box for your total. ACT will be assessed before treatment and at days 15, 30, 60, and 90 in the treatment period. Follow-up visit will be at 3, 6 months after the last treatment session.

Secondary outcomes
Measurement of lung function provides an assessment of the severity, reversibility, and variability of airflow limitation. Forced expiratory volume in 1 s (FEV1) and peak expiratory flow (PEV) will be used in this trial. Attack frequency also will be assessed. These outcomes also will be assessed before treatment and at days 90 in the treatment period. Follow-up visit will be at 3, 6 months after the last treatment session. Adverse event information will be collected at each clinic visit.

Design
A multi-centre, randomized, two parallel arms (group A and B) and assessor blinded, positive controlled trial will be conducted at the twelve centers in China (Table 2).

The study will be sequentially conducted as follows: a run-in period of one week prior to randomization, a treatment period of 90 days, and a follow-up period of six months. At the end of the run-in period, participants will be randomized to the heat-sensitive moxibustion group or the drug group by the central randomization system (Figure 1). This system is provided by China Academy of Chinese Medical Sciences, which adopted the computer telephone integration (CTI) technology to integrate computer, internet and telecom. The random number list will be assigned by interactive voice response (IVR) and interactive web response (IWR) [31]. The success of blinding will be assessed at each participant's last visit. Assessor who did not participate in the treatment and who is blinded to the allocation results will perform the outcome assessment.

Eligibility
Inclusion criteria
According to the guideline of asthma treatment and prevention in China (GATPC) [32], patients are divided into three types, including acute exacerbation, chronic persistent and clinical remission. Severity grade of asthma in GATPC is described in Table 3. Our trial will only choose participants with chronic moderate persistent asthma (Figure 1).

Patients will be required to complete the baseline asthma diary. Written informed consent will be obtained from each participant. Participants 18~65 years of age will be recruited from outpatient and inpatient in 12 centers. Standard of diagnosis listed as follows: (1) Common signs and symptoms of asthma include: recurrent wheezing, coughing, trouble breathing, chest tightness; (2) Symptoms that occur or worsen at night, and symptoms that are triggered by cold air, exercise or exposure to allergens; (3) Scattered or diffuse expiratory wheezing sound could be heard in the lungs in attack; (4) The above symptoms will be relieved or disappear after treatment; (5) Ruling out conditions other than asthma; (6) When typical clinical symptoms can not be observed, lung function tests should be used to confirm, such as positive challenge test, positive bronchodilator test(an increase in FEV1 of ≥12% and ≥200 ml), and mutation rate of PEF≥20% one day/two weeks. Since the research involves moderate asthma (grade III), the inclusion criteria will restrict the following conditions: According to the below GATPC diagnosis standard, meanwhile, heat-sensitivity appears within the rectangle area which consist of two outer lateral lines of dorsal Bladder Meridian of Foot-Taiyang, and two horizontal lines of BL13 (Fei Shu) and BL17 (Ge Shu); 6 inch outer the first and second rib gap of anterior chest. Participants will be instructed to stop asthma symptomatic relief medication

Chen *et al. Trials* 2010, **11**:121
http://www.trialsjournal.com/content/11/1/121

Table 2 List of 12 clinical centers

Name	City	Province
Affiliated Hospital of Jiangxi University of Traditional Chinese Medicine(TCM)	Nanchang	Jiangxi
Guangdong Hospital of Traditional Chinese and Western Medicine	Foshan	Guangdong
Wuhan the First Hospital	Wuhan	Hubei
Guangdong Hospital of TCM	Guangzhou	Guangdong
Guangzhou University of TCM	Guangzhou	Guangdong
Guangdong Disabled Soldier Hospital	Guangzhou	Guangdong
Affiliated Hospital of Shandong University of TCM	Jinan	Shandong
Suzhou Hospital of TCM	Suzhou	Jiangsu
The First Affiliated Hospital of Zhejiang University of TCM	Hangzhou	Zhejiang
The First Affiliated Hospital of Chongqing Medical University	Chongqing	Chongqing
The First Affiliated Hospital of Nanchang University	Nanchang	Jiangxi
Nanchang Hospital of Traditional Chinese and Western Medicine	Nanchang	Jiangxi

during the run-in and treatment periods and will be provided the usual care instruction for asthma.

Exclusion criteria

Participants will be excluded if they have other diseases that also cause breathlessness or dyspnea, such as bronchiectasis, cor-pulmonale, pulmonary fibrosis, tuberculosis, pulmonary abscess, chronic obstructive pulmonary disease and so on. Participants will not be eligible if the female are in the duration of pregnancy or lactation. The following conditions are also excluded items: Complicated with serious life-threatening diseases, such as heart and brain blood vessels, liver, kidney and hematopoietic system disease and psychotic patients; Hormone-dependent type patients, or the people who used adrenal cortical hormone (intravenous, intramuscular injection, subcutaneous injection and oral administration) within 4 weeks before recruiting.

Treatment protocol

Heat-sensitive moxibustion

Moxibustion will be performed by certified acupuncture medical doctors at 12 centers. Qualified specialists of acupuncture in traditional Chinese medicine with at least five years of clinical experience will perform the acupuncture in this study. All treatment regimens will be standardized between 12 centers practitioners via video, hands-on training and internet workshops. Participants will be randomly assigned to the heat-sensitive moxibustion group, or the drug group. In the former group, a 22 mm (diameter) × 160 mm (length) moxasticks (Jiangxi Hospital of Traditional Chinese Medicine, China) will be used. The patient is usually in the comfortable position for treatment, with 24°C~30°C temperature in the room. He should wear loose clothes.

For the heat-sensitive moxibustion group, the moxasticks are lit by the therapist and held over the rectangle area which consist of two outer lateral lines of dorsal Bladder Meridian of Foot-Taiyang, and two horizontal lines of BL13(Fei Shu) and BL17 (Ge Shu);6 inch outer the first and second rib gap of anterior chest. The warming suspended moxibustion about distance of 3 cm above the skin are used to search the acupoint heat-sensitization phenomenon. The following patients sensation will suggest the special heat-sensitization acupoint: diathermanous sensation due to moxa-heat, defining as the heat sensation conducting from the Moxa local skin surface into deep tissue, or even into the thoracic cavity; expand heat sensation due to moxa-heat, defining as the

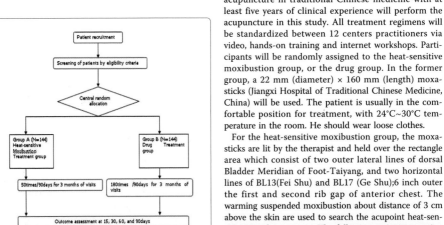

Figure 1 The flow diagram is intended to depict the passage of participants through this RCT.

Chen *et al. Trials* 2010, **11**:121
http://www.trialsjournal.com/content/11/1/121

Table 3 Clinical classification of severity in GATPC

Characteristic	Intermittent (Grade I)	Mild (Grade II)	Moderate (Grade III)	Severe (Grade IV)
symptoms	Less than once week	More than once week, < once a day	Everyday	Everyday
Limitation of activities and sleep	Transient	May be affect activities and sleep	Affect activities and sleep	Frequent
Nocturnal of symptoms/ awakening	Less than twice a month	More than twice a month, < once a week	More than once week	Frequent
Lung function (PEF or FEV1)	≥80% predicted (FEV1)or personal best (PEF); mutation rate < 20%	≥80% predicted (FEV1)or personal best (PEF); mutation rate 20%~30%	60%~79% predicted (FEV1)or personal best (PEF); mutation rate > 30%	< 60% predicted (FEV1)or personal best (PEF); mutation rate > 30%

heat sensation spreading the surrounding little by little around the moxa point; transfer heat sensation due to moxa-heat, defining as the heat sensation transferring along some pathway, or even to the arms. The therapists mark the point as heat-sensitive acupoint. We try our best to seek all the special acupoints in each patient by the repeated manipulation.

The therapists begin to treat patients from the most heat-sensitive intensity acupoint. Treatment sessions end when patients are feel the acupoint heat-sensitization phenomenon disappeared. Generally speaking, we find the time range from 30~60 minutes. In 1st month, patients receive the treatment once a day in the first eight days, and 12 times treatment in the next twenty-two days. Treatments will be given 15 times a month for the remaining two months.

Drug group
In recent years, considerable insight has been gained in to the optimal management of adult asthma. Those with persistent asthma are usually not well controlled without inhaled corticosteroids (ICS). Adding a long-acting beta-agonist (LABA) to ICS appears to be well controlled [33]. The combination of an ICS and LABA is preferred in these patients, and is better than doubling or even quadrupling the dose of ICS to achieve better asthma control and reduce exacerbation risks [34,35]. Two such combinations, salmeterol xinafoate and fluticasone propionate (SFC, Seretide(tm)) and formoterol and budesonide (FBC, Symbicort(tm)) are widely used and have been shown to be effective in controlling asthma of varying severity in adults and children [36-38].

Therefore, we selected the Seretide Accuhaler, containing two medicines, fluticasone propionate and salmeterol xinafoate, which is the mainstay of current asthma treatment. This drug is recommended by GINA as a regular treatment. Our trial uses salmeterol/fluticasone 50 μg/250 μg twice a day. Patients receive the treatment for a total of 180 sessions over 90 days.

Statistical methods
Statistical analysis plan
We will conduct analysis on an intention-to-treat basis, including all randomized participants with at least one measurable outcome report. Analyses will be conducted using 2-sided significance tests at the 5% significance level. An analysis using the Cochran-Mantel-Haenszel procedure will be done to asses center effect. The statistician conducting the analyses will remain blind to treatment group and data will only be unblinded once all data summaries and analyses are completed. All analyses will be conducted in the SAS statistical package program (ver. 9.1.3).

Baseline data
Baseline characteristics will be shown as mean ± standard deviation (SD) for continuous data including age, previous duration, and so on. As for participants' gender, n (%) of male and female in each group will be shown as baseline characteristics. We will conduct between-group comparison in baseline using two-sample t-test or Wilcoxon rank sum test for continuous data and using Chi-square test or Fisher's exact test for gender composition considering $p < 0.05$ as statistically significant.

If any imbalances in baseline characteristics between groups are encountered, we will conduct ANCOVA (analysis of covariance) using these imbalanced variables as covariates and allocated group as fixed factor.

Outcome data
For primary and secondary outcome measures, these will be summarized descriptively (mean, SD, median, minimum and maximum) at each time point by treatment group. The t-test, Mann-Whitney U and Wilcoxon test were used for comparison of variables, as appropriate.

All adverse events reported during the study will be included in the case report forms; the incidence of adverse events will be calculated. The percentage of subjects with adverse events in each group will be calculated and compared using the chi-squared test or Fisher's exact test.

Dropped or missing data Reasons for dropped or missing data will be explored by descriptively. Missing data will be replaced according to the principle of the last observation carried forward.

Follow-up data The primary outcome will be the ACT scores. The primary analysis will compare the two groups in 3 months. A secondary analysis will compare the two groups at 6,9 months to assess if any differences between groups have been maintained over time.

Loss to follow-up is likely to lead to biased estimates of intervention effect. We will try to avoid bias due to attrition by carefully following up the participants in both groups. We will phone participants who fail to complete questionnaires after a second reminder. We anticipate a 20% loss to follow-up in this trial, and will implement procedures to minimize loss to follow-up and patient withdrawal, and where possible, we will collect information on reasons for patient withdrawal.

Data integrity
The integrity of trial data will be monitored by regularly scrutinizing data sheets for omissions and errors. Data will be double entered and the source of any inconsistencies will be explored and resolved.

Sample size
We wished to estimate the sample size according to non-inferiority clinical trial between the heat-sensitive and drug group. Sample size depends on the level of confidence chosen, the risk of type II error (or desired power), and δ. The parameter margin of non-inferiority δ can be specified as a difference in means or proportions. It is often chosen as the smallest value that would be a clinically important effect. To determine δ, we carried out a small sample pilot study previously. The primary endpoint chosen was ACT. The result of outcome showed difference in means between the two groups approximately was 0.45. The choice of δ = 0.15 (30% of Δ) appeared to be reasonable based on clinical relevance and statistical judgment.

If we apply a two-sided 5% significance level(δ = 0.15, α = 0.05, β = 0.2), 95% power the calculated required sample size is approximately 120 participants in each group, according to the following equation. Allowing for a 20% loss to follow up, a total of 144 participants will be required in each group, with 288 participants in total.

$$n = 2 \times \frac{\left(U_\alpha + U_\beta\right)^2}{\delta^2} \times P(1-P)$$

Adverse events
We define adverse events as unfavorable or unintended signs, symptoms or disease occurring after treatment that are not necessarily related to the moxibustion intervention. In every visit, adverse events will be reported by participants and examined by the practitioner.

Ethics
Written consent will be obtained from each participant. This study was approved by all relevant local ethics review boards. Ethics Committee of Affiliated hospital of Jiangxi Institute of Traditional Chinese Medicine had approved this trial: code issued by ethic committee is 2008(13).

Discussion
To our knowledge, the goal of asthma care is to achieve and maintain control of clinical manifestations of the disease for prolong periods. When asthma is controlled, patients can prevent most attacks, avoid troublesome symptoms day and night, and keep physically active [1]. Acupuncture therapy was often perceived as an effective option to control asthma successfully by patients with chronic asthma. The use of acupuncture in asthma patients is increasing as an adjunct and also as a substitute for effective and proven therapies [39]. In China, moxibustion are considered as an ancient treatment to prevent and control asthma, and still widely used today. A number of clinical trial suggested moxibustion as one of traditional acupuncture therapy, should effective in the treatment of asthma. But the methodological problems of published trials haunt us the trust of moxibustion. Therefore, we design this rigorous clinical trials meeting the CONSORT statement and guidelines to guarantee a high internal validity for the results.

At present, various conventional medications are used to slow down and control with the disease. An ICS/LABA combination in a single inhaler represents a safe, effective and convenient treatment option, and recommended by GINA. So, we selected the fluticasone/salmeterol (seretide) as the control treatment in the protocol. Actually, the aim of this trial is to search an effective CAM treatment to control asthma, as good as conventional drug. The focused features of moxibustion are low cost, less adverse event and low risk.

According to the current theory of traditional Chinese medicine, moxibustion resulting from the burning of Moxa produces the radiant heat and drug effects to acupoints. This treatment penetrates deeply into the body, restoring the balance and flow of vital energy or life force through acupoints. So the selected of location for manipulating Moxa plays an important role in obtaining good effects. Generally speaking, the location acupoints are fixed along meridians. The conventional moxibustion is considered as improving general health and treating diseases by stimulating these fixed acupoints. And

Chen et al. Trials 2010, **11**:121
http://www.trialsjournal.com/content/11/1/121

doctors consider hyperemia due to local skin vasodilatation as the indicator of moxibustion's effect. However, our clinical experience and observation in the past suggested that stimulating these fixed acupoints might not the best treatment site for moxibustion. In the human nature, there are two states of acupoints, the stimulated or awake state and the rest state. When the human body suffers form disease, the acupuncture points on the surface of the body are stimulated and sensitive by various stimulants including heat. And acupoint heat-sensitization is a type of acupoint sensitization. Acupoint is more than fixed skin site but external sensitive point reflecting the diseases. Therefore, acupoint is variable and depends on the pathological state. Traditional fixed acupints are thought as indicators to searching specific sensitive acupoint. That is, traditional fixed acupints don not consider the state as the key factor to local the acupoint, so the course of fixing the position is imprecisely.

When we light the Moxa hold over the heat-sensitive acupoints, the patients will produce some heat-sensitization phenomenon. The following patients sensation will suggest the special heat-sensitization acupoint: diathermanous sensation due to moxa-heat, defining as the heat sensation conducting from the moxa local skin surface into deep tissue, or even into the thoracic cavity; expand heat sensation due to moxa-heat, defining as the heat sensation spreading the surrounding little by little around the moxa point; transfer heat sensation due to moxa-heat, defining as the heat sensation transferring along some pathway, or even to the arms.

Acupuncture and moxibustion originated in China several thousands of years ago. The ancient Chinese medical classic *Huáng Dì Nèi Jīng* translated as *'The Yellow Emperor's Inner Classic'* has been treated as the fundamental doctrinal source for Chinese medicine for more than two thousand years. According to the chapter *Annotations on 'The Yellow Emperor's Inner Classic - chapter: jiu zhen shi er yuan'(translated as 'Nine Needles and twelve yuan-primary acupoints")*, it says: *"the so-called joints are the places where Shenqi flows in and out, not just referring to skin, muscles, sinews and bones."* This explains that the acupuncture points are not located according to the flesh and bones, which by definition have a fixed location, but they are alive and have a dynamic state due to the activity of "shen-qi". In the Huáng Dì Nèi Jīng Ling Shu (黄帝内经灵枢) translated as *"Annotations on 'The Yellow Emperor's Inner Classic' - chapter: jiu zhen shi er yuan(translated as 'Nine Needles and twelve yuan-primary acupoints")*, it says: "so the disease of the Five Zang-organs can be treated by needling the twelve Yuan-Primary acupoints. The twelve Yuan-Primary acupoints show how the five Zang-Organs receive the nutrients of food

and water and how Essence-Qi is infused into the three hundred and sixty-five joints. That is why the disease of the Five Zang-Organs are manifested over the twelve Yuan-Primary acupoints which show certain manifestations. Awareness of the twelve Yuan-Primary and observation of the manifestation to know the pathological changes of the Five Zang-Organs". We can learn an important fact from this section of the classical text. It clearly states that acupuncture points reflect the pathological state of the internal diseases and can be stimulated in treatment. Physically, people are not always aware of the existence of the acupuncture points. In contrast, patients can usually feel some changes in the area of the acupuncture point when affected by disease. Through the observation of these changes, the ancient doctors located the acupuncture points. In the *Annotations on 'The Yellow Emperor's Inner Classic - chapter: 'back-shu* acupoints', it states: "The Feishu (BL13) acupoint is located between the third thoracic vertebra. The Xinshu (BL15) acupoint is located below and lateral to the fifth thoracic vertebra. The Geshu (BL17) acupoint is located below and lateral to the seventh thoracic vertebra. The Ganshu (BL18) acupoint is located below and lateral to the ninth thoracic vertebra. The Pishu (BL20) acupoint is located below and lateral to the eleventh thoracic vertebra. The Shenshu (BL23) is located below and lateral to the fourteenth thoracic vertebra. These acupoints are all located beside the spinal column and 3 cun away from the spinal column. The method to locate these acupoints is to press the regions. When pressed, the patient will feel aching and distending or feel that the original pain is relieved." This section of the classical text illustrated that the back shu points are found by founding the sensitive areas on the skin. In the *Annotations on 'The Yellow Emperor's Inner Classic - chapter: 'five xie'* (translated as 'five kinds of pathogenic factor')it says: *"cough involving the shoulder and back, to treat such a disease, acupoints located on the lateral side of the chest and lateral to the third thoracic vertebra can be needled. Before applying acupuncture, the doctor may use his fingers to quickly press the concerned region; the place where the patient feels comfortable when pressed is the acupoint and should be needled".* From this section, we can conclude that the sensitivity of the points is the key factor to locate the position of the acupuncture points.

Among the changes, sensitized status is the common one, described that acupoints on the body surface may be sensitized with various types of sensitization. This sensitized acupoint is not only the pathological phenomenon reflecting the diseases but also stimulating location with acupuncture and moxibustion. Acupoint heat-

Chen *et al. Trials* 2010, **11**:121
http://www.trialsjournal.com/content/11/1/121

sensitization is a type of acupoint sensitization, which derived from our clinical experience and research in past twenty years. The special acupoint makes accordance with the classical thought and theory from the Inner Canon of Huangdi.

Our empirical evidence engaged us to formulate the following hypothesis: selecting the heat-sensitized acupoint may obtain therapeutic effect in asthma. The main aim of this trial is to test and verify the hypothesis. If we can confirm this hypothesis, the results of our trial will be helpful to supply the evidence on searching better safe approach to control asthma.

Acknowledgements
This study was supported by the Major State Basic Research Development Program of People's Republic of China (Grant number: 2009CB522902), the National Key Technology R&D Program (Grant number: 2006BAI12B04-2), the National Natural Science Foundation of China (Grant number: 30760320) and Jiangxi Key R&D Project.

Author details
[1]The Affiliated Hospital of Jiangxi University of TCM, Nanchang, PR China.
[2]Department of Health of Jiangxi Province, Nanchang, PR China.

Authors' contributions
RC and MC obtained funding for the research project and drafted the protocol. JX wrote the final manuscript. RC contributed to the research design and made critical revisions. ZC and BZ were responsible for the statistical design of the trial and wrote portions of the statistical methods, data handling, and monitoring sections. All authors read and approved the final manuscript.

Competing interests
The authors declare that they have no competing interests.

Received: 9 August 2010 Accepted: 15 December 2010
Published: 15 December 2010

References
1. Global Initiative for Asthma (GINA): **Global strategy for asthma management and prevention: NHLBI/WHO Workshop Report**. Bethesda: National Institutes of Health, National Heart, Lung and Blood Institute; 2002.
2. National Asthma Education and Prevention Program: **Guidelines for the diagnosis and management of asthma: expert panel report 2**. Bethesda: National Institutes of Health, National Heart, Lung and Blood Institute; 1997, 97-4051.
3. Masoli M, Fabian D, Holt S: **Beasley Rather global burden of asthma: executive summary of the GINA Dissemination Committee report**. *Allergy* 2005, **59**:469-478.
4. Anderson HR, Gupta R, Strachan DP, Limb ES: **50 years of asthma: UK trends from 1955 to 2004**. *Thorax* 2007, **62**:85-90.
5. World Health Organization Fact Sheet Fact sheet No 307: **Asthma (2009)**. [http://www.who.int/mediacentre/factsheets/fs307/en/print.html], Accessed 08-05-10.
6. Global Initiative for Asthma: **Global strategy for asthma management and prevention**; 2004.
7. Salpeter S, Buckley N, Ormiston T, Salpeter E: **"Meta-analysis: effect of long-acting beta-agonists on severe asthma exacerbations and asthma-related deaths"**. *Ann Intern Med* 2006, **144**:904-912.
8. Blanc PD, Trupin L, Earnest G, Katz PP, Yelin EH, Eisner MD: **"Alternative therapies among adults with a reported diagnosis of asthma or rhinosinusitis: data from a population-based survey"**. *Chest* 2001, **120**:1461-1467.
9. Shenfield G, Lim E, Allen H: **"Survey of the use of complementary medicines and therapies in children with asthma"**. *J Paediatr Child Health* 2002, **38**:252-7.
10. Cho ZH, Hwang SC, Wong EK, Son YD, Kang CK, Park TS, Bai SJ, Kim YB, Lee YB, Sung KK: **Neural substrates, experimental evidences and functional hypothesis of acupuncture mechanisms**. *Acta Neurol Scand* 2006, **113**:370-377.
11. Peng ZF, Zhao JS, Yang F, Wang Y, Zhang LJ, Ran SQ: **Progresses of studies on disease factors influencing the therapeutic effect of acupuncture and moxibustion on bronchial asthma**. *Zhongguo Zhen Jiu* 2009, **29**:72-76.
12. Liu A: **Clinical application of moxibustion over point dazhui**. *J Tradit Chin Med* 1999, **19**:283-286.
13. Zhou D, Yang S: **Effective observation on purulent moxibustion in treating 106 cases of bronchial asthma**. *Zhen Ci Yan Jiu* 1992, **17**:239-241.
14. Hong H: **Analysis to influence of purulent moxibustion on bronchial asthma**. *Zhen Ci Yan Jiu* 1992, **17**:237-239.
15. McCarney RW, Brinkhaus B, Lasserson TJ, Linde K: **Acupuncture for chronic asthma**. *Cochrane Database of Systematic Reviews* 2003, , **3**: CD000008.
16. Jobst KA: **A critical analysis of acupuncture in pulmonary disease: efficacy and safety of the acupuncture needle**. *Journal of Alternative and Complementary Medicine* 1995, **1**:57-84.
17. Linde K, Worku F, Stör W, Wiesner-Zechmeister M, Pothmann R, Weinschütz T: **Randomized clinical trials of acupuncture for asthma - a systematic review**. *Forsch Komplementarmed* 1996, **3**:148-155.
18. Martin J, Donaldson AN, Villarroel R, Parmar MK, Ernst E, Higginson IJ: **Efficacy of acupuncture in asthma: systematic review and meta-analysis of published data from 11 randomized controlled trials**. *European Respiratory Journal* 2002, **20**:846-852.
19. Ayman E, Karl O: **Moxibustion in Breech Version-A Descriptive Review**. *Acupuncture in medicine* 2002, **20**:26-29.
20. Chen RX, Kang MF: **Clinical application of acupoint heat-sensitization**. *Zhongguo Zhenjiu* 2007, **27**:199-202.
21. Chen RX, Kang MF: **Key point of moxibustion, arrival of qi produces curative effect**. *Zhongguo Zhen Jiu* 2008, **28**:44-46.
22. Chen RX, Kang MF, He WL, Chen SY, Zhang B: **Moxibustion on heat-sensitive acupoints for treatment of myofascial pain syndrome: a multi-central randomized controlled trial**. *Zhongguo Zhen* 2008, **28**:395-398.
23. Chen RX, Kang MF: **Acupoint heat-sensitization moxibustion: a new therapy**. Press by People's Medical Publishing House. Beijing in China;, 1 2006.
24. Tang FY, Huang CJ, Chen RX, Xu M, Liu BX, Liang Z: **Observation on therapeutic effect of moxibustion on temperature-sensitive points for lumbar disc herniation**. *Zhongguo Zhen Jiu* 2009, **29**:382-384.
25. Zhang C, Xiao H, Chen Rx: **Observation on curative effect of moxibusting on heat-sensitive points on pressure sores**. *China Journal of Traditional Chinese Medicine and Pharmacy* 2010, **25**:478-488.
26. Kang MF, Chen RX, Fu Y: **Observation on curative effect of moxibusting on heat-sensitive points on knee osteoarthritis**. *Jiangxi Journal of Traditional Chinese Medicine and Pharmacy* 2006, **18**:27-28.
27. Global Initiative for Asthma (GINA): **Pocket guide for asthma management and prevention**. Bethesda: National Institutes of Health, National Heart, Lung, and Blood Institute; Publication No. 95-3659B; 1998.
28. Eric DBateman, Homer ABoushey, Jean Bousquet, William WBusse, Clark JHTim, Romain APauwels, Søren E, Pedersen for the GOAL. Investigators Group: **Can Guideline-defined Asthma Control Be Achieved? The Gaining Optimal Asthma Control Study**. *Am J Respir Crit Care Med* 2004, **170**:836-844.
29. US Department of Health and Human Services, National Institutes of Health, National Heart, Lung and Blood Institute: **Expert Panel Report 3: Guidelines for the Diagnosis and Management of Asthma (EPR-3 2007)**. NIH Item No. 08-4051.[http://www.nhlbi.nih.gov/guidelines/asthma/asthgdln.htm], Accessed September 10, 2007.
30. Lababidi H, Hijaoui A, Zarzour M: **Validation of the Arabic version of the asthma control test**. *J Allergy Clin Immunol* 2004, **113**:59-65.
31. Liu B, Wen T, Yao C, Yan S, He L, Xie Y, Mu Z: **The central randomization system in multi-center clinical trials**. *Chin J New Drugs Clin Rem* 2006, **12**:931-935.
32. Asthma group of Chinese Society of Respiratory Diseases: **The guideline of asthma treatment and prevention**. *Clin J Tuberc Respir Dis* 1997, **20**:261-267.
33. Greening AP, Ind PW, Northfield M, Shaw G: **Added salmeterol versus higher-dose corticosteroid in asthma patients with symptoms on**

Chen *et al. Trials* 2010, **11**:121
http://www.trialsjournal.com/content/11/1/121

existing inhaled corticosteroid. Allen & Hanburys Limited study group. *Lancet* 1994, **344**:219-24.

34. Condemi JJ, Goldstein S, Kalberg C, Yancey S, Emmett A, Rickard K: The addition of salmeterol to fluticasone propionate versus increasing the dose of fluticasone propionate in patients with persistent asthma. *Ann Allergy Asthma Immunol* 1999, **82**:383-9.

35. Pauwels TA, Lofdahl C-G, Postma DS, Pride NB, Ohlsson SV: Effect of inhaled formoterol and budesonide on exacerbations of asthma. *N Engl J Med* 1997, **337**:1405-11.

36. Vanden Berg NJ, Ossip M, Hederos CA, Antilla H, Ribeiro BL, Davies PI: Salmeterol/fluticasone propionate (50/100 mcg) in combination in a Diskus inhaler (Seretide) is effective and safe in children with asthma. *Paed Pulmonol* 2000, **30**:97-105.

37. Zetterström O, Buhl R, Mellem H, Perpina M, Hedman J, O'Neill S, Ekstrom T: Improved asthma control with budesonide/formoterol in a single inhaler, compared with budesonide alone. *Eur Respir J* 2001, **18**:262-8.

38. Tal A, Simon G, Vermeulen JH, Petru V, Cobos N, Everard ML, De Boeck K: Budesonide/formoterol in a single inhaler versus inhaled corticosteroids alone in the treatment of asthma. *Pediatr Pulmonol* 2002, **34**:342-50.

39. Ernst E: Complementary therapies for asthma: what patients use? *J Asthma* 1998, **35**:667-71.

doi:10.1186/1745-6215-11-121
Cite this article as: Chen *et al.*: Comparison of heat-sensitive moxibustion versus fluticasone/salmeterol (seretide) combination in the treatment of chronic persistent asthma: design of a multicenter randomized controlled trial. *Trials* 2010 **11**:121.

Chen *et al. BMC Complementary and Alternative Medicine* 2010, **10**:32
http://www.biomedcentral.com/1472-6882/10/32

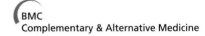

BMC
Complementary & Alternative Medicine

STUDY PROTOCOL   **Open Access**

The design and protocol of heat-sensitive moxibustion for knee osteoarthritis: a multicenter randomized controlled trial on the rules of selecting moxibustion location

Rixin Chen*, Mingren Chen, Mingfei Kang, Jun Xiong, Zhenhai Chi, Bo Zhang and Yong Fu

Abstract

Background: Knee osteoarthritis is a major cause of pain and functional limitation. Complementary and alternative medical approaches have been employed to relieve symptoms and to avoid the side effects of conventional medication. Moxibustion has been widely used to treat patients with knee osteoarthritis. Our past researches suggested heat-sensitive moxibustion might be superior to the conventional moxibustion. Our objective is to investigate the effectiveness of heat-sensitive moxibustion compared with conventional moxibustion or conventional drug treatment.

Methods: This study consists of a multi-centre (four centers in China), randomised, controlled trial with three parallel arms (A: heat-sensitive moxibustion; B: conventional moxibustion; C: conventional drug group). The moxibustion locations are different from A and B. Group A selects heat-sensitization acupoint from the region consisting of Yin Lingquan(SP9), Yang Lingquan(GB34), Liang Qiu(ST34), and Xue Hai (SP10). Meanwhile, fixed acupoints are used in group B, that is Xi Yan (EX-LE5) and He Ding (EX-LE2). The conventional drug group treats with intra-articular Sodium Hyaluronate injection. The outcome measures above will be assessed before the treatment, the 30 days of the last moxibustion session and 6 months after the last moxibustion session.

Discussion: This trial will utilize high quality trial methodologies in accordance with CONSORT guidelines. It will provide evidence for the effectiveness of moxibustion as a treatment for moderate and severe knee osteoarthritis. Moreover, the result will clarify the rules of heat-sensitive moxibustion location to improve the therapeutic effect with suspended moxibustion, and propose a new concept and a new theory of moxibustion to guide clinical practices.

Trial Registration: The trial is registered at Controlled Clinical Trials: ChiCTR-TRC-00000600.

Background

Osteoarthritis (OA) is the most common form of arthritis [1] and the leading cause of disability among older adults [2,3]. As one part of weight-bearing peripheral and axial joints, knee is the most commonly affected by osteoarthritis [4]. Among adults aged 30 years, symptomatic knee OA occurs in 6% and symptomatic hip OA in about 3%[4].Knee osteoarthritis (KOA) is associated with symptoms of pain and functional disability. Physical disability arising from pain and loss of functional capacity reduces

the quality of life and increases the risk of further morbidity and mortality [5]. The prevalence, disability, and associated costs of KOA are expected to steadily increase over the next 25 years because of aging in the population [6]. After adjusting for age, sex, and comorbidity, KOA is responsible for a higher percentage of disability than any other medical condition for the following activities: stair climbing, walking a mile, and housekeeping.

The underlying disease processes of KOA involve cartilage degeneration, proliferation and remodeling of subchondral bone structure. Recently there is no cure for KOA [7]. Therefore, the treatment of KOA is primarily focused on managing the condition by minimizing mor-

* Correspondence: chenrixin*123@yahoo.com.cn
† Affiliated Hospital with Jiangxi University of TCM, Nanchang, PR China
Full list of author information is available at the end of the article

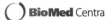

Chen et al. BMC Complementary and Alternative Medicine 2010, **10**:32
http://www.biomedcentral.com/1472-6882/10/32

bidity. The current conventional treatment of KOA symptoms and analgesics, such as NSAIDS, glucosamine, topical analgesics, intra-articular (Sodium Hyaluronate, Synvisc) and surgical treatment[8,9]. Substantial numbers of patients with KOA are not satisfied with conventional drug treatment and repeatedly experience side effects [10,11]. As a result, a large number of patients with KOA are turning to complementary and alternative treatments. Non-pharmacological treatments such as acupuncture are therefore attractive. Acupuncture is often used for KOA. For example, it is gaining popularity among KOA patients in the US and about 1 million consumers utilize acupuncture annually which has musculoskeletal disorders [12].

Acupuncture is a safe treatment that has a low risk for serious side effects. Moxibustion is a traditional Chinese method of acupuncture treatment, which utilizes the heat generated by burning Moxa (it is also called Mugwort or Moxa) to stimulate the acupuncture points. The technique consists of lighting a moxa stick and bringing it close to the skin until it produces hyperaemia due to local vasodilatation. The intensity of moxibustion is just below the individual tolerability threshold. Moxibustion has anti-inflammatory or immunomodulatory effects against chronic inflammatory conditions in humans [13]. Moreover, the heat of moxa treatment improves microcirculation in the knee. Therefore, these Arthritis substances may be reduced and weakened by moxibustion. Then Elimination of swelling and pain relief also may be achieved. Especially for swell type KOA, which derived from surrounding tissues strain, moxibustion may get a better effect. Further deterioration of cartilage is set back, as a result of pathological chain of KOA is cut in treatment of moxibustion. That is to say, moxibustion does not make osteophyte disappeared in short treatment, but its therapeutic effects relieve the main symptoms, and minimizing morbidity of new osteophyte by avoiding pathological product of stimulus and mechanical structural imbalance.

Although firm evidence has not been established, the results of some systematic review and meta-analysis suggest that acupuncture and moxibustion may effective in the treatment of KOA [14-16].Such as the latest meta-analysis concluded that sham-controlled trials showed clinically irrelevant short-term benefits of acupuncture for treating knee osteoarthritis. Waiting list controlled trials suggested clinically relevant benefits, some of which may be due to placebo or expectation effects [16]. However, these reviews do not confirm the efficacy of acupuncture and moxibustion. This may be because all relevant RCTs were limited by methodological defects, including inappropriate sample size, variability of acu-

puncture and sham protocols, and missing information. Therefore, rigorous high-quality randomised controlled trials are needed.

Thinking about moxibustion itself, the selection of location for manipulating Moxa plays an important role in obtaining good effects [17]. In our opinion, the nature of acupoint is not location , but status. In the human being there are two functional states, sensitization state and rest state. When the human body has disease, acupoints on the body surface may be sensitized with various types of sensitization, and acupoint heat-sensitization is a type of acupoint sensitization. The sensitized acupoints show acupoint-specific "small stimulation inducing large response" for external relative stimulation. The Inner Canon of Huangdi or Yellow Emperor's Inner Canon is an ancient Chinese medical text that has been treated as the fundamental doctrinal source for Chinese medicine for more than two millennia and until today. According with its core viewpoint and theory, acupoint is described and understood with the state , which is certain area of the skin in the course of diseases. Among the changes, sensitized status is the common one, described that acupoints on the body surface may be sensitized with various types of sensitization. This sensitized acupoint is not only the pathological phenomenon reflecting the diseases but also stimulating location with acupuncture and moxibustion. Acupoint heat-sensitization is a type of acupoint sensitization.

Our research term found that the heat-sensitized phenomenon was a new type of acupoint sensitized features in pathological state [18-20]. We applicated the acupoint heat-sensitization phenomenon and rule in the past twenty years. The past experiential evidences in our research indicated that the functional state might jump from the rest state to the heat-sensitized state suffering from diseases. Its characteristic was thought that these special acupoints might produce heat response and farther warm sensation, as a result of stimulation of moxibustion heat. If we can search out these heat-sensitized acupoints associating with pathological state, good effect will be achieved. Therefore, selecting the heat-sensitized acupoint may obtain therapeutic effect far better than acupuncture and moxibustion at acupoints of routine rest state. We carried our many clinical trials to test and verify the efficacy heat-sensitized acupoint, such as myofascial pain syndrome [21], lumbar disc herniation[22], pressure sores[23] and KOA[24]. The result of clinical trials almost suggested superiority effect of heat-sensitized acupoint and encouraged us to proceed.

With these constraints, we planned a rigorous multi-centre randomised controlled trial with a large sample size.

Chen *et al. BMC Complementary and Alternative Medicine* 2010, **10**:32
http://www.biomedcentral.com/1472-6882/10/32

Method/design

Objective

The aim of this study is to investigate the effectiveness of heat-sensitive moxibustion compared with conventional moxibustion or conventional drug treatment (intra-articular Sodium Hyaluronate injection) in patients with moderate to severe KOA in China.

Outcome

Ministry of Health of the People's Republic of China (MHPRC) has proposed a series of criteria to define patient response in the context of clinical trials of KOA, known as the guiding principle of clinical research on new drugs (GPCRND) [25]. According to these criteria, a patient with KOA is assessed including pain, the relation between activity and pain, function impairment, and special exams (Table 1). This scoring system was previously validated. The degree of KOA is divided into three level: mild- < 5 score;moderate-5 ~ 9 score; severe-> 9 score.

Therapeutic effect was assessed by comparing baseline and final conditions reported by the patient. Four categories were listed as below: clinical response-no symptom, normal function activity, clinical symptom score reduction ≥ 95%; markedly effective-no obvious symptom, normal joint function activity, able to participate in activity and work, clinical symptom score reduction 70 ~ 95%; improved-no pain, normal joints' flexion and extension, improvement in activity and work, clinical symptom score reduction 30 ~ 70%; ineffective-not arrived at the above standard involving with symptom and function impairment, clinical symptom score reduction < 30%.

This trial also records adverse effects reported by patients during treatment. The outcome measures above will be assessed before the treatment, the 30 days of the last moxibustion session and 6 months after the last moxibustion session.

Design

A multi-centre (four centers in China), randomised, subject blinded(group A and B) and assessor blinded, positive controlled trial will be conducted at the Jiangxi Traditional Chinese Medicine Hospital in Nanchang, The first Affiliated Hospital with Anhui University of TCM in Hefei, Jiangsu Traditional Chinese Medicine Hospital in Nanjing, and Shanxi Traditional Chinese Medicine Hospital in Xian. The study will be sequentially conducted as follows: a run-in period of one week prior to randomisation, a treatment period of 30 days (5 sessions per week), and a follow-up period of six months. The total study period will be eight months. At the end of the run-in period, participants will be randomised to the heat-sensitive moxibustion group, the conventional moxibustion group, or the conventional drug treatment group by the central randomization system (Figure 1).This system is provided by China Academy of Chinese Medical Sciences, which adopted the computer telephone integration (CTI) technology to integrate computer, internet and telecom. The random number list will be assign by interactive voice response (IVR) and interactive web response (IWR)[26]. The success of blinding will be assessed at each participant's last visit. Researchers who did not participate in the treatment and who are blinded to the allocation results will perform the outcome assessment

Eligibility

Inclusion criteria

Eligible participants will be those previously diagnosed with moderate to severe KOA, according to the GPCRND-KOA criteria(> 5 score). Patients will be required to complete the baseline KOA diary. Written informed consent will be obtained from each participant. , Participants 38 ~ 70 years of age will be recruited from outpatient and inpatient in four centers. Standard of diagnosis listed as follows:(1) Keen pain almost occurred in the past one month; (2)Osteophyma at the edge of joints are all well demonstrated in X-ray; (3)Laboratory examinations of arthritis support the diagnosis of osteoarthritis;(4) Morning stiffness continued less than 30 minutes;(5) Bone sound existed when joints was taking flexion and/or extension. If a patient accord with (1), (2), or (1), (3), (4), (5), we can diagnose. Since the research involves moderate to severe KOA or severe KOA, the inclusion criteria will restrict the following conditions: According with the below KOA diagnosis standard, meanwhile, knee joints appear die Schwellung; Floating patella test is negative; Patients accept the treatment protocol in this trial; Acupoint heat-sensitization phenomenon exists in the region consisting of Yin Lingquan(SP9), Yang Lingquan(GB34), Liang Qiu(ST34), and Xue Hai (SP10).

Participants will be instructed to stop KOA symptomatic relief medication during the run-in and treatment periods and will be provided the usual care instruction for KOA.

Exclusion criteria

Participants will be excluded if they suffer from serious life-threatening disease, such as disease of the heart and brain blood vessels, liver, kidney and hematopoietic system, and psychotic patients. Participants will not be eligible if the female are in the duration of pregnancy or lactation. The following conditions are also excluded items: acute knee joint trauma or ulceration in its local skin; complicated with serious genu varus/valgue and flexion conttration.

Chen *et al. BMC Complementary and Alternative Medicine* 2010, **10**:32
http://www.biomedcentral.com/1472-6882/10/32

Table 1: List of GPCRND-KOA

Item	Grade/Classification		Score
Pain or discomfort in night when lying in bed	No		0
	Pain in activity or some position		1
	Pain in non-activity		2
Morning stiffness or pain worse when getting out of bed	No		0
	< 30 minutes		1
	≥ 30 minutes		2
Pain or discomfort in walk	No		0
	After walking in some distance		1
	Pain at beginning of walk or worse		2
Arise from seat	Independent		0
	Need assistance		1
The maximum walk distance(accompany with pain)	Unrestricted		0
	Restricted, > 1 km		1
	300 m ~ 1 km		2
	< 300 m		3
Daily Activities	Board standard airstairs		
		Independent	0
		Difficulty	1
		Unable	2
	Step down standard airstairs		
		Independent	0
		Difficulty	1
		Unable	2
	Squat or bend knees		
		Independent	0
		Difficulty	1
		Unable	2
	Walk over rough terrain		
		Independent	0
		Difficulty	1
		Unable	2

Treatment protocol

Heat-sensitive moxibustion

Moxibustion will be performed by certified acupuncture medical doctors at four centers. Qualified specialists of acupuncture in traditional Chinese medicine with at least five years of clinical experience will perform the acupuncture in this study. All treatment regimens will be standardized between four centers practitioners via video, hands-on training and internet workshops. Participants will be randomly assigned to the heat-sensitive moxibus-

tion group, the conventional moxibustion group, or the conventional drug group. In the former groups, a 22 mm (diameter) × 160mm (length) moxa-sticks (Jiangxi Traditional Chinese Medicine Hospital, China) will be used. The patient is usually in the comfortable supine position for treatment, with 24°C ~ 30°C temperature in the room. He should be wearing loose trousers, especially making his knee joints exposed.

For the heat-sensitive moxibustion group, the moxa-sticks are lit by the therapist and held over the region

Chen *et al. BMC Complementary and Alternative Medicine* 2010, **10**:32
http://www.biomedcentral.com/1472-6882/10/32

Page 5 of 9

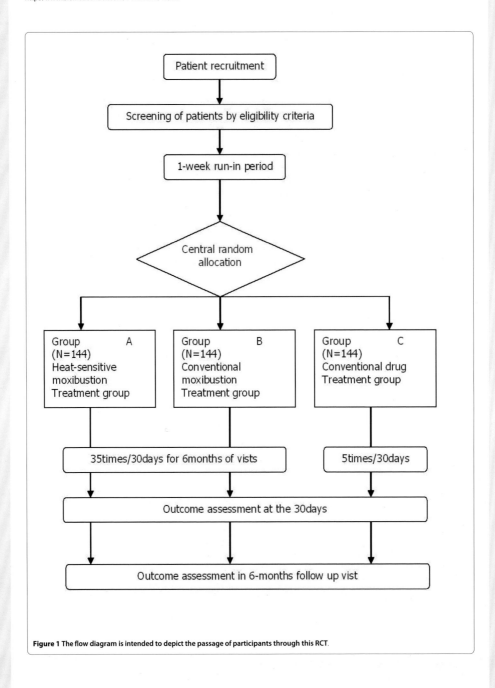

Figure 1 The flow diagram is intended to depict the passage of participants through this RCT.

Chen *et al. BMC Complementary and Alternative Medicine* 2010, **10**:32
http://www.biomedcentral.com/1472-6882/10/32

consisting of Yin Lingquan(SP9), Yang Lingquan(GB34), Liang Qiu(ST34), and Xue Hai (SP10). The warming suspended moxibustion about distance of 3cm are used to search the acupoint heat-sensitization phenomenon. The following patients sensation will suggest the special heat-sensitization aupoint: diathermanous sensation due to moxa-heat, defining as the heat sensation conducting from the moxa local skin surface into deep tissue, or even into the joint cavity; expand heat sensation due to moxa-heat, defining as the heat sensation spreading the surrounding little by little around the moxa point; transfer heat sensation due to moxa-heat, defining as the heat sensation transferring along some pathway or direction, even to the ankle or hip conduction; non-heat sensation due to moxa-heat. When some acupoint exists one below sensation at least, the therapists mark the point as heat-sensitive acupoint. We try our best to seek all the special acupoints in each patient by the repeated manipulation.

The therapists begin to treat patients from the most heat-sensitive intensity acupoint. Treatment sessions end when patients are feel the acupoint heat-sensitization phenomenon disappeared. Generally speaking, we find the time range from 30 ~ 60 minutes.Patients receive the treatment two times/day in 1st week(two times/day from 2nd week) for a total of 35 sessions over 30 days.

Conventional moxibustion group
Patients assigning in conventional moxibustion group will receive fixed acupoint moxibustion. Common practices are similar with the first group. The different manipulation is that the therapists carry out warming moxibustion in traditional acupoint, selecting Xi Yan (EX-LE5) and He Ding (EX-LE2). One point is treated 15minutes a time. Three points are treated by suspended moxibustion at the same time. In the treatment, the therapists make patients the same intensity of local warm sensation as the former group. The sensation of acupoint heat-sensitization phenomenon is not pursued and not avoided in the treatment. Patients receive the treatment two times/day in 1st week (two times/day from 2nd week) for a total of 35 sessions over 30 days.

Conventional drug group
Now, intra-articular hyaluronan (HA) or hylan is popular approved for the treatment of KOA [27]. A number of systematic reviews have published positive evidence of efficacy and safety of intra-articular HA for KOA. For example, a recent review proved HA to be an effective, safe, and tolerable treatment for symptomatic KOA [28]. Therefore, this protocol selected Sodium Hyaluronate Injection Intra-articula as the conventional drug. The injection will be used six days a time (2ml) as a total of five times.

Statistical methods
Analysis
We will conduct analysis on an intention-to-treat basis (significance level p < 0.05) using the SAS statistical pack-

age program (ver. 9.1.3).The analysis of center effect will be used Cochran-Mantel-Haenszel. Baseline characteristics will be shown as mean ± standard deviation (SD) for continuous data including age, previous duration, and GPCRND-KOA criteria. As for participants' gender, n (%) of male and female in each group will be shown as baseline characteristics. We will conduct between-group comparision in baseline using ANCOVA (analysis of covariance) for continuous data and using Chi-square test or nonparametric test for gender composition considering p < 0.05 as statistically significant.

For outcome measures, the mean differences from baseline values to the end of treatment will be compared using ANCOVA. If any imbalances in baseline characteristics between groups are encountered, we will conduct ANCOVA (analysis of covariance) using these imbalanced variables as covariates and allocated group as fixed factor.

Data integrity
The integrity of trial data will be monitored by regularly scrutinizing data sheets for omissions and errors. Data will be double-entered and the source of any inconsistencies will be explored and resolved.

Sample size
We wished to estimate the sample size that would suffice to detect GPCRND-KOA between the heat-sensitive and conventional moxibustion groups. In our previous pilot study, the effective rate in heat-sensitive moxibustion group is 70%, and 50% in the other group. If we apply a two-sided 5% significance level, 95% power the calculated required sample size is approximately 120 participants in each group, according to the following equation. Allowing for a 20% loss to follow up, a total of 144 participants will be required in each group, with 432 participants in total.

$$n = \frac{p_1 \times (1-p_1) + p_2 \times (1-p_2)}{(p_2-p_1)^2} \times f(\alpha, \beta)$$

Adverse events
We define adverse events as unfavorable or unintended signs, symptoms or disease occurring after treatment that are not necessarily related to the moxibustion intervention. In every visit, adverse events will be reported by participants and examined by the practitioner.

Ethics
Written consent will be obtained from each participant. This study was approved by all relevant local ethics review boards. Ethics Committee of Affiliated hospital of Jiangxi Institute of Traditional Chinese Medicine had approved this trial: code issued by ethic committee is 2008(9).

Discussions

To our knowledge, although there is no cure for KOA, current kinds of therapies focus on the relief of pain and stiffness and maintenance or improvement in functional status and quality of life as important goals. A number of clinical trial suggested moxibustion as one of traditional acupuncture therapy, should effective in the treatment of KOA. But the methodological problems of published trials haunt us the trust of moxibustion. Therefore, we design this rigorous clinical trials meeting the CONSORT statement and guidelines to guarantee a high internal validity for the results. In view of the special nature of the KOA itself, positive control should be selected to solve the patient's pain, swell, and impairment. At present, various conventional medications are used to slow down and control with the disease. Although Anesthetic and NSAIDS can relive the pain and inflammation, patients are not considered it as priority options because of multiple adverse reactions. Sodium Hyaluronate acid injections may give you more pain relief than oral medicines, and less adverse reactions. Therefore, we used the Sodium Hyaluronate acid injections as drug treatment in the protocol.

Actually, the aim of this trial contains two parts: "Is moxibustion treatment superior to Sodium Hyaluronate acid injections for KOA? And is heat-sensitive moxibustion superior to conventional moxibustion for KOA?" The latter one is our more interesting goal. According to the current theory of traditional Chinese medicine, moxibustion resulting from the burning of moxa, produces the radiant heat and drug effects to acupoints. This treatment penetrates deeply into the body, restoring the balance and flow of vital energy or life force through acupoints. So the selected of location for manipulating Moxa plays an important role in obtaining good effects. Generally speaking, the location acupoints are fixed along meridians. The conventional moxibustion is promoted for improving general health and treating diseases by stimulating these fixed acupoints. And doctors consider hyperaemia due to local skin vasodilatation as the indicator of moxibustion's effect. However, our clinical experience and observation in the past suggested that stimulating these fixed acupoints might not the best treatment site for moxibustion. In the human being there are two functional states, sensitization state and rest state. When the human body has disease, acupoints on the body surface may be sensitized with various types of sensitization, and acupoint heat-sensitization is a type of acupoint sensitization. acupoint is more than fixed skin site but external sensitive point reflecting the diseases. Therefore, acupoint is variable and depends on the pathological state. Traditional fixed acupints are thought as indicators to searching specific sensitive acupoint. That is, traditional fixed acupints don not consider the state as the key factor

to local the acupoint, so the course of fixing the position is imprecisely.

When we light the moxa hold over the heat-sensitive acupoints, the patients will produce some heat-sensitization phenomenon. The following patients sensation will suggest the special heat-sensitization aupoint: diathermanous sensation due to moxa-heat, defining as the heat sensation conducting from the moxa local skin surface into deep tissue, or even into the joint cavity; expand heat sensation due to moxa-heat, defining as the heat sensation spreading the surrounding little by little around the moxa point; transfer heat sensation due to moxa-heat, defining as the heat sensation transferring along some pathway or direction, even to the ankle or hip conduction; non-heat sensation due to moxa-heat.

It is well-known that acupuncture and moxibustion originated from China several thousands years ago. The Inner Canon of Huangdi or Yellow Emperor's Inner Canon is an ancient Chinese medical text that has been treated as the fundamental doctrinal source for Chinese medicine for more than two millennia and until today. According with its core viewpoint and theory, acupoint is described and understood with the state , which is certain area of the skin in the course of diseases. "*Said section (acupoint) who shen-qi out of the procession itself, not flesh bones* "(Huang Di Neijing, Lingshu, Chapter: jiu zhen shi er yuan).That is, acupoints are not flesh bones, which have their particular morphology and fixed location, but dynamic functional state due to shen-qi's activity. "*when five internal organs are suffering from diseases, we can use 12 yuan-acupoints to treat. These acupoints are derived from five internal organs intrinsic nature. Five internal organs are diagnosed by 12 yuan-acupoints. Different organs accord with relative yuan-acupoint. We can observe and distinguish the acupoint response to external stimulation. Then, the disease from five internal organs can be diagnosed and treated by 12 yuan-acupoints*" (Huang Di Neijing, Lingshu, Chapter: jiu zhen shi er yuan).So an important view was expressed by this sentence, that is, acupoints reflect the internal diseases and can be operated in treatment of disease with the functional role. In physiological status, people do not always become aware of the existence of acupoint. In contrast, patients can feel some changes from acupoint involving with diseases in pathological state. So the ancient persons located the acupoints through the state changes. "*Lung shu-acupoints locate nearby the third vertebrae; Heart shu-acupoints locate nearby the fifth vertebrae; Ge shu-acupoints locate nearby the seventh; Liver shu-acupoints locate nearby the ninth vertebrae; Spleen shu-acupoints locate nearby the eleventh vertebrae; Kindey shu-acupoints locate nearby the fourteenth vertebrae. These acupoints are far from about three-inch by spinal crest. If you want to search our acupoints exactly, the finger's touch* and press are must be use above the skin and we obtain the sensation from patients, such as pain. " (Huang Di Neijing, Lingshu, Chapter: back shu). Back shu acupoints are searched by doctor through external stimulation. "If a patient is coughing with shoulder, we can select the lateral chest shu acupoints to treat. The shu acupoints are nearby from *the third vertebrae to the fifth vertebrae. Press the location, patients will be comfortable at once. Then we needle the location, which is acupoint actually.*" (Huang Di Neijing, Lingshu, Chapter: five xie) *We conclude that* sensitized status is key factor to locate the position of acupoints.

Among the changes, sensitized status is the common one, described that acupoints on the body surface may be sensitized with various types of sensitization. This sensitized acupoint is not only the pathological phenomenon reflecting the diseases but also stimulating location with acupuncture and moxibustion. Acupoint heat-sensitization is a type of acupoint sensitization, which derived from our clinical experience and research in past twenty years. The special acupoint makes accordance with the classical thought and theory from the Inner Canon of Huangdi.

Our empirical evidence engaged us to formulate the following hypothesis: selecting the heat-sensitized acupoint may obtain therapeutic effect far better than acupuncture and moxibustion at acupoints of routine rest state. The main aim of this trial is to test and verify the hypothesis. If we can confirm this hypothesis, promoting moxibustion clinical efficacy would be carried our in this extraordinary way. It is of great significance to develop the theory of acupuncture and moxibustion.

Therefore, the purpose of this trial is more than discuss the efficacy of moxibustion as treatment. The results of our trial will be helpful to supply the evidence on the rules of heat-sensitive moxibustion location in China.

Competing interests
The authors declare that they have no competing interests.

Authors' contributions
RC and MC obtained funding for the research project and drafted the protocol. JX wrote the final manuscript. MK contributed to the research design and made critical revisions. ZC, BZ and YF were responsible for the statistical design of the trial and wrote portions of the statistical methods, data handling, and monitoring sections. All authors read and approved the final manuscript.

Acknowledgements
This study was supported by the National Natural Science Foundation of China and the Major State Basic Research Development Program of People's Republic of China (Grant number: 2009CB522902).

Author Details
Affiliated Hospital with Jiangxi University of TCM, Nanchang, PR China

Received: 30 April 2010 Accepted: 25 June 2010
Published: 25 June 2010

References
1. Scott JC, Hochberg MC: **Arthritic and other musculoskeletal diseases.** In *Chronic disease epidemiology and control* 2nd edition. Edited by: Brownson RC, Reminton PL, Davis JR. Washington (DC): American Public Health Association; 1993:465-489.
2. Peat G, McCarney R, Croft P: **Knee pain and osteoarthritis in older adults: a review of community burden and current use of primary health care.** *Ann RheumDis* 2001, **60**:91-97.
3. Prevalence of self-reported arthritis or chronic joint symptoms among adults United States, 2001. *MMWR Morb Mortal Wkly Rep* 2002, **51**:948-950.
4. Felson DT, Zhang Y: **An update on the epidemiology of knee and hip osteoarthritis with a view to prevention.** *Arthritis Rheum* 1998, **41**:1343-1355.
5. Jordan KM, Arden NK, Doherty M, *et al.*: **EULAR Recommendations 2003 an evidence based approach to the management of knee osteoarthritis report of a Task Force of the Standing Committee for International Clinical Studies Including Therapeutic Trials (ESCISIT).** *Ann Rheum Dis* 2003, **62**:1145-1155.
6. Lethbridge CM, Schiller JS, BerLethbridg CM, Schiller JS, Bernadel L: Summary health statistics for U.S. adults: National Health Interview Survey, 2002. *Vital Health Stat 10* 2004:1-151.
7. American College of Rheumatology Subcommittee on Osteoarthritis Guidelines. Recommendations for the medical management of osteoarthritis of the hip and knee 2000 update. *Arthritis Rheum* 2000, **43**:1905-1915.
8. Felson DT, Lawrence RC, Hochberg MC, *et al.*: Osteoarthritis new insights Part 2 treatment approaches. *Ann Intern Med* 2000, **133**:726-737.
9. Hamburger MI, Lakhanpal S, Mooar PA, Oster D: **Intra-articular hyaluronans a review of product-specific safety profiles.** Semin. *Arthritis Rheum* 2003, **32**:296-309.
10. McGettigan P, Henry D: **Cardiovascular risk and inhibition of cyclooxygenase a systematic review of the observational studies of selective and nonselective inhibitors of cyclooxygenase 2.** *JAMA* 2006, **296**:1633-1644.
11. Blower AL, Brooks A, Fenn GC, Hill A, Pearce MY, Morant S: **Emergency admissions for upper gastrointestinal disease and their relation to NSAID use.** *Aliment Pharmacol Ther* 1997, **11**:283-291.
12. Paramore LC: **Use of alternative therapies estimates from the 1994 Robert Wood Johnson Foundation National Access to Care Survey.** *J Pain Symptom Manage* 1997, **13**:83-89.
13. Cho ZH, Hwang SC, Wong EK, Son YD, Kang CK, Park TS, Bai SJ, Kim YB, Lee YB, Sung KK: **Neural substrates, experimental evidences and functional hypothesis of acupuncture mechanisms.** *Acta Neurol Scand* 2006, **113**:370-377.
14. Ezzo J, Victoria V, Stephen S, Lixing L, Gary G, Marc M, Brian B: **Acupuncture for Osteoarthritis of the Knee: A Systematic Review.** *Arthritis & Rheumatism* 2001, **44**:819-825.
15. Terry KS, Ann GT: **Acupuncture and Osteoarthritis of the Knee: A Review of Randomized Controlled Trials.** *Fam Community Health* 2008, **31**:247-254.
16. Eric M, Klaus L, Lixing L, Lex M, Brian M: **Meta-analysis: Acupuncture for Osteoarthritis of the Knee.** *Ann Intern Med* 2007, **146**:868-877.
17. Ayman E, Karl O: **Moxibustion in Breech Version-A Descriptive Review.** *Acupuncture in medicine* 2002, **20**:26-29.
18. Chen RX, Kang MF: **Clinical application of acupoint heat-sensitization.** *Zhongguo Zhen* 2007, **27**:199-202.
19. Chen RX, Kang MF: **Key point of moxibustion, arrival of qi produces curative effect.** *Zhongguo Zhen Jiu* 2008, **28**:44-46.
20. Chen RX, Kang MF, He WL, Chen SY, Zhang B: **Moxibustion on heat-sensitive acupoints for treatment of myofascial pain syndrome a multi-central randomized controlled trial.** *Zhongguo Zhen* 2008, **28**:395-398.
21. Chen RX, Kang MF: **Acupoint heat-sensitization moxibustion an new therapy.** 1st edition. Press by People's Medical Publishing House. Beijing in China; 2006.
22. Tang FY, Huang CJ, Chen RX, Xu M, Liu BX, Liang Z: **Observation on therapeutic effect of moxibustion on temperature-sensitive points for lumbar disc herniation.** *Zhongguo Zhen Jiu* 2009, **29**:382-384.
23. Zhang C, Xiao H, Chen Rx: **Observation on curative effect of moxibusting on heat-sensitive points on pressure sores.** *China Journal of Traditional Chinese Medicine and Pharmacy* 2010, **25**:478-488.

Chen *et al. BMC Complementary and Alternative Medicine* 2010, **10**:32
http://www.biomedcentral.com/1472-6882/10/32

24. Kang MF, Chen RX, Fu Y: **Observation on curative effect of moxibusting on heat-sensitive points on knee osteoarthritis.** *Jiangxi Journal of Traditional Chinese Medicine and Pharmacy* 2006, **18**:27-28.
25. **The Guideline of the latest Chinese herbs to Clinical Research.** 1st edition. Edited by: Zhen XY. Beijing: Medicine Science and Technology Press of China; 2002.
26. Liu B, Wen T, Yao C, Yan S, He L, Xie Y, Mu Z: **The central randomization system in multi-center clinical trials.** *Chin J New Drugs Clin Rem* 2006, **12**:931-935.
27. Brzusek D, Petron D: **Treating knee osteoarthritis with intra-articular hyaluronans.** *Curr Med Res Opin* 2008, **24(12)**:3307-3322.
28. Bannuru RR, Natov NS, Obadan IE, Price LL, Schmid CH, McAlindon TE: **Therapeutic trajectory of hyaluronic acid versus corticosteroids in the treatment of knee osteoarthritis a systematic review and meta-analysis.** *Arthritis Rheum* 2009, **61(12)**:1704-1711. 15

Pre-publication history
The pre-publication history for this paper can be accessed here:
http://www.biomedcentral.com/1472-6882/10/32/prepub

doi: 10.1186/1472-6882-10-32
Cite this article as: Chen *et al.*, The design and protocol of heat-sensitive moxibustion for knee osteoarthritis: a multicenter randomized controlled trial on the rules of selecting moxibustion location *BMC Complementary and Alternative Medicine* 2010, **10**:32

Chen *et al. Trials* 2011, **12**:226
http://www.trialsjournal.com/content/12/1/226

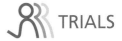 TRIALS

STUDY PROTOCOL   **Open Access**

Effectiveness of heat-sensitive moxibustion in the treatment of lumbar disc herniation: study protocol for a randomized controlled trial

Mingren Chen[1], Rixin Chen[1*], Jun Xiong[1], Fan Yi[2], Zhenhai Chi[1] and Bo Zhang[1]

Abstract

Background: Lumbar disc herniation is a common and costly problem. Moxibustion is employed to relieve symptoms and might therefore act as a therapeutic alternative. Many studies have already reported encouraging results in heat-sensitive moxibustion for lumbar disc herniation. Hence, we designed a randomized controlled clinical trial to investigate the effectiveness of heat-sensitive moxibustion compared with conventional moxibustion.

Methods: This trial is a multicenter, prospective, randomized controlled clinical trial. The 316 eligible patients are randomly allocated to two different groups. The experimental group is treated with heat-sensitive moxibustion (n = 158); while the control group (n = 158) is treated with conventional moxibustion. The moxibustion locations are different for the groups. The experimental group selects heat-sensitization acupoints from the region which consists of bilateral Da Changshu (BL25) and Yao Shu (Du2). Meanwhile, fixed acupoints are used in control group; patients in both groups receive 18 sessions in 2 weeks.

Discussion: The study design guarantees a high internal validity for the results. It is one large-scale randomized controlled trial to evaluate the efficacy of heat-sensitive moxibustion compared to conventional moxibustion and may provide evidence for this therapy as a treatment for moderate and severe lumbar disc herniation. Moreover, the result may uncover the inherent laws to improve the therapeutic effect with suspended moxibustion.

Trial Registration: The trial is registered at Chinese Clinical Trials Registry: ChiCTR-TRC-09000604. The application date was 27 November 2009. The first patient was randomized on the 16 June 2011.

Background

Lumbar disc herniation (LDH) is one of the most common causes of nerve root pain, and become a painful, debilitating disorder in working adults [1]. In the majority of patients, experiencing their first episode of sciatica due to LDH, the symptoms recede to a non-disabling level within a period of six weeks [2].

LDH most typical symptoms are low back pain, accompanied by one or both lower extremity pain, numbness, pain, mostly by lumbosacral, buttocks, posterolateral to the lower limbs and feet, back radiation when bending, cough worse with movements. Herniated discs also often occur without symptoms, as revealed by magnetic resonance imaging studies in asymptomatic people. They are only clinically relevant when they impinge on a nerve root, causing radiculopathy [3,4].

In general, LDH is due to disc degeneration or trauma leading to nucleus, annulus fibrosis to the vertebral canal prominent, spinal cord or nerve root compression. As a result, conventional treatments including physical therapy, pain medication, anti-inflammatory drugs and surgery, are provided by physicians. Most patients with low back pain respond well to conservative therapy [5,6]. Recently, a large number of patients with LDH are turning to complementary and alternative treatments. Complementary and alternative treatments such as acupuncture are therefore attractive. Acupuncture is often used for LDH. For example, it is gaining popularity among LDH patients in the US and about 1 million consumers with musculoskeletal disorders utilize acupuncture annually [7].

Moxibustion is a traditional Chinese method that uses the heat generated by burning herbal preparations

---

* Correspondence: chenrixin123@yahoo.com.cn
[1]The Affiliated Hospital of Jiangxi University of TCM, Nanchang, Jiangxi, PR China
Full list of author information is available at the end of the article

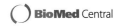

containing Artemisia vulgaris to stimulate acupoints [8]. Moxibustion has anti-inflammatory or immunomodulatory effects against chronic inflammatory conditions in humans [9,10]. Different moxibustion methods for treatment of LDH and their mechanism may be due to moxibustion can improve local blood circulation, eliminate nerve root inflammation and edema, loosen adhesions and improve protrusion and nerve root relations or the promotion of nerve injury repair [11,12]. Moreover, the heat of moxa treatment improves microcirculation in the lumbar vertebra.

Therefore, these arthritis substances may be reduced and weakened by moxibustion. Especially for acute LDH, moxibustion may have a good effect. Severe low-back pain with leg pain (sciatica) may be caused by a herniated intervertebral disc exerting pressure on the nerve root in this stage. Nerve root inflammation and the surrounding edema aggravate the pain. The role of moxibustion may manage the pathological process.

There are many factors influencing therapeutic effect in moxibustion. But the selection of location for manipulating moxa should deserve the greatest attention [13]. Our previous studies suggested that the dominating factor in selecting the location of acupoints is associated with the area on the body surface which is affected by disease, not only the standardized fixed position [14]. In humans, acupoints contain two states: stimulated and resting. When people get sick, the acupoints on the body surface area are activated and sensitized. The sensitive areas are susceptible to heat stimulation and called "heat-sensitized acupoints". A feature of these areas is that they are specific or closely relevant to acupoints and produce the same clinical effect as "a small stimulation induces a large response". This sensitized acupoint is not only the pathological phenomenon reflecting the diseases but also an effective stimulating location with acupuncture and moxibustion [15].

Our research found that the heat-sensitive phenomenon to acupoint or an area is a new type of reaction in a pathological state [16-19]. A lot of observations and research were used to confirm this phenomenon in the 1990s [16]. We summarized the experiential evidence and found that the state of acupoints might change from the rest state to the heat-sensitized state in patients when suffering from diseases. These special acupoints might bring out further heat sensation and response in the stimulation of moxibustion heat. If we can search out these heat-sensitized acupoints associating with pathological state, good effects may be achieved. Therefore, selecting the heat-sensitized acupoint may obtain therapeutic effect far better than acupuncture and moxibustion at acupoints of the routine resting state [14]. So the heat-sensitive moxibustion is a medical technique usually involving suspended moxibustion on the heat-sensitized acupoint. A great many

physicians utilized heat-sensitive moxibustion therapy in different kinds of diseases in China. Moreover, several articles and research have documented the effectiveness and safety of heat-sensitive moxibustion, such as myofascial pain syndrome [18], LDH [20], pressure sores [21] and knee osteoarthritis [22]. Together these findings suggest a superiority effect of heat-sensitized acupoints. However, the results do not provide convincing evidence. This may be because of inappropriate sample size, variability of acupuncture and sham protocols, and missing information which were frequent methodological problems [19]. Therefore, well-designed randomized controlled clinical trials are needed to establish the efficacy of heat-sensitive moxibustion for LDH.

Method/design
Objective
The aim of this study is to investigate the effectiveness of heat-sensitive moxibustion compared with conventional moxibustion in patients with acute LDH in China.

Outcome
The improvement Japanese Orthopedic Association has proposed a series of criteria to define patient response in the context of clinical trials of LDH. M-JOA scale is known as the modified edition of JOA Back Pain Evaluation Questionnaire [23]. According to these criteria, a patient with LDH is assessed including pain, the activities of daily life and work, function impairment, and special exams (Table 1). This scoring system was previously validated [23]. The degree of LDH is divided into three levels: mild: < 10, moderate: 10 to 20, severe: > 20.

Therapeutic effect is assessed by comparing baseline and final conditions reported by the patient. This trial also records adverse effects reported by patients during treatment. The outcome measures above will be assessed before treatment, the 14 days after the last moxibustion session and 6 months after the last moxibustion session.

To evaluate the improvement of severity, we will make use of M-JOA score and take the secondary analysis. Improvement rate = [(scores before treatment - after treatment score)/pretreatment score] × 100%. Definition are listed below: Clinically important improvement as ≥ 75%, markedly effective improvement as 50 to 75%, improved as 30 to 50% and ineffective as < 30%. The numbers in the four categories will be calculated respectively at every time point.

Design
A multi-center (four centers in China), randomized, subject blinded(group A and B) and assessor blinded, parallel positive controlled trial will be conducted at the affiliated Hospital of Jiangxi University of TCM in Nanchang, The

Chen *et al. Trials* 2011, **12**:226
http://www.trialsjournal.com/content/12/1/226

Table 1 List of M-JOA

Item	Grade/Classification	Score
Subjective symptoms		
Lumbar and leg pain	No	0
	Mild pain or occasional moderate pain	1
	Usual moderate pain or occasional severe pain	2
	Frequent or continuous severe pain	3
Numbness	No	0
	Occasional	1
	Frequent but relief may be on their own	2
	Continuous, not alleviated	3
Objective signs		
Paravertebral tenderness	No	0
	Mild	1
	Moderate	2
	Severe	3
Myodynamia	Grade V	3
	Grade IV	2
	Grade III	1
	Grade 0 to II	0
Straight let raising test	> 70°, straight leg drive up (-)	0
	> 45°, straight leg drive up (+)	1
	> 30°, straight leg drive up (+)	2
	< 30°, straight leg drive up (+)	3
Radiating pain	No	0
	Hip/thigh	1
	Shank	2
	Foot	3
Activities of daily life and work		
Stoop and lift heavy things	Normal stoop, lift weight > 3 kg	0
	Able to stoop, lift weight ≤ 3 kg	1
	Unable to stoop	2
	Serious difficulties in bending and lifting	3
Walking distance/time	Walking ≥ 1 km or 60 min	0
	Walking ≥ 500 m or 30 min	1
	Walking ≥ 100 m or 10 min	2
	Serious difficulties in walking	3
Daily time in bed(h)	< 10	0
	10 to 12	1
	12 to 16	2
	> 16	3
Ability to work	Full-time to do as before	0
	Although able to work, occasionally need a break	1
	Although able to work, usually need a break	2
	Unable to work	3

first Affiliated Hospital of Anhui University of TCM in Hefei, Jiangsu TCM Hospital in Nanjing, and Shanxi TCM Hospital in Xian. The study will be sequentially conducted as follows: a recruitment period prior to randomization, a treatment period of 14 days (5 sessions per week), and a follow-up period of six months. Participants will be randomized to the heat-sensitive moxibustion group or the conventional moxibustion group by the central randomization system (Figure 1). This system is provided by China Academy of Chinese Medical Sciences, which adopted the computer telephone integration (CTI) technology to integrate computer, internet and telecom. The random number list will be assigned by interactive voice response (IVR) and interactive web response (IWR)

Chen *et al. Trials* 2011, **12**:226
http://www.trialsjournal.com/content/12/1/226

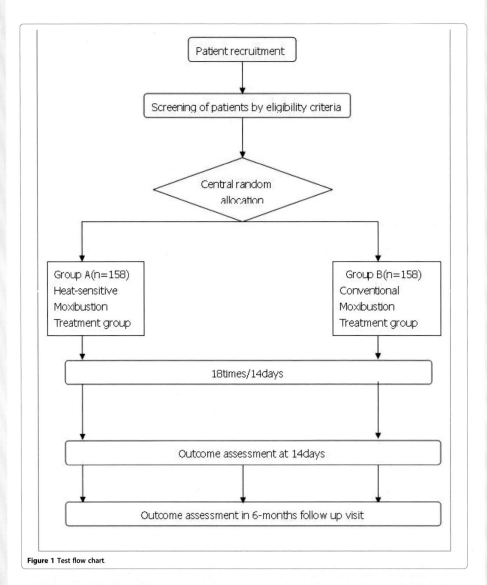

Figure 1 Test flow chart.

[24]. The success of blinding will be assessed at each participant's last visit. Researchers who did not participate in the treatment and who are blinded to the allocation results will perform the outcome assessment. Patients meeting the inclusion criteria were randomly assigned in a 1:1 ratio to the two groups. We used the parallel controlled design and did not stratify by center or block within center.

Chen *et al. Trials* 2011, **12**:226
http://www.trialsjournal.com/content/12/1/226

Eligibility

Inclusion criteria

Eligible participants will be those previously diagnosed with moderate to severe LDH, according to the M-JOA criteria(> 10 score). Patients will be required to complete the baseline LDH diary. Written informed consent will be obtained from each participant. Participants 18 to 65 years of age will be recruited from outpatient and inpatient in four centers. Standard of diagnosis listed as follows:

① Pain occurred in lower back and radiated to the lower limb; ② Limitations of tender point; ③ Straight leg raising test and it's strengthen test are positive; ④ Skin sensation, muscle strength and tendon reflex have some changes; Changes in spinal posture; ⑤ CT suggestive of disc herniation. The above standard mainly originated from the guiding principle of clinical research on new drugs (GPCRND) [23]. Since the research involves moderate to severe LDH or severe LDH, the inclusion criteria will restrict the following conditions: According to the below LDH diagnosis standard, meanwhile, the triangle region formed with bilateral Da Changshu (BL 25)and Yao Shu (Du 2) of patients (Da Changshu- Yao Shu -contralateral Da Changshu intra-region) appear heat-sensitive points.

Participants will be instructed to stop LDH symptomatic relief medication during the run-in and treatment periods and will be provided the usual care instruction for LDH.

Figure 1 The flow diagram is intended to depict the passage of participants through this RCT.

Exclusion criteria

Participants will be excluded if they suffer from serious life-threatening disease, such as disease of the heart and brain, blood, vessels, liver, kidney and hematopoietic system, and psychotic patients. Participants will not be eligible if they are female and whether pregnant or lactating. The following conditions

are also excluded items: appeared a single nerve palsy, or cauda equina nerve palsy, manifested as muscle paralysis or have rectum or bladder problems; complicated with lumbar spinal canal stenosis and space-occupying lesions or for other reasons; complicated with lumbar spine tumors, infections, tuberculosis; moxibustion syncope and unwilling to be treated with moxibustion; do not sign informed consent.

Treatment protocol

Heat-sensitive moxibustion

Moxibustion will be performed by certified acupuncture medical doctors at four centers. Qualified specialists of acupuncture in traditional Chinese medicine with at least five years of clinical experience will perform the acupuncture in this study. All treatment regimens will be standardized between four centers practitioners via video, hands-on training and internet workshops. Participants will be randomly assigned to the heat-sensitive moxibustion group, the conventional moxibustion group. In the former groups, a 22 mm (diameter) × 120 mm (length) moxa-sticks (Jiangxi Traditional Chinese Medicine Hospital, China) will be used. The patient is usually in the comfortable supine position for treatment, with 24°C to 30°C temperature in the room.

For the heat-sensitive moxibustion group, the moxa-sticks are lit by the therapist and held over the region consisting in two Da Changshu (BL 25) and Yao Shu (Du 2) of patients. The warming suspended moxibustion about distance of 3 cm are used to search for the acupoint heat-sensitization phenomenon. The following patient sensation will suggest the special heat-sensitization aupoint: diathermanous sensation due to moxa-heat, defined as the heat sensation conducting from the moxa local skin surface into deep tissue; expand heat sensation due to moxa-heat, defined as the heat sensation spreading to the surrounding little by little around the moxa point; transfer heat sensation due to moxa-heat, defined as the heat sensation transferring along some pathway or direction. When some acupoint exists one below sensation at least, therapists mark the point as a heat-sensitive acupoint. We try our best to seek all the special acupoints in each patient by the repeated assessment.

The therapists begin to treat patients from the most heat-sensitive intensity acupoint. Treatment sessions end when patients feel the acupoint heat-sensitization phenomenon has disappeared. Generally speaking, we select one point each time. One point is treated 45 minutes. Patients receive the treatment for two times daily in the first four days and for one time daily in remaining ten days. The full treatment contains 18 sessions over 14 days.

Conventional moxibustion group

Patients assigned to the conventional moxibustion group will receive fixed acupoint moxibustion. Common practices are similar with the first group. The different manipulation is that the therapists carry out warming moxibustion in traditional acupoint, selecting Da Changshu (BL 25), Wei Zhong (BL40) and A-shi Xue. One point is treated 15 minutes a time. The total time is 45 minutes as well. Three points are treated by suspended moxibustion at the same time. In the treatment, the therapists try to give patients the same intensity of the local warm sensation as the experimental group. The sensation of acupoint heat-sensitization phenomenon is not pursued and not avoided in the treatment. Patients receive the treatment for two times daily in the first four days and for one time daily in remaining ten days. The full treatment contains 18 sessions over 14 days.

Chen *et al. Trials* 2011, **12**:226
http://www.trialsjournal.com/content/12/1/226

Page 6 of 8

Statistical methods

Statistical analysis plan

We will conduct analysis on an intention to treat basis, including all randomized participants. Analyses will be conducted using 2-sided significance tests at the 5% significance level. The analysis of center effect will be used logistic regression method. The statistician conducting the analyses will remain blind to treatment group and data will only be unblinded once all data summaries and analyses are completed. All analyses will be conducted in the SAS statistical package program (ver. 9.1.3).

Baseline data

Baseline characteristics will be shown as mean, standard deviation (SD) for continuous data including age, previous duration, and so on. The first step of analysis is to check for integrity of randomization. The unbalanced analysis in baseline characteristics will use ANCOVA.

Outcome data

These will be summarized descriptively (mean, SD, median, minimum and maximum) at each time point by treatment group. The t-test, Mann-Whitney U and Wilcox on test were used for comparison of variables, as appropriate. When the data do not fit a normal distribution, we will consider more general tests such as ANOVA and possible transformations.

All adverse events reported during the study will be included in the case report forms; the rates of adverse events will be calculated. The percentage of subjects with adverse events in each group will be calculated and compared using the chi-squared test or Fisher's exact test. The outcomes will be analyzed using linear mixed and logistic regression models that will include their respective baseline scores as covariates, subjects as a random effect and treatment conditions as fixed factors. Regression diagnostics will be used to check for normality of the measures and homogeneity of variance as appropriate.

Dropouts or missing data Reasons for dropout or missing data will be explored descriptively. Multiple imputation will be used to make sure that dropouts do not impact the conclusions [25].

Follow-up data The primary outcome will be the M-JOA scores. The primary analysis will compare the two groups at 14 days. A secondary analysis will compare the two groups at 6 months to assess if any differences between groups have been maintained over time.

Loss to follow-up is likely to lead to biased estimates of intervention effect. We will try to avoid bias due to attrition by carefully following up the participants in both groups. We will phone participants who do not complete questionnaires after a second reminder. We anticipate a 20% loss to follow-up in this trial, and will implement procedures to minimize loss to follow-up and patient withdrawal, and where possible we will collect information on reasons for patient withdrawal.

Data integrity

The integrity of trial data will be monitored by regularly scrutinizing data sheets for omissions and errors. Data will be double-entered and the source of any inconsistencies will be explored and resolved.

Sample size

We wished to estimate the sample size that would suffice to detect M-JOA between the heat-sensitive and conventional moxibustion groups. If we apply a two-sided 5% significance level, 90% power the calculated required sample size is approximately 126 participants in each group, according to the equations in [26]. Allowing for a 20% loss to follow up, a total of 158 participants will be required in each group, with 316 participants in total.

Adverse events

We define adverse events as unfavorable or unintended signs, symptoms or disease occurring after treatment that are not necessarily related to the moxibustion intervention. In every visit, adverse events will be reported by participants and examined by the practitioner.

Ethics

Written consent will be obtained from each participant. This study was approved by all relevant local ethics review boards. Ethics Committee of Affiliated hospital of Jiangxi Institute of Traditional Chinese Medicine had approved this trial: code issued by ethic committee is 2008(11).

Discussion

Currently, although different therapeutic methods can be used in patients with LDH, the treatments can be divided into two categories, conservative (or non-surgical) and surgical. Conservative treatments mainly avoid painful positions and relieve symptoms in nine out of 10 people with a herniated disk, according to the American Academy of Orthopedic Surgeons [27]. Many clinical trials held that moxibustion should be effective in the treatment of LDH. But the evidence obtained from these trials was quite limited because of methodology defects. Therefore, we designed this clinical trial to meet the CONSORT statement and guidelines to improve the chances of high internal validity for the results [28]. On the basis of the classical notion of traditional Chinese medicine, moxibustion caused by the burning of moxa leads to the radiant heat and bring drug-like effects to acupoints. Practitioners use moxa to warm acupoints with the intention of stimulating circulation through the acupoints and inducing a smoother flow of blood and qi. So the selection of moxa locations has an important impact on obtaining good effects. It is widely believed that the acupoint locations are fixed along meridians. The conventional moxibustion

Chen et al. Trials 2011, **12**:226
http://www.trialsjournal.com/content/12/1/226

applies moxa to get the desired results by stimulating these fixed acupoints. Doctors regard hyperemia due to local skin vasodilatation as the indicator of moxibustion effect. However, we support the notion that these fixed acupoints might not be the best stimulating sites for moxibustion.

In humans, acupoints contain two states: stimulated and resting. When people get sick, the acupoints on the body surface area are activated and sensitized. The sensitive areas are susceptible to heat stimulation and are called "heat-sensitized acupoints". Acupoints are more than fixed skin sites but externally sensitive reflecting diseases. Therefore, acupoint is variable and determined by the pathological state. Heat-sensitive moxibustion is a therapeutic method through heat-sensitized acupoints [14].

Acupuncture and moxibustion is a form of therapy derived from Traditional Chinese Medicine (TCM). It is well known that *Huáng Dì Nèi Jīng (黄帝内经)* is the source of theoretical and academic foundation in TCM. According to core theory in this classic,

pathological state of the internal diseases can be manifested through the acupoints. It is very difficult for persons to experience the existence of the acupoints in a normal physical state. However, patients can usually feel some changes in the area of the acupoints when they are sick.

With the state transition and change, sensitized status is often observed. Acupoints on the body surface may be sensitized with various types of sensitization under the circumstances. On the one hand, these sensitized acupoints are supposed to be the pathological phenomena reflecting the diseases; on the other hand, acupuncture and moxibustion treat diseases by stimulating these acupoints [14,15]. Our clinical experience and research in the 1990s pointed out that acupoint

heat-sensitization was a type of acupoint sensitization. The features of acupoints heat-sensitization correspond with the classical thought and theory from the Inner Canon of Huangdi, according to the previous analysis in the above paragraphs [29]. Therefore, it would be valuable to know whether heat-sensitized acupoints is superior to fixed points.

It is hypothesized that selecting the heat-sensitized acupoint may obtain therapeutic effect far better than moxibustion at acupoints of routine resting states. Our purpose is to test and verify the hypothesis. The study outcomes will facilitate the development of the theory of acupuncture and moxibustion. Therefore, the primary aim of this project is more than providing the efficacy of heat-sensitive moxibustion as a treatment modality in patients with LDH. The results of our trial will be helpful to disclose inherent law of moxibustion and present

evidence for better therapeutic options to enhance the efficacy of moxibustion in China.

Acknowledgements
This study was supported by the Major State Basic Research Development Program of People's Republic of China (Grant number: 2009CB522902), the National Natural Science Foundation of China (Grant number: 30760320) and Jiangxi Key R&D Project.

Author details
[1]The Affiliated Hospital of Jiangxi University of TCM, Nanchang, Jiangxi, PR China. [2]Department of Health of Jiangxi Province, Nanchang, Jiangxi, PR China.

Authors' contributions
RC and MC obtained funding for the research project and drafted the protocol. JX wrote the final manuscript. FY contributed to the research design and made critical revisions. ZC and BZ were responsible for the statistical design of the trial and wrote portions of the statistical methods, data handling, and monitoring sections. All authors read and approved the final manuscript.

Competing interests
The authors declare that they have no competing interests.

Received: 10 January 2011 Accepted: 13 October 2011
Published: 13 October 2011

References
1. Keller RB, Atlas SJ, Singer DE, Chapin AM, Mooney NA, Patrick DL, Deyo RA: The Maine lumbar spine study, Part I. Background and concepts. *Spine* 1996, 21(15):1769-76.
2. Luijsterburg PA, Verhagen AP, Ostelo RW, van den Hoogen HJ, Peul WC, Avezaat CJ, Koes BW: Physical therapy plus general practitioners' care versus general practitioners' care alone for sciatica: a randomized clinical trial with a 12-month follow-up. *Eur Spine J* 2008, 17(4):509-517.
3. Gibson JNA, Waddell G: Surgical interventions for lumbar disc prolapsed. *Cochrane Database of Systematic Reviews* 2007, 2.
4. Andersson GB, Brown MD, Dvorak J, Herzog RJ, Kambin P, Malter A, McCulloch JA, Saal JA, Spratt KF, Weinstein JN: Consensus summary of the diagnosis and treatment of lumbar disc herniation. *Spine* 1996, 21(24 Suppl):S75-78.
5. Peul WC, van Houwelingen HC, van den Hout WB, Brand R, Eekhof JA, Tans JT, Thomeer RT, Koes BW, Leiden-The Hague Spine Intervention Prognostic Study Group: Surgery versus prolonged conservative treatment for sciatica. *N Engl J Med* 2007, 356(22):2245-2256.
6. Chae KH, Ju CI, Lee SM, Kim BW, Kim SY, Kim HS: Strategies for Noncontained Lumbar Disc Herniation by an Endoscopic Approach: Transformational Suprapedicular Approach, Semi-Rigid Flexible Curved Probe, and 3-Dimensional Reconstruction CT with Discogram. *J Korean Neurosurg Soc* 2009, 46(4):312-316.
7. Paramore LC: Use of alternative therapies: estimates from the 1994 Robert Wood Johnson Foundation National Access to Care Survey. *J Pain Symptom Manage* 1997, 13(2):83-89.
8. Lee DH, Kim JI, Lee MS, Choi TY, Choi SM, Ernst E: Moxibustion for ulcerative colitis: a systematic review and meta-analysis. *BMC Gastroenterol* 2010, 10:36.
9. Cho ZH, Hwang SC, Wong EK, Son YD, Kang CK, Park TS, Bai SJ, Kim YB, Lee YB, Sung KK, Lee BH, Shepp LA, Min KT: Neural substrates, experimental evidences and functional hypothesis of acupuncture mechanisms. *Acta Neurol Scand* 2006, 113(6):370-377.
10. Chen W, Yang AT, Dai MT, Fu QL: [Observation on therapeutic effect of electroacupuncture under continuous traction for treatment of lumbar disc herniation]. *Zhongguo Zhen Jiu* 2009, 29(12):967-9, [Chinese].
11. Chen HL, Qiu XH, Yan XC: [Observation on therapeutic effect of electroacupuncture plus blood-letting puncture at Weizhong (BL 40) on acute lumbar disc herniation]. *Zhongguo Zhen Jiu* 2009, 29(2):123-5, [Chinese].

Chen *et al. Trials* 2011, **12**:226
http://www.trialsjournal.com/content/12/1/226

12. Peng KZ, Xiang KW, Cui J: [Observation on therapeutic effect of intradermal needle combined with Tuina on lumbar disc herniation]. *Zhongguo Zhen Jiu* 2008, **28**(12):894-6, [Chinese].
13. Ewies A, Olah K: Moxibustion in Breech Version-A Descriptive Review. *Acupuncture in medicine* 2002, **20**(1):26-29.
14. Chen RX, Chen MR, Xiong J, Yi F, Chi ZH, Zhang B: **Comparison of heat-sensitive moxibustion versus fluticasone/salmeterol (seretide) combination in the treatment of chronic persistent asthma: design of a multicenter randomized controlled trial.** *Trials* 2010, **11**:121.
15. Chen RX, Chen MR, Kang MF, Xiong J, Chi ZH, Zhang B, Fu Y: **The design and protocol of heat-sensitive moxibustion for knee osteoarthritis: a multicenter randomized controlled trial on the rules of selecting moxibustion location.** *BMC Complement Altern Med* 2010, **10**:32.
16. Chen RX, Kang MF: [Clinical application of acupoint heat-sensitization]. *Zhongguo Zhen Jiu* 2007, **27**(3):199-202, [Chinese].
17. Chen RX, Kang MF: [Key point of moxibustion, arrival of qi produces curative effect]. *Zhongguo Zhen Jiu* 2008, **28**(1):44-46, [Chinese].
18. Chen RX, Kang MF, He WL, Chen SY, Zhang B: [Moxibustion on heat-sensitive acupoints for treatment of myofascial pain syndrome: a multi-central randomized controlled trial]. *Zhongguo Zhen Jiu* 2008, **28**(6):395-398, [Chinese].
19. Chen RX, Kang MF: **Acupoint heat-sensitization moxibustion: a new therapy.** Press by People's Medical Publishing House. Beijing in China;, 1 2006.
20. Tang FY, Huang CJ, Chen RX, Xu M, Liu BX, Liang Z: [Observation on therapeutic effect of moxibustion on temperature-sensitive points for lumbar disc herniation]. *Zhongguo Zhen Jiu* 2009, **29**(5):382-384, [Chinese].
21. Zhang C, Xiao H, Chen Rx: [Observation on curative effect of moxibusting on heat-sensitive points on pressure sores]. China Journal of Traditional Chinese. *Medicine and Pharmacy* 2010, **25**(4):478-488, [Chinese].
22. Kang MF, Chen RX, Fu Y: [Clinical Research on Ostioarthritis of Knee Treated with Moxibustion to Heat Sensitivity Point]. *Journal of Jiangxi university of TCM* 2006, **18**(2):27-28, [Chinese].
23. Fukui M, Chiba K, Kawakami M, Kikuchi S, Konno S, Miyamoto M, Seichi A, Shimamura T, Shirado O, Taguchi T, Takahashi K, Takeshita K, Tani T, Toyama Y, Wada E, Yonenobu K, Tanaka T, Hirota Y: **JOA back pain evaluation questionnaire: initial report.** *J Orthop Sci* 2007, **12**(5):443-50.
24. Liu B, Wen T, Yao C, Yan S, He L, Xie Y, Mu Z: [The central randomization system in multi-center clinical trials]. *Chin J New Drugs Clin Rem* 2006, **12**(2):931-935, [Chinese].
25. Wayman JC: **Multiple Imputation For Missing Data: What Is It And How Can I Use It?**[http://www.csos.jhu.edu/contact/staff/jwayman_pub/wayman_multimp_aera2003.pdf], Accessed on August 1 2011.
26. Wu SX, Wang CX: **Clinical studies estimate sample size.** Press by People's Medical Publishing House. Beijing in China;, 1 2008.
27. Snelling NJ: **Spinal manipulation in patients with disc herniation: A critical review of risk and benefit.** *International Journal of Osteopathic Medicine* 2006, **9**(3):77-84.
28. Moher D, Hopewell S, Schulz KF, Montori V, Gøtzsche PC, Devereaux PJ, Elbourne D, Egger M, Altman DG, Consolidated Standards of Reporting Trials Group: **CONSORT 2010 Explanation and Elaboration: updated guidelines for reporting parallel group randomized trials.** *BMJ* 2010, **63**(8):e1-37.
29. Veith I, translator (1972): **The Yellow Emperor's Classic of Internal Medicine.** Berkeley, CA: University of California Press;, Revised paperback.

doi:10.1186/1745-6215-12-226
Cite this article as: Chen *et al.*: Effectiveness of heat-sensitive moxibustion in the treatment of lumbar disc herniation: study protocol for a randomized controlled trial. *Trials* 2011 **12**:226.

六、陈日新热敏灸悟言

灸之钥

艾灸之要，气至有效；
奇特灸感，穴位深妙；
灸在皮部，热在深处；
灸在局部，热在远处；
以快为腧，有感就灸；
大道至简，返璞归真；
穴位诚贵，得气价高；
重视灸感，经穴全貌。

　　穴位是疾病在体表敏化态的反映点与治疗点。换句话说，穴位是在疾病过程中出现在身体表面的敏化部位，同时也是调控人体脏腑功能达到防病治病目的的针灸刺激部位。

　　穴位有状态之别，即敏化状态与静息状态。穴位敏化的类型多种多样，穴位热敏是一种新发现的敏化类型。热敏穴位对艾热刺激产生"小刺激大反应"，是我们采用探感定位方法准确找到穴位的依据，也是辨敏选穴、提高疗效的突破口。

　　灸感，指施灸时被灸者的自我感觉。提高灸疗疗效的规律隐藏于灸感密码之中。破译热敏灸感密码是提高艾灸疗效的关键！

　　敏化状态的穴位对外界的适宜刺激呈现"小刺激大反应"特征，从而体现"四两拨千斤"的疗效；热敏态穴位在艾热刺激下极易激发得气，气至病所，气至而有效。

　　灸之要，气至而有效。灸法的核心是得气，是人体正气激发的表现，是人体内源性调节功能被激活的标志，它的产生预示着能显著提高艾灸疗效。

　　热敏灸通过对穴位的热刺激，激发体内固有的调节系统（即经气系统）功能，使失调、紊乱的生理生化过程恢复正常。因此热敏灸作用并不是艾热刺激直接产生的，而是通过体内调节系统所产生，这就决定了热敏灸作用是调节作用，并具有双向调节、整体调节、品质调节及自限调节的特点。

热敏灸激发得气,"经气所过,主治所及,调节所至",因此热敏灸对寒证、热证、表证、里证、虚证与实证均有效。

自然规律是和谐统一的,医学规律也应是和谐统一的。灸材、灸位、灸法和灸量是影响灸疗疗效的四个关键环节,其规律一直扑朔迷离,繁杂纷纭。灸疗热敏规律能一线贯穿之,和谐统一之。

热敏灸疗法与传统悬灸疗法都是对准穴位"悬空"而灸的疗法,但存在五个本质的不同:灸感不同、灸位不同、灸法不同、灸量不同、灸效不同。